Military Chemical And Biological Agents

Military Chemical And Biological Agents

Chemical and Toxicological Properties

James A. F. Compton

THE TELFORD PRESS
Caldwell, NJ

DEDICATION

Dr. Shayne C. Gad

Diligent toxicologist, old friend, and tolerant observer of life's foibles.

Introduction

This book is written to fill a few gaps in a general awakening of interest in chemical and biological warfare both by professionals and the public at large. The purpose of this small treatise is to acquaint the reader with some of the chemical specifics of the subject as they are put into their proper historical significance.

I do not propose to make a chemist out of anyone. Nothing new is proposed. The formulations in this book are well known by the professional toxicologist and may be simplified to the point of boredom as regards that worthy branch of pharmacology. On the other hand there should be enough to interest industrial hygienists, safety professionals, civil and military defense planners, and perhaps a social scientist or two. Anyone even mildly interested in the struggle of nation states and ideologies might be well advised to read a page or two. Chemical weapons work. They are undergoing revolutionary developments which make them, and a new generation of biological substances as well, practical and very lethal participants in those human affairs which are ultimately resolved with blood and iron. Be ignorant and be damned, and condemn your children as well.

James A.F. Compton
September, 1987.

Table of Contents

Why the emphasis on military codes?

Those chemical substances which are, or have been, a standardized military agents have a two or three letter code printed in **BOLDFACE** beside the structural diagrams. By United Nations agreement, these (NATO) codes have become part of international convention. They refer to specific war chemicals and are recognized in military and diplomatic parlance worldwide. To say *pinacolyl methyl phosphonofluoridate* in any defense ministry in the world would only elicit blank stares. Only one person in ten thousand would know what you meant, and even he or she might get the name confused with several hundred other chemicals with similar names. However, if you say *GD* or *Soman*, even recruits and second lieutenants will know exactly what you're talking about.

The book was not written for the professional chemist so much as it was written for the person who has heard or read about chemical warfare and who wants to go beyond abstract arguments and examine the actual substances. To study chemical warfare you *must* study it in its own particular terminology.

And, in final retrospect, whereas a specific compound may have a host of acceptable chemical names, it will have only *one* legitimate code designation.

Can I use this book to make nerve gas in my bathtub?

The answer is no. Complex organic chemical compounds can not be taken apart and reassembled as if they were tinker-toys. To change the location of a single crucial atom is more likely to collapse a molecular structure than to transform it. Crucial temperature and pressure gradients are involved and those will not be discussed, nor will any of the "alchemist's tricks" be hinted at. Finally, many of the chemical agents in this book are shown with the often harmless substances they owe their "ancestery" to. Be mindful that the derivation came to pass on paper and not in the lab. As any second-year chemistry student knows, quite often "you can't get there from here."

Chapters one through four

C A S U A L T Y

A G E N T S

Official definition

A [Casualty] agent is a chemical compound that is used in military operations to kill, incapacitate, or seriously injure personnel through its chemical properties.

FM 3-9

Casualty agents are what commonly come to mind in the general literature of chemical warfare. The four subtypes of casualty agents are taught to most military personnel, who are not specialists in military chemistry, as being the "four types" of chemical agents.

Casualty agents, which are the principal types that would be deployed in battle, fulfill a number or tactical objectives:

- To cause casualties (injury or death).
- To decrease an opponent's effectiveness.
- To restrict and channel the use of terrain.
- To delay an opponent's advance.
- To contaminate avenues of approach.
- To attack hardened targets.
- To deny the use of structures.
- To deny the use of material or equipment.
- To attack an opponent's reserves.
- To attack an opponents fire support (artillery).
- To attack an opponent's logistical train (supply and maintenance).

Casualty agents are divided into four types: blister, blood, choking, and nerve. Each of these four types form specific families, and each family has its unique pathology, field characteristics, decontamination procedures and medical treatment. These are covered in detail under their individual types.

Chapter One

Blister Agents

official definition

The blister agents are used primarily for casualty effects. They may also be used to restrict the use of terrain, to slow movements, and to hamper the use of material and installations. These agents affect the eyes and lungs and blister the skin.

During World War I mustard was the only blister agent in major use. It was recognized by a distinctive odor and had a fairly long duration of effectiveness under normal weather conditions. Since then, blister agents have been developed which are odorless and vary in duration of effectiveness.

Most blister agents are insidous in action; there is little or no pain at the time of exposure except with lewisite (L) and phosgene oxime (CX), which cause immediate pain on contact. The development of casualties is somewhat delayed. CX produces a wheal (similar to a bee sting) rather than a water blister which the other blsiter agents produce.

Protection from blister agents is extremely difficult.

FM 3-9

Blister agents may be divided into five catagories, each explained under its own heading. The total list, in order of historical development, consists of:

Mustards

- HD distilled mustard

Arsenicals

- MD methyldichloroarsine
- PD phenyldichloroarsine
- ED ethyldichloroarsine
- L lewisite [dichloro (2-chlorovinyl) arsine]

Nitrogen Mustards

- HN-1 2,2'-dichlorotriethylamine
- HN-2 2,2'-dichloro-N-methyldiethylamine
- HN-3 2,2',2''-trichlorotriethylamine

Oximes

- CX phosgene oxime (dichloroformoxime)

Mixes

- HL mustard-lewisite mix: 63% L and 37% HD, by weight
- HT mustard-T mix: 60% HD and 40% T, by weight (see section, Code-designated blister agents not in production)

Code-designated blister agents not in production

- T
- Q sesquimustard

The Mustards

One agent of importance remains in this catagory, distilled mustard (HD). Two other agents, coded Q and T were developed but then dropped from production as being either redundant or tactically superceded by newer agents. See *code-designated blister agents not in production.*

Mustards got their name from their smell. Early production mustard (H), or unrefined distilled mustard (HD), in particiualr had a pungent mustard-garlic stench. "Mustard" was an obvious nickname which soon became an official designation.

bis (2-chloroethyl) sulfide

Distilled Mustard

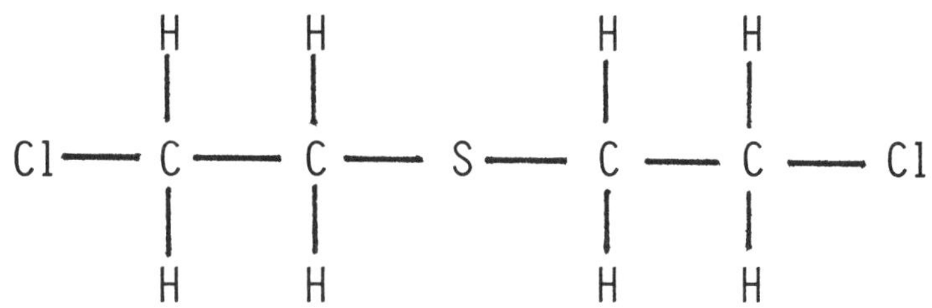

HD

Standard NATO agreement (STANAG) code: HD

Chemical name: bis (2-chloroethyl) sulfide
Common name: distilled mustard*
Formula: $Cl(CH_2)_2S(CH_2)_2Cl$

Family: casualty agent
Type: blister agent (mustard)

An amber brown liquid with an odor similar to that of burning garlic, the odor becoming more pronounced with impurities in the solution. Creates a low-laying colorless vapor around the splashed liquid.

* during WWI HD was variously known as HS (Britain), das Lost (Germany), and Yprite (France). International codes became standardized by convention after 1919-1920.

History

Distilled mustard (HD) was known as early as the late 1880s as a by-product of the dye industry whose toxic effects might be of use in both treating minor tumors and in killing warehouse pests.

Origionally investigated by the British and rejected as not being lethal enough, it was first used against them. At 10 PM on the evening of July 12th, 1917 the British 15th and 55th infantry divisions came under an artillery barrage in their positions near Ypres, France. Mixed in with high explosives was a significant quantity of distilled mustard. Other than a stench "like garlic" of "like mustard" (which is how the compound gets its name) there was little nuisance beyond eye irritation like diluted phosgene. Many troops did not bother to put their gas masks on. By the following afternoon the British field hospitals were clogged and on the next evening the first deaths began.

Distilled mustard, the first of the major blister agents, became the chemical compound by which all others have been judged since. According to a British army study, the Foulkes Papers, 16½% of all encountered casualties in the last eighteen months of that war were due to chemicals, mainly distilled mustard. In 1920 about 19,000 British veterans drew permanent disability, mainly from mustard. A 1927 Porton Down study of HD victims found pre-cardiac conditions common, and typical conjunctivitis, laryngitis, bronchitis, and reoccuring skin burns. A Porton Down study of 1929 of 29 severe cases showed fibrosis, respiratory and spinal TB, persistent laryngitis, anaemia, conjunctivitis, aphonia, and pulmonary fibrosis. By 1930, 80% of known survivors suffered chronic bronchitis.

After the first world war limited production continued in Great Britain and France. Production began in Italy and the

Soviet Union by 1925, and in Japan in 1928.

HD was allegedly used against the Afgans by the British in 1919 It was known to be used against Moroccans by the French and Spanish in 1925, against Ethopians by the Italians after 1935, and by the Japanese against China after 1934 and ending by 1944.

The late 1920s through the 1930s were a time a chemical warfare experimentation as the older agents were adapted to fit new methods and tactics of war. New munitions, especially those for aerial sprays and bombs, were developed. It was assumed that chemicals would be used in the the "next war" to the same extent they had been used in 1915-1918. As German rearmament beginning in 1934 started a general trend, chemical munitions plants were upgraded.

Great Britain built new facilities such as those at Sutton Oak-St Helens, Lancashire. France opened a HD and CG plant at Clancy. The USSR built new HD-L-CG plants at Brandyuzhsky, Kuibyshev, and Karaganda. Germany built plants at Munster, Wunsdorf, and List. The US reluctantly reopened Pine Bluff Arsenal (in production by 1942) and built new facilities such as Rocky Mountain Arsenal (near Denver) and opened the Dugway, Utah, Proving Grounds for the express purpose of testing chemical agents.

Casualty agent use in the second world war, outside of China through 1943-1944, was virtually non-existent. The only known incident in the west occured in Bari harbor on the Italian Adriatic.

An American merchantman, the S.S. John Harvey, carried the bulk of US chemical munitions for the Mediterranean area, in the form of 2000 M47A1 aerial bombs, containing a total of about 100 tons of HD. The S.S. John Harvey's cargo was known only to SHAFE in London and a few junior Army Ordinance officers on board. On 7:30 PM, July 2nd, 1943, the John Harvey was sunk in a German air raid. Her cargo of HD had all been made by the quick-but-dirty Levinstein process. Thus it had hydrogen and ethane gas impurites in the HD mix. The John Harvey blew up and flooded the harbor. By the following morning it was Ypres all over again, except nobody knew why the massive blistering was happening, especially among sailors soaked in oil and some smelly stuff from the harbor waters. About 630 serious military cases occured and over a thousand Italian civilians died within a few days.

Allegations of the use of distilled mustard surface from time to time. Yemen and Afganistan are often mentioned in this regard, as are Laos and Cambodia. Allegations they remain. New chemical and biological technologies have produced whole new variations and nobody's bragging about what they may or may not be doing.

A known area of occasional distilled mustard use is in the Iran-Iraq war which began in 1979. When Iraq was pushed back to its starting point by the early 1980s, it is alleged to have begun the use of chemical agents as an effective weapon against Iranian human wave attacks consisting of untrained volunteer levies begging for death and recieving it in spades.

Structure

Distilled mustard has a simple structure, consisting of two ethyl ($C_2H_5^-$) groups bound together around an atom of sulphur. The outer two hydrogen bonds along the central axis have been replaced by chlorine bonds.

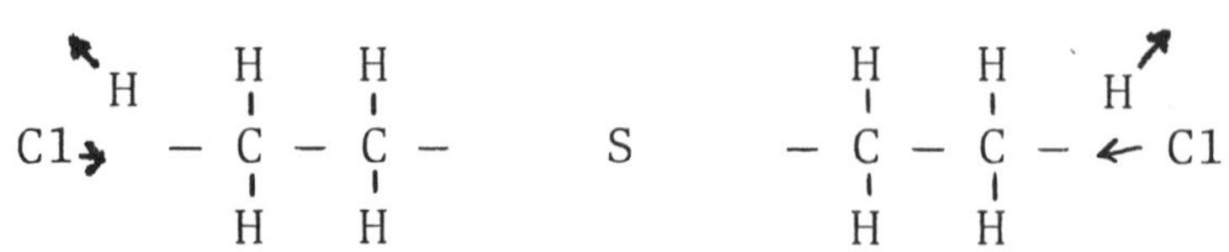

The old Levinstein process consisted of treating ethylene with sulphur chloride.

Pathology

Both distilled mustard and its vapors create an extreme hazard. The greater the absorbed dose of either the greater the damage.

Vapors of this agent will cause temporary blindness and inflammation of the entire respiratory tract. Further heavy vapor exposure will make the blindness permanent and will strip the bronchial tubes of their mucus membrane lining. Any concentration will cause a severe choking effect.

Distilled mustard liquid is corrosive to human tissue both locally and systematic. Local effects include immediate inflammation of the tissues around the eyes and pronounced reddening of exposed skin. If not decontaminated, reddened skin will ulcerate into waterish boils within four to six hours. These blisters, if crudely broken, will reblister. Systemic effects from prolonged exposure may include internal inflammation and blistering (ulceration) of the throat and lungs, resulting in what is termed "dry land drowning," in which the windpipe clogs from bottom to top. Ingestion will cause nausea and vomiting within the same time frame. Absorption into the blood results in white blood cell destruction. Long term exposures may promote bone marrow destruction and subsequent damage to the immune system. Currently listed by NIOSH/RTECS as being mutagenic in all mammals in solution concentrations above 750 m/liter.

Field behavior

Distilled mustard is among the most commonly listed military casualty agents. It is used to deny terrain and to contaminate equipment and stores.

The delayed effects of distilled mustard necesitate constant chemical survey and monitoring. The human body slowly detoxifies this agent, so prolonged toxic exposures may slowly build up without initial warning symptoms. The vapors are heavier than air and may persist as long as one month in winter weather. They will seek lower elevations in open terrain and substructures, tunnels, and conduits in man-made terrain.

With a flash point of 105°C (221°F) distilled mustard, and particularly its vapors, may explode if exposed to fire or munitions detonations.

Decontamination must be immediate and thorough when this agent is discovered. Exposed personnel should recieve immediate personal decontamination and medical examination.

Slightly soluble in cold water, although volatile in steam. Soluble in most organic solvents.

Specific data

median lethal dosage (LCt_{50})

(Inhalation) 1500 mg-min/m^3 or 23 ppm/10 molar.
(Skin absorption) 10,000 mg-min/m^3 or 34 mg/kg.

median incapacitating dosage (ICt_{50})

(Eye injury) 200 mg-min/m^3.
(Skin absorption) 2000 mg-min/m^3.

eye toxicity

Very susceptible to low concentrations (see above). Damage is accumulative to tissue and blood vessels, causing blindness or permanent impairment if untreated.

skin toxicity

Less susceptible to concentrations, but accumulative and irritating. Severe blistering is possible and permanent damage to skin tissues may result even from delayed treatment. HD dissolved in sweat is of great danger to areas of skin like the face, underarms, knees, elbows, and crotch!

rate of action

Delayed. Major pathological symptoms commonly do not appear until at least four hours after exposure. However, do to the accumulative effect of this compound, symptoms may manifest perhaps a week or more after a series of incremental exposures. Effects from ingestion and eye exposure may be more immediate.

protection required

Protective mask/respirator, with full protective overclothing under all conditions.

rate of detoxification

Very low natural detoxification in the body makes the dosages (and effects) accumulative.

decontaminants

Strong bleach solutions and caustic soda (sodium hypochlorite) for personnel and terrain. For the decontamination of buildings and substructures live steam may also be used. Under combat conditions fire may be used as a field expedient decontaminant, mindful of an explosive hazard.

vapor density

5.4 times heavier than air.

vapor pressure

0.072 mm Hg at 20°C (68°F).

liquid density

1.27 g/cc.

persistency

Heavily splashed liquid may last several days in temperate climates. May last up to a month under winter conditions.

volatility

(Solid) 75 mg/m^3 at 0°C (32°F), (liquid) 610 mg/m^3 at 20°C (68°F), 2680 mg/m^3 at 40°C (104°F).

latent heat of vaporization

94 calories per gram

melting point

14.45°C (58.1°F).

boiling point

217°C (422.6°F) with decomposition.

decomposition point

Begins at 149°C (300°F).

flash point

105°C (221°F).

rate of hydrolysis

Hydrolyses within 17 minutes in distilled water at 25°C (77°F) and two hours in salt water at the same temperature.

hydrolysis products

Hydrochloric acid and thiodiglycol.

stability in storage

Stable in steel or aluminum canisters.

actions on metals or other materials

Little corrosive property when pure. Electrostatic properties in electrical equipment.

molecular weight

159.08

Warning

The above specific data refer to distilled mustard in its traditional form of a pure chemical. Microencapsulation techniques could make this into a highly persistent poison presenting a profoundly greater hazard.

The Arsenicals

MD methyldichloroarsine
PD phenyldichloroarsine
ED ethyldichloroarsine
L lewisite

The arsenicals are a series of blister agents based around a chloroarsine ($AsCl_3$) molecule in which one of the chlorine atoms is replaced by an organic radical.

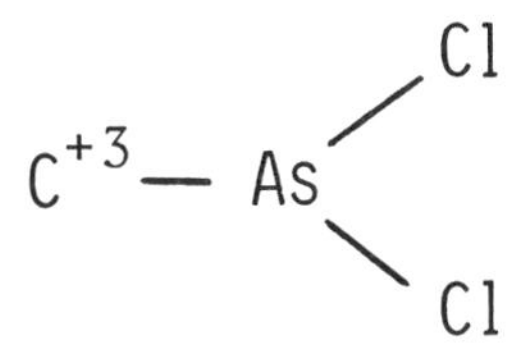

In and of itself chloroarsine, like arsine (AsH_3) are effective cytochrome oxidase destroyers, or blood agents. Arsenic seeks to replace calcium in the bones, thus causing bone marrow destruction as the endocrine system is concurrently attacked. Many organic radicals penetrate the human skin, carrying their compounds with them. Chloroarsines, most importantly, are destructive to human tissue such as is found in the throat and lungs. Chloroarsine compounds tend to hydrolyse rapidly.

These agents represent a pre-nerve agent technology attempt to create a usable non-persistent casualty agent.

Methyldichloroarsine

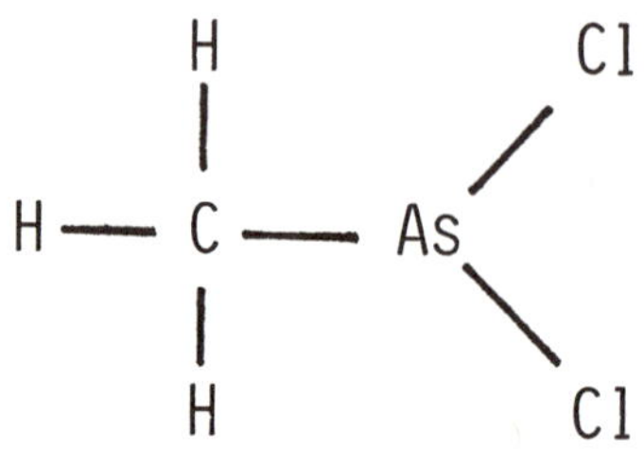

MD

Standard NATO agreement (STANAG) code: MD

Chemical name: methyldichloroarsine
Common name: methyldichloroarsine
Formula: CH_3AsAl_2

Family: casualty agent
Type: blister agent (arsenical)

A colorless liquid which (if impure) has a colorless vapor smelling similar to rotting fruit. It is always irritating to the eyes and nasal membranes, to which the splashed liquid may cause severe injury. A rare but not entirely obsolete agent.

History

Chloroarsines first made their appearence in the dyes and fumigants studies of the mid to late 19th century, done principally in Germany and France. First thought of as impurities in arsine production, they were developed in their own right as fumigants. Combining a chloroarsine radical with a methyl radical proved to be an efficient means of liquification.

Distilled mustard (HD) was efficient enough for trench warfare until the German army developed new tactics by the fall of 1917. A semi-persistent agent was required, and as the choking agents were by then easily dealt with, the blood agents still a theory, and the nerve agents unborn, chloroarsines were brought into use. Methyldichloroarsine was the first of three to be field tested by the German army.

Methyldichloroarsine was first used in the late fall of 1917. Not as effective as distilled mustard, it did serve as an effective agent on the forward edge of battle. Superceeded by phenyl, then ethyldichloroarsine, all three became somewhat passe when replaced by the nerve agents. However, since these lightweight blister agents are relatively easy to manufacture and are quite effective against unprotected personnel, it could be fatal to disregard them.

Structure

The structure of methyldichloroarsine is extremely simple. It consists of a trichloroarsine ($ASCl_3$) molecule combined through catalysation with a methyl (CH_3^-) group.

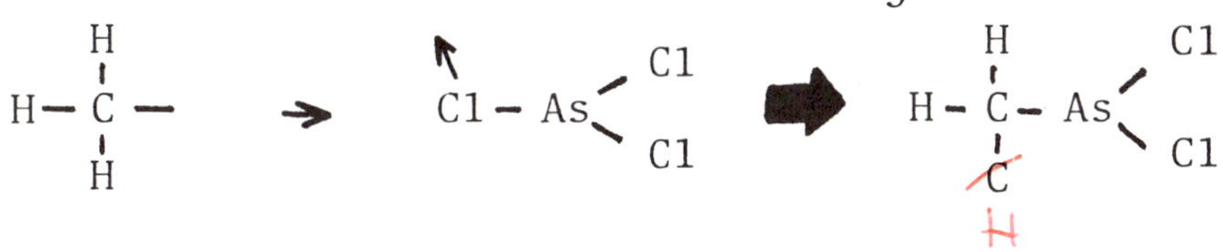

Alternately, methyldichloroarsine may be produced from methylization of any chlorinated arsenite or arsenate salt or in reductions of arsenious oxide, As_4O_6, an insecticide dating back to antiquity.

Pathology

Methyldichloroarsine's chlorine bonds give it its blistering qualities. The methyl group simply aids in its assimilation into the human body, in particular into the blood. The arsenic atom acts mainly as a central molecular bond, its own toxicity being almost an afterthought.

Chlorine reactivity causes severe respiratory pain and damage to the membranes of the lungs. This same mechanism will cause severe eye discomfort and, in the case of even lightly splashed liquid, permanent corneal damage. The methyl arsenic group will readily penetrate the skin as a liquid, and prolonged exposure to the arsenic component will lead to systemic damage through bone calcium displacement and subsequent bone marrow destruction. Vapor concentration in open areas , given MD's high volatility (74,000 mg/m^3 at 68°F), is not enough to cause Cl^- induced blistering although liquid contamination will give rise to blistering similar to that of distilled mustard within several hours. "Dry-land drowning" can occur as the lungs flood with water and mucous and the victim dies a combination of blood poisoning and asphyxiation.

Field behavior

Methyldichloroarsine evaporates very quickly, almost four times as rapidly as ethyldichloroarsine, and over 192 TIMES as rapidly as phenyldichloroarsine. It would disperse quickly in open terrain and would present a continuous hazard only within tightly closed buildings, where its density (5.5 x air) might cause it to seek refuge in substructures, conduits, tunnels, or caves. With its fast hydrolysis rate, MD would not persist for any militarily significant period of time.

Like all arsenic-based compounds, MD does have an ability to break down protective filters based on cellulose fibers. This, and MD's stabilty in storage (as opposed to arsine and arsenic trichloride) were its selling points in 1917.

Specific data

median lethal dosage (LCt_{50})

3,000 mg-min/m^3.

median incapacitating dosage (ICt_{50})

25 mg-min/m^3 (inhalation).

skin toxicity

Exposure of skin to liquid MD will cause blistering similar to that of HD within several hours. Vapor exposure is unlikely to cause blistering as sufficient concentration is unlikely in open areas.

eye toxicity

Exposure to even the slightest amount is highly irritating. At exposures above 300 mg-min/m^3 permanent corneal damage is almost assured.

rate of action

Immediate eye, respiratory tract irritation.

protection required

Protective mask and respirator. Protective overclothing must be worn as a protection against liquid MD.

rate of detoxification

Sublethal dosages are rapidly detoxified, although arsenic poisoning may be accumulative if untreated.

decontaminants

Bleaches and alkaline solutions such as sodium hydroxide (NaOH) for the liquid. Live steam is also field effective.

vapor density

5.5 times as heavy as air.

vapor pressure

2.17 mm Hg at 0°C(32°F); 7.76 mm Hg at 20°C(68°F).

liquid density

1.836 g/cc at 20°C(68°F).

persistency

Very short duration in humid climates due to high volatility and rapid hydrolysis. In dry, cold climates MD can persist up to several hours.

volatility

74,900 mg/m^3 at 20°C(68°F).

latent heat of vaporization

49 calories per gram.

freezing point

-55°C(-67°F).

boiling point

133°C(271°F) with decomposition.

decomposition point

133°C(271°F).

flash point

No imminent hazard of explosion or fire.

rate of hydrolysis

Rapid.

hydrolysis products

Hydrochloric and methylarsenic acids.

stability in storage

stable in steel.

action on metals and other materials

None on ferrous alloys. Slight oxidation to copper-based alloys.

molecular weight

160.86

Warning

The above specific data refer to methyldichloroarsine in its traditional form as a pure chemical. Microencapsulation techniques could make this into a highly persistent poison presenting profoundly greater hazards.

Phenyldichloroarsine

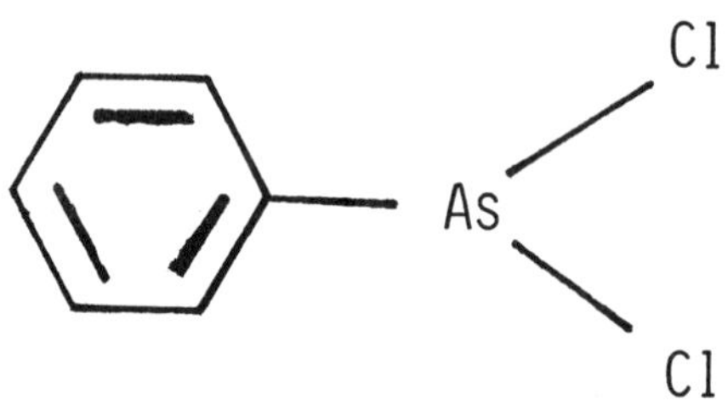

PD

Standard NATO agreement (STANAG) code: PD

Chemical name: phenyldichloroarsine
Common name: phenyldichloroarsine
Formula: $C_6H_5AsCl_2$

Family: casualty agent
Type: blister agent (arsenical)

A clear liquid with little or no odor. Creates a colorless vapor irritating and damaging to the eyes and nasal membranes. PD vapors will induce vomiting within one to two minutes. A rare but not entirely obsolete agent.

History

Phenyldichloroarsine (PD) was developed for war potential at the Kaiser Wilhelm Institute in Berlin under the direction of Dr Fritz Haber during the final trials of methyldichloroarsine(MD). It was suspected that MD would prove too volatile and too prone to hydrolysis for practical field use. The rains of November, 1917 proved this to be true and the new compound replaced MD. Then within months PD showed flaws of its own. First, by inhalation it was less lethal than distilled mustard. Secondly, it wasn't much more volatile than mustard. Thirdly, in sheltered, dry areas it could be highly persistent, thus offering a hazard to friendly assalt troops who reached their target objectives. On the other hand, PD's phenyl ($C_6H_5^-$) radical did make PD an effective vomiting compound. Phenyldichloroarsine served as inspiration for the first of the British "D" series vomiting agents, diphenylchloroarsine (DA) that appeared in the late spring of 1918.

With its two chlorine atoms per molecule, PD is an effective blister agent, its benzyl group allowing for efficient penetration of the human skin. Although unlikely to be found in quantity in the arsenals of the major powers, PD is fairly easy to manufacture by countries having their own pesticide production capability.

Structure

Phenyldichloroarsine has a very simple structure, that of a benzene ring grafted onto a molecule of arsenic trichloride:

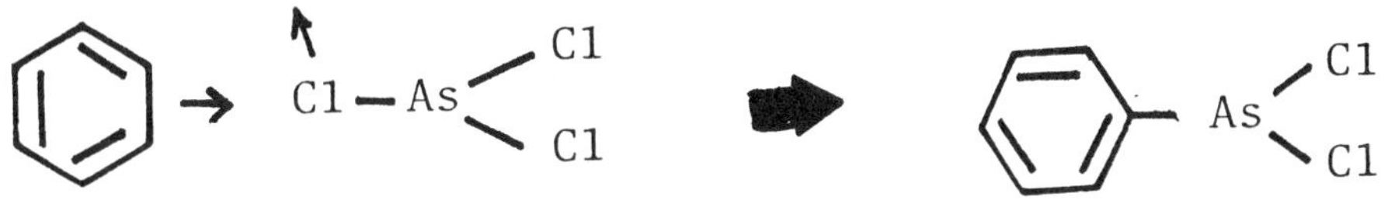

Phenyldichloroarsine would be most easily manufactured from methyldichloroarsine. Alternately, it might be produced by benzene reduction of various chlorinated arsenite or arsenate salts, or reductions involving arsenious oxide, As_4O_6, an naturally occuring compound long used as an insecticide.

Pathology

Phenyldichloroarsine's chlorine bonds give it its blistering qualities, its ability to damage the throat and lungs, and its severe lacrimatory and corneal damaging abilities.

PD's Phenylarsenic group aids in its penetration into the body and its absorption into the bloodstream. PD's persistency when not hydrolyzed increases the danger of systemic damage through arsenic-calcium replacement and bone marrow destruction.

PD's liquid persistency gives it significant blister-producing qualities akin to light amounts of distilled mustard. Blistering may be expected, following skin rash, in four to six hours. Blistering by PD, assuming the casualty survives and is detoxified, may cause permanent skin discoloration where blistering occured.

PD may cause "dry-land drowning" as damaged lungs secrete blood and mucous. The victim will die of a combination of asphyxiation and blood poisoning. Survivors may suffer permannet damage to the lungs, digestive, and endocrine systems.

Field behavior

Phenyldichloroarsine was designed for use in a wet environment (specifically the winter of 1917-1918) and was meant to have a slow but noticable hydrolysis rate. In dry climates, especially in cool, shady areas, PD may persist for several days. Under average conditions, concentrations should evaporate and hydrolyze within the same day of dissemination. Mediocre volatility (390 mg/m^3 at 77°F) and low vapor pressure (0.033 mm Hg at 77°F) would make PD little more than a nuisance in open terrain, were it not for PD's profound vomiting inducing capabilities. However, its extreme vapor density (7.7 times as heavy as air) make it highly effective against persons inside enclosed structures, especially in basements and tunnels. Terrain such as gullies and caves would become thickly infested with this agent. Likewise it would be expected to flow down through utility conduits and culverts. PD is highly effective as an aircraft-delivered aerosol.

Specific data

median lethal dosage (LCt_{50})

2600 mg-min/m^3 (inhalation).

median incapacitating dosage (ICt_{50})

1800 mg-min/m^3 (inhalation); 633 mg-min/m^3 (eyes); 16 mg-min/m^3 (for vomiting).

skin toxicity

Very toxic. About 90% the blistering effect of HD, although decomposed by wet clothing. See Pathology.

eye toxicity

Very toxic. Immediate stinging at low dosages, and permanent corneal damage at around 633 mg-min/m3 vapor concentration — or from any splashed liquid.

rate of action

Immediate on the eyes. Skin rash may first appear with 30 minutes. See Pathology.

protection required

Protective mask/respirator and protective overclothing under all conditions.

rate of detoxification

Rapidly detoxified in non-lethal dosages. Eye damage and systemic poisoning may be permament.

decontaminants

Bleaches and other oxidizers, and alkaline solutions such as sodium hydroxide (NaOH). May be used with live steam against liquid concentrations, especially those in closed or confined spaces.

vapor density

7.7 times as heavy as air.

vapor pressure

0.033 mm Hg at 25°C(77°F); 0.113 mm Hg at 40°C(104°F).

liquid density

1.65 g/cc at 20°C(68°F).

persistency

Up to one day under average conditions. Several days in cool, dry areas. Very short in wet, humid places.

volatility

390 mg/m^3 at 25°C(77°F).

latent heat of vaporization

69 calories per gram.

freezing point

-20°C(-40°F).

boiling point

252°C(485.6°F).with decomposition.

decomposition point

252°C(485.6°F).

flash point

No imminent hazard of explosion or fire.

rate of hydrolysis

Rapid.

hydrolysis products

Hydrochloric and phenylarsenious acids.

stability in storage

Very stable.

actions on metals and other materials

None of significance.

molecular weight

222.91

Warning

The above specific data refer to phenyldichloroarsine (PD) in its traditional form as a pure chemical. Microencapsulation techniques would make this into a highly persistent poison presenting profoundly greater hazards.

Ethyldichloroarsine

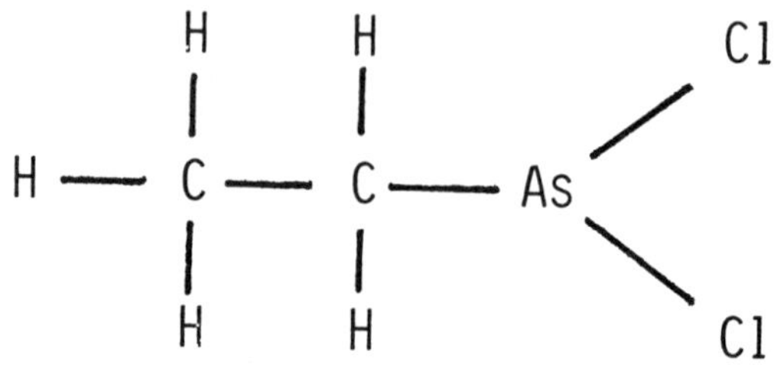

ED

Standard NATO agreement (STANAG) code: ED

Chemical name: ethyldichloroarsine
Common name: ethyldichloroarsine
Formula: $C_2H_5AsCl_2$

Family: casualty agent
Type: blister agent (arsenical)

A colorless liquid which gives off a colorless vapor smelling similar to rotting fruit and highly irritating to the eyes and nasal membranes. A rare but not entirely obsolete agent.

History

Ethyldichloroarsine (ED) was the third, and last, of the three blistering arsenicals developed in the late fall of 1917 and the winter of 1918 for the German army. This formula succeeded in being both quick acting and non persistent enough so as to not interfere with the newer tactics designed to break the trench warfare stalemate. In this regard, ED played an important role in the Somme Offensive in March of 1918, in which one sector of the front was pushed about forty miles west within a week.

ED was the state-of-the-art quick-acting agent until dichloro (2-chlorovinyl) arsine, based on the German arsenicals, was developed by at team at the Catholic University, Washington, DC, in April/May of 1918.

In military terms, ED is just as much an antique as are MD and PD (qv). However, this agent is highly lethal and can be easily manufactured in any country having basic pesticide manufacturing capacity.

Structure

Ethyldichloroarsine has an extremely simple structure. It consists of a trichloroarsine ($AsCl_3$) molecule combined through catalysation with a methyl ($C_2H_5^-$) group.

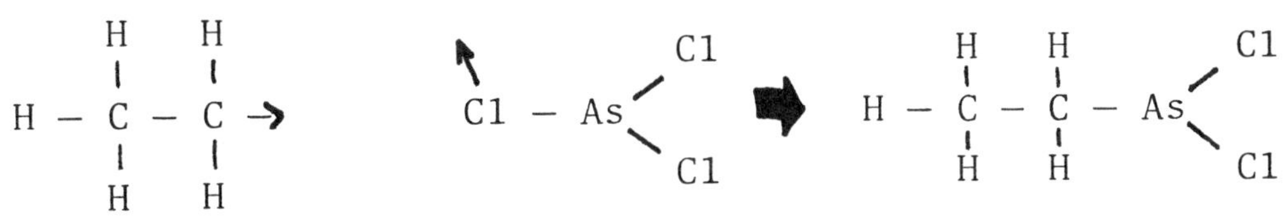

Production of ED is similar to that of methyldichloroarsine (MD), involving the ethylization of a chlorinated arsenite or arsenate salt, or in reductions of arsenious oxide, As_4O_6, a naturally occuring compound.

Pathology

Ethyldichloroarsine's chlorine bonds give it its blistering, lacrimatory, and harsh respiratory effects. Dosages as low as 5 mg-min/m^3 may cause severe discomfort to the eyes and throat. Sublethal dosages detoxified by the body.

ED's ethylarsenic group may cause systemic damage to bone marrow (as arsenic replaces calcium in bone structures) and to the digestive and endocrine systems if significant quantities are absorbed over an extended period.

Blistering may appear within two to four hours following skin redness or rash, although ED typically does not cause the severe subcutaneous damage of the sulfur-based mustards. However, like the mustards ED actively attacks lung tissue. Lethal dosages will cause "dry-land drowning," in which a victim's lungs will clog with mucous, dead tissue, water and blood causing death simultaneously from asphyxiation and blood poisoning. Like all the other blister agents, damage to lung tissue is permanent to its survivors and presents a hazard area for future infections and tumors.

ED is highly poisonous to the eyes. It may cause permanent corneal damage.

Field behavior

Ethyldichloroarsine was designed specifically for the climate of northern Europe and as part of a tactics/weapons package. Its requirements: lethality, residual effects and non-persistency were not met until twenty years later with the advent of the nerve agents.

ED is about half as volatile as diphosgene (20,000 vs 45,000 mg-min/m^3), which it temporarily replaced in 1918 and its vapors are six times as heavy as air. It main foible is its tendency to rapidly hydrolyse. Thus, humid or wet climatic conditions would cause liquid concentrations to both evaporate and break down rapidly. Again, ED was designed to fulfill a tactical need that the later non-persistent nerve agents better served.

Ethylchloroarsine would be expected to flow to the lowest possible terrain. It would also present a great hazard within buildings, especially underground structures, tunnels, caves, utility conduits, and stagnant sewer lines. Of least hazard in forests and jungles, of greater hazard in shaded desert areas, or in such dry climates in the cooler hours preceding sunrise.

Specific data

median lethal dosage (LCt_{50})

Between 3,000 and 5,000 mg-min/m^3 (inhalation).

median incapacitating dosage (ICt_{50})

5 to 10 mg-min/m^3 (inhalation). Profound pain to throat and lungs, and to the eyes.

skin toxicity

Rapid advent of blistering (possible within one hour in dense concentrations), although only 1/20th the capacity of lewisite or distilled mustard. Tends not to have the extreme residual toxicity of the latter two, either.

eye toxicity

ED vapors are highly irritating but not generally toxic. Splashed liquid may cause permanent corneal damage.

rate of action

Immediate effects on eyes and respiratory tract. Skin rash leads to blistering within one to two hours (see above).

protection required

Protective mask/respirator and full protective overclothing.

rate of detoxification

Rapid for non-lethal dosages (see above).

decontaminants

Bleaches and other oxidizers, and strong alkalines such as sodium hydroxide (NaOH) against liquid concentrations. Should be used with live steam to decontaminate massed concentrations in closed or confined spaces.

vapor density

6.0 times as heavy as air.

vapor pressure

2.09 mm Hg at 20°C(68°F); 15.1 mm Hg at 50°C(122°F).

liquid density

1.66 g/cc at 20°C(68°F).

persistency

Short. High volatility with rapid hydrolyzation gives ED an average persistency of less than an hour in temperate climates.

volatility

6500 mg-min/m^3 at 0°C(32°F); 20,000 mg-min/m^3 at 20°C (68°F); 27,200 mg-min/m^3.

latent heat of vaporization

52.5 calories per gram.

melting point

-65°C(-85°F).

boiling point

156°C(312.8°F) with decomposition.

decomposition point

156°C(312.8°F).

flash point

No immediate hazard of fire or explosion.

rate of hydrolysis

Rapid. Principal cause of ED's non-persistency.

hydrolysis products

Hydrogen chloride and ethylarsenious oxide.

stability in storage

Stable in steel canisters.

actions on metals and other materials

Very destructive to rubber and plastics, including those used in protective masks. Corrodes brass at temperatures above 122°F. No effect on ferrous alloys.

molecular weight

174.88

Warning

The above specific data refer to ethyldichloroarsine (ED) in its traditional form as a pure chemical compound. Microencapsulation could make this into a very persistent poison presenting profoundly different types of hazards.

Lewisite

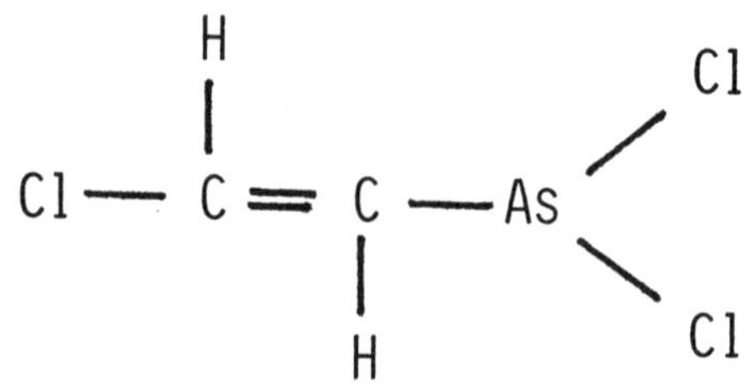

L

Standard NATO agreement (STANAG) code: L

Chemical name: dichloro (2-chlorovinyl) arsine
Common name: Lewisite
Formula: $ClCH{:}CHAsCl_2$

Family: casualty agent
Type: blister agent (arsenical)

A light amber brown liquid with a colorless vapor smelling like fresh-cut geraniums. The vapors cause immediate pain to the eyes and nasal membranes.

History

Lewisite (L) is named after its inventor, the head of a research team at the Catholic University, Washington DC where the agent was formulated in April/May of 1918. This agent was a research effort to produce a semi-persistent blister agent using the basic structure of the German arsenicals (MD, PD, and ED) fielded earlier that winter. The result was a casualty agent rivaled only by distilled mustard in terms of quantity and length of production.

Dr Lewis[1] forwarded the formulation to the newly built Edgewood Arsenal where details of manufacture and munitions were completed. First production began in mid-summer of 1918, with sufficient stocks available for shipment by October.

150 tons of lewisite-filled munitions were on their way to France at the time of the Armistice.

Lewisite was never intended to be a replacement for distilled mustard (HD), but rather to complement it as an all-purpose non/semi-persistent agent to replace the phosgenes.

Production technology was established, post-war, in Great Britain and France in 1918-1919. Italy and the Soviet Union established production by the mid 1920s. Japan began manufacture in 1928. In all these cases lewisite and distilled mustard were produced concurrently within the same plant complexes. Only the United States cut back on chemical agents production with the closure of the lewisite facility at Edgewood Arsenal.

The late 1920s and 1930s saw a revolution in the theory of war. The European powers and Japan added mechanization and aviation to their doctrines. Chemicals had been part of the last war, so they were assumed to be a part of the next one. New munitions, such as aerial sprays and bombs were developed and more factories were built to make them.

1. Dr W. Lee Lewis, Ph D, 1879-1943.

Britain built a new mustard-lewisite plant at Sutton Oak, Lancashire. Japan expanded its Tandanoumi arsenal. The USSR built a series of plants, at Brandyuzhsky, kuibyshev, and Karaganda devoted to mustard, lewisite, and phosgene. Germany's opening of plants in Munster, Wunsdorf (SW or Berlin), and List, concurrent with Japan's first use of chemicals against the Chinese in 1934 started a pre-war chemical arms race. Italy used lewisite against the Ethop-ians after 1935.

Chemical weapons were virtually non-existent in the 1939-1945 war except for China, and use there tapered off sharply after 1943. That they were not used was more an accident of misunderstanding and misapprehension. Had they been used the outcome(s) of the war would have been strangely different. Typical of non-use was the US reopening of Edgewood Arsenal and the establishment of other production plants and testing grounds. The US produced $500 million's worth of mustard and lewisite. Most of the mustard and virtually all the lewisite was mixed with sodium hypochlorate and dumped into the Gulf of Mexico by 1946.

With the discovery of the German army developed nerve agents, the western interest in lewisite tapered off. It is, however, a highly effective agent in its own right and any nation posessing simple pesticides technology can easily produce it. The odds are that lewisite is stockpiled in more than one place in this world.

Structure

It is interesting to make a simple comparison between ethylchloroarsine and lewisite.

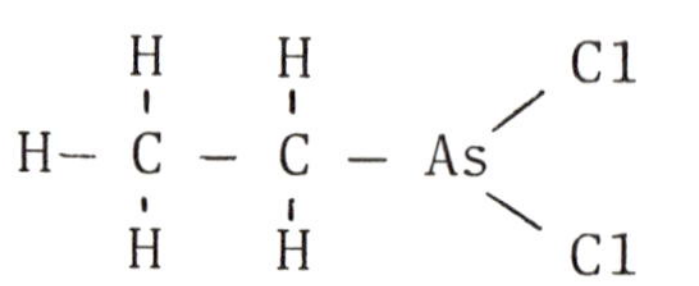

ED

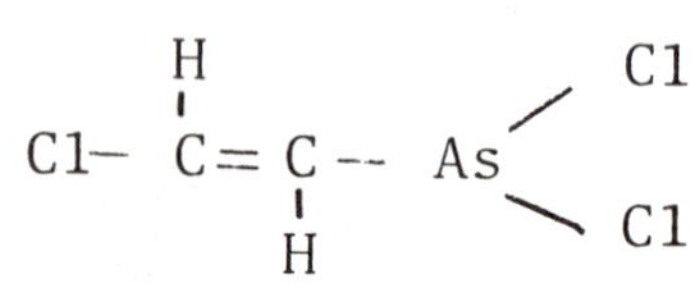

L

Replacing the ethyl bond (-C-C-) with a vinyl bond (-C=C-) accounts for lewisite's low solubility in water and lower volatility (4480 mg-min/m^3 vs 20,000 mg-min/m^3 at 68°F) than lewisite. This and the low hydrolysis of lewisite in liquid form make it a semi-persistent agent, so in a sense Dr Lewis' formulation never lived up to its origional expectations. Lewisite survived mainly due to its absolute nonflammability, which made it ideal as an aircraft delivered aerosol. It can be thinned better in light organic solvents than the sulfur-based distilled mustard and still be effective under all climatic conditions.

Lewisite involves rather sophisticated processes in its manufacture, although it can easily be produced by any country having pesticide production facilities. It is commonly obtained upon passing acetylene into a mixture of arsenic trichloride and aluminum chloride. The product must be fractionated in moving hydrogen chloride gas. The results will be lewisite [dichloro(2-chlorovinyl)arsine], bis(2-chlorovinylchloroarsine, and tris(2-chlorovinyl)arsine. Lewisite will form the lighter portion at the top of the liquid mass. All three compounds are toxic as are the vapors above the liquid, mandating, as with everything else in this book, a completely closed production cycle.

Lewisite's chlorovinyl structure gives it an ability to attack all natural and many synthetic rubbers.

Pathology

Lewisite attacks human tisue. In a pure liquid form it will cause blindness , immediate destruction of lung tissue, and systemic blood poisoning (including both red and T-cell destruction and destruction of cytochrome oxidase) should it enter either through the lungs of breaks in the skin. Absorption through the skin is similar to that of distilled mustard and like mustard blistering may take up to 13 hours, although blistering is only a symptom of subcutaneous cell destruction. Lewisite is much more toxic to the skin than distilled mustard: liquid and vapor mist on the skin will cause immediate pain with a rash forming within 30 minutes, with severe chemical burns possible. Lewisite will not dissolve in human sweat but will co-mingle with it enough to flow into such danger areas as the inner arm, elbow, ~~and~~ knee joints and ~~to~~ around the buttocks and crotch.

Inhalation death comes within 10 minutes and is more a direct effect of dry-land drowning than of systemic damage, when lethal dosage has been reached. The lungs and throat fill with mucus, blood, and dead tissue, causing asphyxiation.

The vinyl bond is not readily broken down in the human body. Lewisite accumulates in the body and for all purposes is not naturally detoxified. Dosages, especially those by some form of direct blood absorption, may accumulate and not show outward symptoms such as blistering or lung damage.

2 ml of pure liquid absorbed into a 150 lb adult through any means would probably prove fatal.

A last footnote must be made concerning hydrolysis of lewisite both to clear up a misconception and to voice a warning. Hydrolysis is dependent on surface area exposure to water vapor and air. Water will float on lewisite and prevent hydrolysis. Lewisite *vapor* or *mist* will, through the presence of oxygen and nitrogen, hydrolyze rapidly.

Among survivors symptoms of systemic poisoning may continue for an indefinate period. Including: pulmonary edema, neural disorders, subnormal temperatures, low blood pressure, and permanent damage to the endocrine system.

Field behavior

Lewisite creates vapors that are about seven times as

heavy as air. These would be expected to flow into lower portions of the terrain, and into caves, culverts, sewers, and conduits. Employed in the top floors of buildings, especially sealed buildings, lewisite would pour in a steady torrent down to the sub-basement. Lewisite lasts least in warm, humid conditions. Vaporization means hydrolysis. Used in snowy winter conditions it might last for months. Presense of water does not mean hydrolysis. Under average field conditions (68°F, partly cloudy, mild humidity) lewisite would last about a day.

Lewisite penerates many types of rubber. It presents a hazard to personnel even with protective clothing, and may damage a multitude of field equipment with rubber parts, fittings, gaskets and hoses. It will corrode many rubber-base paints and protective coatings

Specific data

median lethal dosage (LCt_{50})

1200 to 1500 mg-min/m^3 (inhalation); 100,000 mg-min/m^3 (vapor through skin: hard to build up). Accumulative.

median incapacitating dosage (ICt_{50})

Below 300 mg-min/m^3 for severe eye injury; 1500 mg-min/m^3 (inhalation). Accumulative.

skin toxicity

Immediate irritation. Toxic through subcutaneous tissue destruction in a manner identical to that of distilled mustard.

eye toxicity

Immediate searing pain with possibility of permanent corneal damage.

rate of action

Rapid.

protection required

Full mask/respirator and full protective clothing under all conditions.

rate of detoxification

Accumulative. The human body does not naturally detoxify lewisite.

decontaminants

Strong oxidizers, bleaches, and caustic soda (sodium hypochlorate). Closed or confined spaces should be treated with alkalai solutions and live steam.

vapor density

7.1 times as heavy as air.

vapor pressure

0.087 mm Hg at 0°C(32°F); 0.394 mm Hg at 20°C(68°F).

liquid density

1.89 g/cc at 20°C(68°F).

persistency

Heavily splashed liquid will persist up to a day under temperate conditions. Vapor hydrolyzation in hot, humid climates. Long duration in snow.

volatility

1060 mg/kg at 0°C(32°F); 4480 mg/kg at 20°C(68°F); 8620 mg/kg at 30°C(86°F).

latent heat of vaporization

58 calories per gram (32°F-374°F).

freezing point

-18 to 0°C(0.4 to 32°F) depending on purity.

boiling point

190°C(374°F).

decomposition point

Above 100°C (212°F).

flash point

None. Lewisite doesn't burn.

rate of hydrolysis

Low solubility in water. Rapid hydrolysis for vapor.

hydrolysis products

Hydrochloric acid. Chlorovinylarsenious oxide (a mildly toxic and blistering compound destroyed by alakaline solutions).

stability in storage

Stable in steel or glass canisters.

Actions on metals and other materials

None on ferrous alloys. May attack some forms of rubber.

molecular weight

207.35

Warning

The above specific data refer to lewisite (L) in its traditional form as a pure compound. Microencapsulation techniques could make this into a highly persistent poison presenting profoundly greater hazards.

The Nitrogen Mustards

The nitrogen mustards represent an effort to create new chemical agents from scratch in the late 1920s-1930s before the advent of nerve agents. Distilled mustard was an effort to throw a stabilized waste product at an enemy, The German arsenicals were a chance effort at making stabilized chloroarsine under a deadline. Lewisite was a two month gamble to make a better German arsenical. Nitrogen mustard was a well thought out project.

These agents were developed by accident in the German and Czech drug industries by the chloronation of triethylamine, $(C_2H_5)_3N$, used in the preparation of quaternary ammonium compounds, and related to triethanolamine $N(CH_2CH_2OH)_3$, used as an alkalizing agent in pharmaceutical therapies.

Nitrogen Mustard One

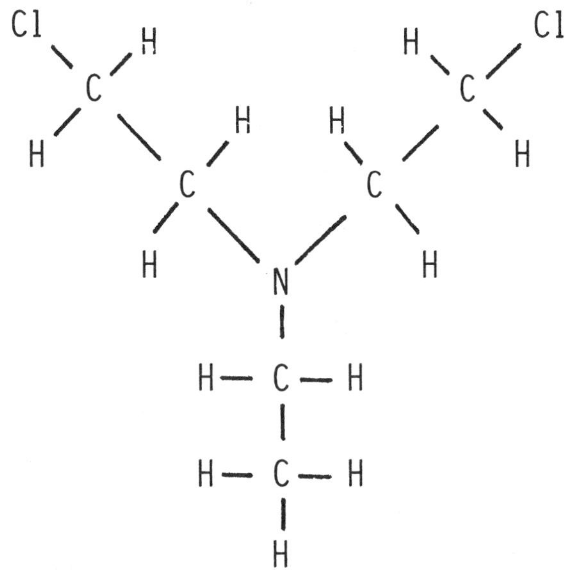

HN-1

Standard NATO agreement (STANAG) code: HN-1

Chemical name: 2, 2′-dichlorotriethylamine
Common name: nitrogen mustard one
Formula: $(ClCH_2CH_2)_2NC_2H_5$
Family: casualty agent
Type: blister agent (nitrogen mustard)

A pale amber liquid which produces a colorless vapor with an odor often described as resembling fish left out in the sun too long, or otherwise something musty. The vapors are irritating to the eyes and nasal membranes even in low concentrations.

History

Nitrogen mustard 1, HN-1 (2,2'-dichlorotriethylamine) was the first successful ammonia derivative of this series. Its war potentials first came under consideration when laboratory reports observed that blistering similar to distilled mustard and lewisite could occur with other characteristics such as respiratory damage, degenerative changes in the digestive tract, and inhibition of cell mitosis. This compound was first developed to remove warts. Subsequent studies showed that minute concentrations (typically 0.4mg in 1 kg distilled water) in direct injection would kill certain malign growths and tumors. Whole system toxic effects occured among pharmacologists and laboratory workers. From this point forward began nitrogen mustard's split personality: antineoplastic and antianthropomorphic.

Nitrogen mustard 1 is slightly less toxic than the other two agents under discussion here. Both it and nitrogen mustard 2 (HN-2) lack the stability in storage of nitorgen mustard 3 (HN-3) and so both of the former have been superseded by the latter. However, HN-1 is an extremely deadly poison and is easier (and quicker) to manufacture than HN-3, and any country having basic pesticide or pharmacological production capacity could easily make it from scratch.

Structure

Nitrogen mustard 1 has a simple structure, in which the hydrogen bonds of simple ammonia (NH_3) have been replaced with an ethyl group and two chloroethyl groups:

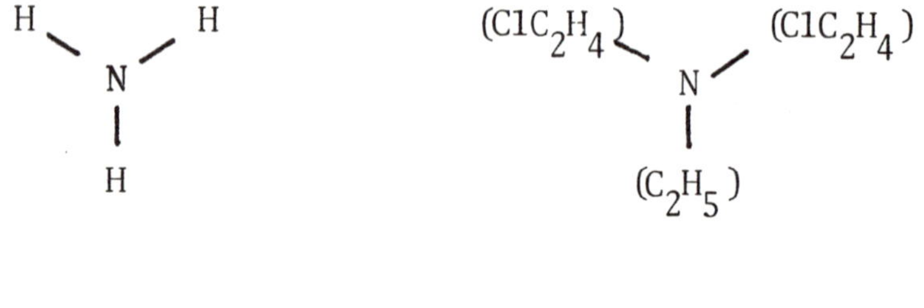

Nitrogen mustard 1's ancestry is best explained in direct comparison with its precursors, triethylamine and triethanolamine:

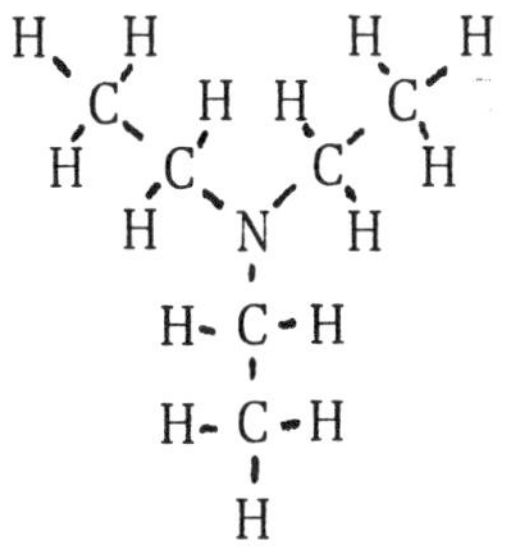

triethylamine

$(C_2H_5)_3N$

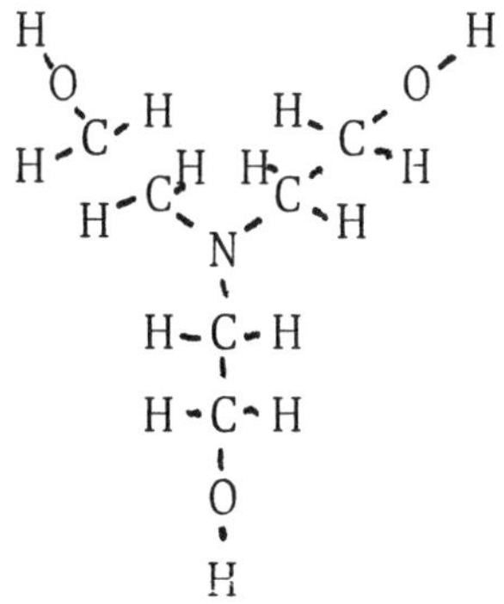

triethanolamine

$N(C_2H_4OH)_3$

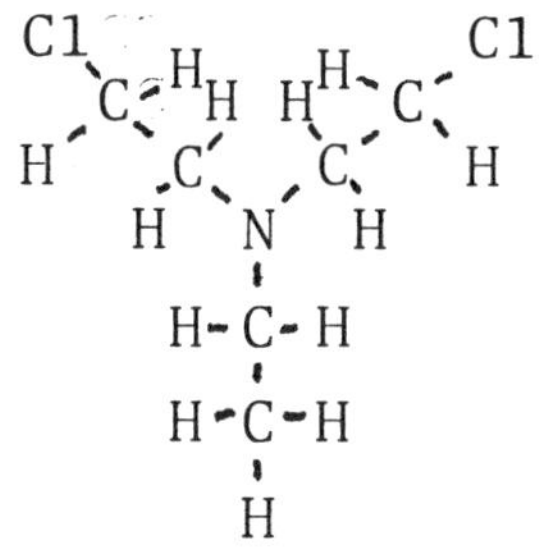

nitrogen mustard 1

$(ClC_2H_4)_2N(C_2H_5)$

Pathology

Nitrogen mustard 1 is a cumulative poison which is highly irritating to the eyes and throat. Permanent corneal damage is possible through vapor alone in concentrations of about 200 mg-min/m^3, whereas single vapor exposure probably will not cause blistering of the skin. Multiple vapor exposures, as the human body does not detoxify HN-1 in appreciable quantities, may cause skin rash within 30 minutes to an hour although full blistering may not occur for more than 12 hours. Within that twelve hour period, a progressive irritation of the respiratory tract should occur, especially if further dosages are recieved.

HN-1 penetrates the lung-blood barrier to inhibit the formation of new blood cells within the marrow and would degrade blood oxidase function. Dry-land drowning syndrome

syndrome might not be as pronounced as with distilled mustard or the chloroarsines, but bronchial pneumonia would occur in survivors after the first 24 hours.

HN-1 attacks the digestive tract, forming lesions in the small intestines, and a general necrosis with degenerative changes to all mucous membranes. Severe bloody diarrhea is a common symptom.

Field behavior

At about 6 times the weight of surrounding air, HN-1 would be expected to seek the lower levels of terrain and would flow into caves, culverts, conduits, sewers and such. Likewise, employed in the upper floors of sealed buildings, HN-1 would slowly creep downstairs to the sub-basement.

HN-1 is very slightly soluable in water (although it will suspend in water enough to be of medical use), although miscible in many organic solvents and oils, so that low hydrolysis gives it a mild persistency. Decomposition comes through slow change into quaternary ammonium salts. HN-1 will persist up to a day under moderate climatic conditions (68°F, semi-cloudy). May persist up to a week under snow, although the lower the ambiant temperature the less its vaporization becomes.

Specific data

median lethal dosage (LCt_{50})

1500 mg-min/m^3 (inhalation); 20,000 mg-min/m^3 (skin).

median incapacitating dosage (ICt_{50})

9,000 mg-min/m^3 (skin); 200 mg-min/m^3 (eyes).

skin toxicity

Toxic to subcutaneous tissue. Rashes quickly but blisters slowly (blister rate similar to HD). Worst effects are to underarms, behind knees and elbows, and around the buttocks and crotch.

eye toxicity

Eye injury possible with low concentrations. The nitrogen mustards have the greatest immediate effects on the eyes of all the blister agents.

rate of action

Immediate effect on eyes. Skin rash will appear within an hour from liquid or very heavy vapor. Blistering delayed an average of 12 hours (replacing rash) and systemic poisoning may not become apparent for days.

protection required

Protective mask/respirator and full protective clothing against the hazard of liquid, mist, or heavy vapor.

rate of detoxification

Essentially no natural detoxification. Effects will be accumulative.

decontaminants

Strong bleaches and oxidizers. Sodium hydroxide (NaOH); caustic alcohol, and other strong alkalai solutions must be used against liquid infestation. Alkalies with live steam recommended for use in closed or confined spaces.

vapor density

5.9 times as heavy as air.

vapor pressure

0.24 mm Hg at 25°C(77°F).

liquid density

1.09 g/cc at 25°C(77°F).

persistency

Mildly persistent. Up to a day in moderate climate, less in dry, arid conditions. May last for about a week under snowy conditions. Delivered effectively as an aerial spray, a la HD.

volatility

127 mg/m^3 at -10°C(14°F); 308 mg/m^3 at 0°C(32°F); 1520 mg/m^3 at 20°C(68°F); 3100 mg/m^3 at 30°C(86°F). Compare with HD as basis.

latent heat of vaporization

77 calories per gram.

freezing point

-34°C.

boiling point

194°C(381°F) with decomposition.

decomposition point

Below 194°C(381°F).

flash point

No immediate danger of fire or explosion.

rate of hydrolysis

Slow. HN-1 hydrolyzes very slowly.

hydrolysis products

Hydroxyl derivatives and condensation products.

stability in storage

Polymerizes slowly, so munitions would be effective for several years. HN-1 is obsolete, this being one of the prime reasons.

actions on metals and other materials

Corrosive to ferrous alloys beginning at 65°C(149°F).

molecular weight

170.08

Nitrogen Mustard Two

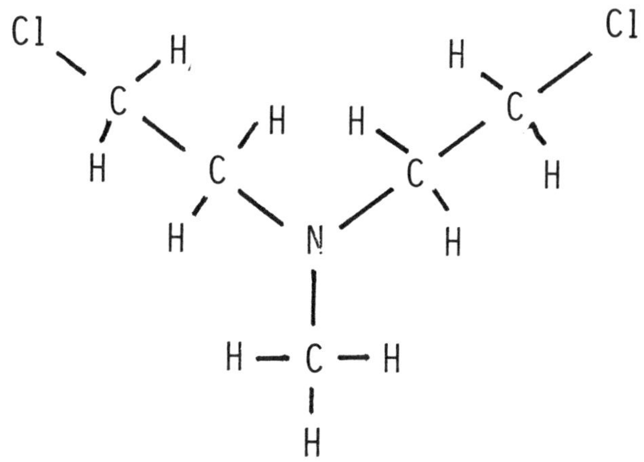

HN-2

Standard NATO agreement (STANAG) code: HN-2

Chemical name: 2,2'-dichloro-N-methylethylamine
Common name: nitrogen mustard two; mustine
Formula: $(ClCH_2CH_2)_2 NCH_3$

Family: casualty agent
Type: blister agent (nitrogen mustard)

A pale amber liquid which produces a colorless vapor smelling somewhat like old-fashioned lye soap and which is immediately damaging to the eyes and respiratory tract. Unlikely to be encountered due to its tendency to break down within its munitions.

History

Nitrogen mustard two (HN-2; 2,2′ dichloro-N-methyldiethylamine) appears to have been formulated about the same time as nitrogen mustard one (HN-1). Whereas HN-1 was a pharmaceutical experiment that became a military agent, HN-2 was a prospective military agent that became a pharmaceutical substance known as *mustine* (or HN-2).

The nitrogen mustards are ammonia derivatives dating from the early 1930s. Their immediate chemical ancestors include triethylamine $[(C_2H_5)_3N]$ and triethanolamine $[N(C_2H_4OH)_3]$.

There were several reasons for the development of this series of agents. First, they are more immediately toxic than the sulfur mustards, especially to the eyes. Secondly, they tended to break down the cellulose-based filter elements of the day. Thirdly, they are effective systemic poisons, their use causing an enemy's medical facilities to be streached to the limit.

An HN-2 molecule is asymmetrical, causing it to break down in storage through polymerization, forming numerous condensation products. Otherwise this is a very dangerous compound creating high vapor pressure, having an appreciable vapor density, and being highly volatile.

HN-2's reactivity makes it a good antineoplastic, a substance for destroying tumors if injected directly into them. As a pharmaceutical it is mixed with water at a ratio of 0.4 mg HN-2 to 1 kg distilled water. The maxim has it that one molecule of HN-2 kills one tumor cell. However, since the human body by itself does not detoxify HN-2, such therapy is a very complicated process.

Although not considered seriously as a military agent by the major powers, HN-2 can be manufactured by any country having pharmaceutical production capacity and used as a last-ditch effort.

Structure

Nitrogen mustard two has a simple structure, being formed around a simple ammonia (NH_3) structure in which two of the hydrogen bonds are replaced by chloroethyl (ClC_2H_4-) groups and the third replaced by a methyl (CH_3) group.

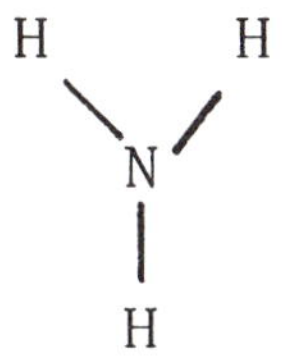

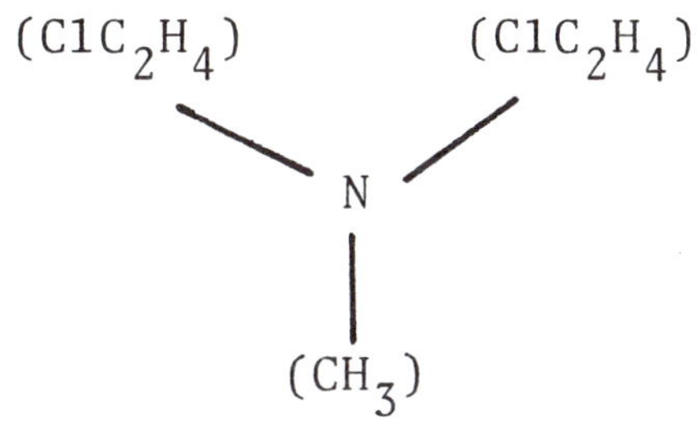

The asymetry of NH-2 is obvious when the structural diagram pages of the three nitorgen mustards are compared.

The production process of HN-2 involves preparation by the action of thionyl chloride on 2,2' -(methylamino) diethanol in trichloroethylene.

Pathology

Nitrogen mustard two is a cumulative poison. It is highly irritating to the eyes and throat and in high enough concentrations can cause blindness. Absorbed into the bloodstream it will seriously interfere with the functioning of hemoglobin and will eventually damage the endocrine system. High volatility and vapor pressure give HN-2 an ability to create blistering through vapor absorption exceeding that of HN-1 and HN-3. In liquid toxicity it falls halfway between HN-1 and HN-3. The skin is attacked in the subcutaneous layers, forming an epidermal rash within an hour or so following exposure or build-up of sub-dosages within the skin to significant levels. Actual blistering may not occur for about twelve hours following the beginning of a skin rash. As with all of the blister agents, insdiious effects are possible when vapor or liquid mixes with sweat and flows down to tender skin areas. Common would be under the armpits, knee and elbow joints, and around the buttocks and crotch. Pulmonary effects may not be as spectacular as those evidenced by distilled mustard. although dry-land drowning syndrome is possible as the lungs flood with mucus, dead tissue and blood and a victim dies of asphyxiation and heart failure.

Field behavior

Nitrogen mustard is highly unlikely to ever appear under wartime conditions. However, production and laboratory incidents can occur.

HN-2, at 5.4 times the weight of air would seek the lower terrain and structural elevations. The greater the ambiant temperature the greater HN-2's volatility, and thus the greater its diffusion. Between 80°F and 100°F HN-2's volatility increases dramatically. It would further flow into substrcutures and thence into conduits, culverts, service corridors and into sewage systems.

Under temperate conditions (68°F, moderate humidity) heavily splashed HN-2 may last perhaps a day in open areas and longer in enclosed or confined spaces. It will precipitate into polymeric quaternary ammonium salts (dark brown crystalline solids) which present their own health hazards.

Specific data

median lethal dosage (LCt_{50})

3000 mg-min/m^3 (inhalation)

median incapacitating dosage (ICt_{50})

9500 mg-min/m^3 (skin absorption, est); 100 mg-min/m^3 (eyes) *skin toxicity*

Toxic. See Pathology. Accumulative.

eye toxicity

Toxic. Eye effects are very pronounced, and more rapidly produced than with distilled mustard. Permanent corneal damage possible. Accumulates in system.

rate of action

Immediate effects on eyes. Skin rash may be possible within 30 minutes if significant doage is recieved or builds up. Actual blistering and pulmonary effects may be delayed about 12 hours.

protection required

Protective mask/respirator. Full protective clothing should be worn, especially in presence of liquid or mist.

rate of detoxification

Not naturally detoxified by the body.

decontaminants

Strong bleaches and other oxidizers; strong alkalies (eq, sodium hydroxide, NaOH). Liquid infestation should be dealt with using strong alkalai solutions and live steam.

vapor density

5.4 times as heavy as air.

vapor pressure

0.29 mm Hg at 20°C(68°F); 1.25 mm Hg at 40°C(104°F).

liquid density

1.15 g/cc at 20°C(68°F).

persistency

Heavily splashed liquid may last up to one day in moderate weather and for about four or five days under extreme cold. HN-2 polymerizes of its own accord.

volatility

3580 mg/kg at 25°C(77°F); 5100 mg/kg at 30°C(86°F); 10,000 mg/kg at 40°C(104°F).

latent heat of vaporization

78.8 calories per gram.

freezing point

-65°C(-85°F).

boiling point

75°C(167°F). Decomposes before boiling.

decomposition point

Below boiling point. Polymerized components will present an explosion hazard in open air.

flash point

No immediate danger of fire or explosion. See decomposition point, above, for warning.

rate of hydrolysis

Slow, except in present of alkalais (which make effective decontaminants). Breaks down in water with an hour.

hydrolysis products

Complex polymeric quaternary ammonium salts.

stability in storage

Unstable due to tendency to polymerize under all conditions. This includes spray tanks as well as artillery and rocket rounds. Pharmaceutical solutions tend to have a short shelf life.

action on metals and other materials

None of significance.

molecular weight

156.07

Nitrogen Mustard Three

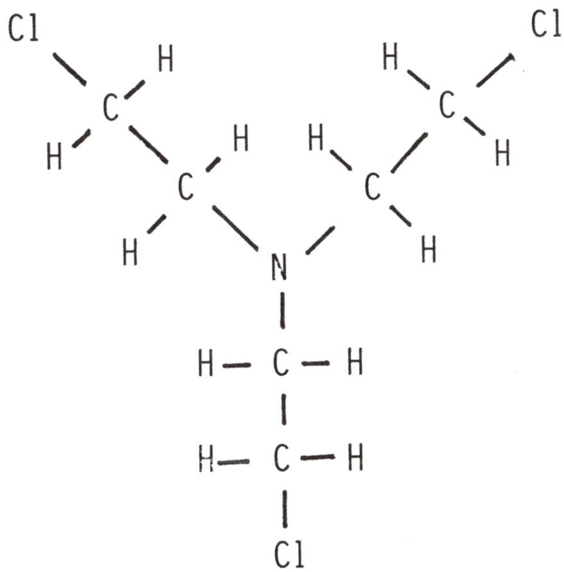

HN-3

Standard NATO agreement (STANAG) code: HN-3

Chemical name: 2,2',2''-trichlorotriethylamine

Common name: nitrogen mustard three

Formula: $N(CH_2CH_2Cl)_3$

Family: casualty agent

Type: blister agent (nitrogen mustard)

A pale amber liquid which produces a colorless and odorless (when pure) vapor which produces immediate eye irritation, eye photosensitivity, and respiratory tract damage.

History

Nitrogen mustard 3 (2,2',2'' trichlorotriethylamine) was the last of the three nitrogen based blister agents standardized under an HN code. Whereas HN-1 was designed as a pharmaceutical and became a military agent, and HN-2 was designed as a military agent and became a pharmaceutical, HN-3 was designed as a military agent and remained such. It is the only one of the three that remains anywhere as a military agent, notably in the east block nations.

The nitrogen mustards do not store well, due to a tendency to polymerize into quaternary ammonium salts which are not reabsorbed into solution. Although HN-3 is the most stable of the series, it too will decompose while in munitions. For this reason HN-3 never superceded distilled mustard (HD) in NATO inventories. Toxicologically, HN-3 and HD are similar, save that HN-3 has a pronounced lacrimatory effect and rapidly produces skin rash.

Any nation with pesticide production capacity can produce this agent.

Structure

Nitrogen mustard 3 has a simple structure, in which the hydrogen bonds of simple ammonia (NH_3) have been replaced with three chloroethyl ($ClC_2H_4^-$) groups.

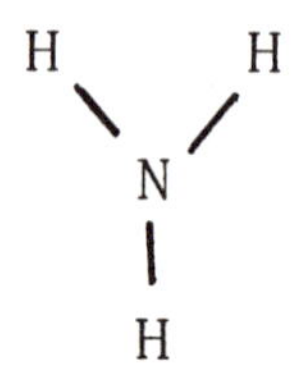

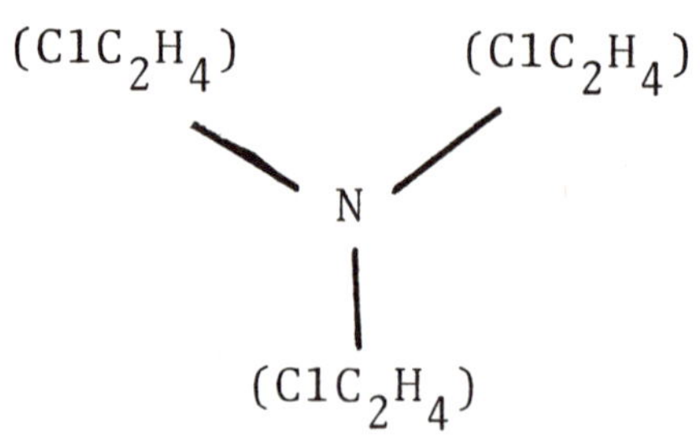

Nitrogen mustard 3 may be considered a purification of nitrogen mustard 1 $(ClC_2H_4)_2N(C_2H_5)$ in which the latter ethane group is replaced with a chloroethane (ClC_2H_4) group producing a symmetrical molecule less prone to internal reaction than the parent compound. HN-3 is the least volatile of the HN series.

The HN series developed from nitrogen compounds developed in the pharmaceutical industries of Czechoslovakia, Germany, and France in the late 1920s and early 1930s. The immediate parent coumpounds were triethylamine, $(C_2H_5)_3N$, and triethanolamine, $N(C_2H_4OH)_3$.

Pathology

Nitrogen mustard 3 is a cumulative poison which is highly irritating to the eyes and throat. Permanent corneal damage is possible through vapor exposure alone in concentrations of about 200 mg-min/m^3, as with the other HN agents. HN-3, as a drawback to its relative stability, does not create sufficient vapor density to cause rash and blistering from single exposures. Blistering may result from either splashed liquid, multiple or persistent exposure, or vapor condensation in sweat. The latter may have insidious effects as sweat tends to accumulate in tender areas such as the armpits, the back of knee and elbow joints, and around the buttocks and crotch. A rash will develop from liquid contamination within about an hour, replaced by blistering anywhere between six and twelve hours. Toxic effects on the eyes are immediate.

HN-3 penetrates the lung-blood barrier with ease. It will interfere with hemoglobin functioning in the blood and upon reaching bone marrow will hinder the production of new blood cells. It will destroy white blood cells, thus damaging the body's immune system.

Dry-land drowning may occur following lethal dosage

absorption. In this syndrome the lungs become clogged with mucus, dead tissue and blood. The victim dies of asphyxiation and concurrent pulmonary endema.

Survivors may suffer permanent damage to the immune and endocrine systems. Damages to the lungs and throat would also be permament.

Field behavior

Nitrogen mustard 3 presents the least vapor hazard of these three HN agents, even under tropical or desert conditions. Its vapor density of about 7 times the weight of air would, however, make a danger within substructures of buildings and lower laying terrain.

HN-3 is far more persistent than distilled mustard, perhaps by a factor of two to three, depending on conditions. HN-3 has low water solubility in addition to low vapor mass. Its freezing point is slightly below that of water and it would remain for considerable periods in extreme weather conditions, adhering to passing equipment and personnel.

Soviet doctrine emphasizes the use of this type agent to contaminate ("deny use of") enemy stores and equipment far behind the lines, and to deny the use of terrain to an opponent for extended periods.

Specific data

median lethal dosage (LCt_{50})

1500 mg-min/m^3 (inhalation); 10,000 mg-min/m^3 (skin absorption).

median incapacitating dosage (ICt_{50})

200 mg-min/m^3 (eye injury); 2500 mg-min/m^3 (skin absorption).

skin toxicity

Toxic. Subcutaneous damage via liquid. See Pathology.

eye toxicity

Toxic. Immediate irritation, with permament eye damage possible through liquid or dose accumulation.

rate of action

Eye effects are immediate. Skin rash will appear within an hour or so, with blistering delayed for as much as ten to twelve hours, assuming non immediate lethal dosage.

protection required

Protective mask/respirator with full protective overclothing against liquid.

rate of decontamination

Not naturally detoxified by the body. Effects are cumulative.

decontaminants

Strong bleaches or oxidizers. Strong liquid infestations may be decontaminated by strong alkalis such as caustic soda (sodium hydroxide, NaOH) and live steam. Also DS2 (caustic alcohol).

vapor density

7.1 times as heavy as air.

vapor pressure

0.0109 mm Hg at 25°C(77°F).

liquid density

1.24 g/cc at 25°C(77°F).

persistency

Considerably longer than HD (without HD's vapor hazard). May last for several days under temperate weather conditions and for an indefinate time in extreme winter situations.

volatility

Low: 13 mg-min/m^3 at 0°C(32°F); 121 mg-min/m^3 at 25°C(77°F); 180 mg-min/m^3 at 30°C(86°F); 390 mg-min/m^3 at 40°C(104°F).

latent heat of vaporization

74 calories per gram.

freezing point

-3.7°C(25.3°F).

boiling point

256°C(492.8°F), calculated.

decomposition point

Below 256°C(492.8°F).

flash point

No immediate hazard of fire.

rate of hydrolysis

Slow. HN-3 has low water solubility.

hydrolysis products

Trietholamine [$N(C_2H_4OH)_3$] and hydrochloric acid (HCl).

stability in storage

Slow but steady polymerization. Munitions effective for severla years, with gradual formation of dark amber polymeric quaternary ammonium salts not resoluble in their parent compound.

action on metals and other materials

None of significance.

molecular weight

204.54

Warning

The above specific data refer to nitorgen mustard 3 in its usual form as a pure chemical. Microencapsulation techniques could make this a poison presenting profoundly greater hazards.

The Oximes

• CX

Phosgene oxime (CX) is the only extant member of this class. It appears to have origionated in the Soviet Union as a by-product of research into insecticides for cockroaches.

Much of the information regarding this agent has come from East block military manuals, such as those produced by East Germany (the DDR).

Phosgene Oxime

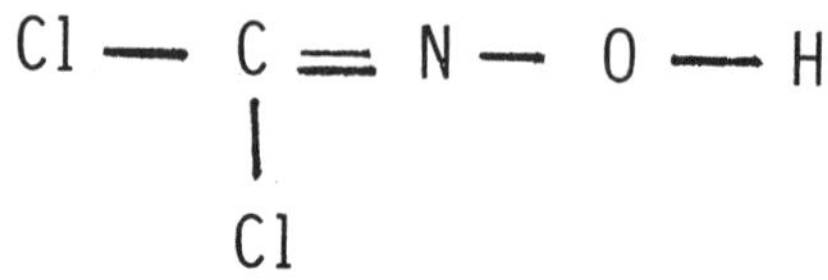

CX

Standard NATO agreement (STANAG) code: CX

Chemical name: dichloroform oxime
Common name: phosgene oxime
Formula: CCl_2NOH

Family: casualty agent
Type: blister agent (oxime)

In pure form a white solid. When melted, burned, or dissolved it emits a clear musty, pepperish vapor causing violent irritation to the eyes and nasal membranes.

History

Nothing of this compound exists in any of the standard chemical or pharmaceutical texts. Passing references are made to it in chemical warfare literature in terms of its effects, and to the fact that samples were taken in central and northern Laos in the 1980s.

Commonly confused with phosgene in some popular sources, although that compound ($COCl_2$) is probably the aldehyde from which this compound is formed (see below).

Phosgene oxime has developed a reputation for being a very nasty systemic poison whose effects are prone to reoccur up to a year after exposure. It produces ulcerating sores which feel like elongated bee stings. One wag has put it that the "bees" that dropped "yellow rain" in Laos also left some of this, their venom.

Structure

Oximes are compounds containing an NOH^{+2} radical, formed as a condensation product of hydroxylamine (N_3OH) with aldehydes or keytones. Phosgene (carbonyl chloride, $COCl_2$) fits the catagory of a keytone by virtue of its (C:O) bond, so the following would seem feasible:

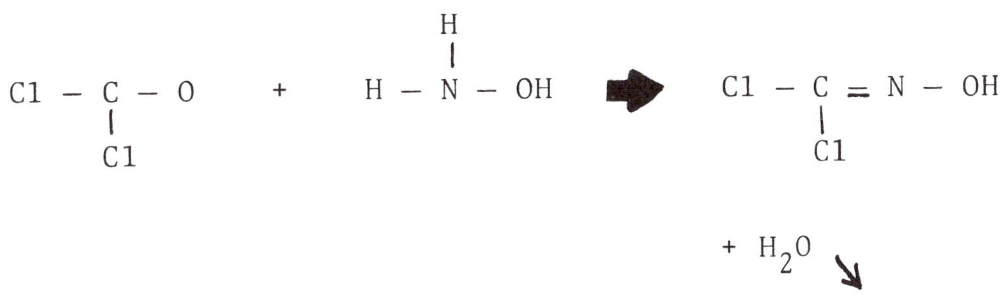

The result would be an anhydrous solid, phosgene oxime.

Pathology

Phosgene oxime represents an entirely new concept in blister agents. The previous agents in this chapter all attack the human system to produce toxic effects *under* the skin with the result that oxidation-reduction reactions in living tissue produce water blisters containing concentrations of unutilized chemical agent form on the surface. In this manner the body attempts to detoxify a systemic poison which has entered through the skin.

Phosgene oxime acts a bit different. It simply attacks whatever tissue it comes in contact with, skin, muscle and nerve alike. Its neuro-destructiveness can cause intense, unremitting pain. The human body detoxifies this agent very slowly. The mechanism of expulsion appears to be through the skin, hence the reappearence of initial symptoms. Being anhydrous in nature, this compound even prevents water-blisters common to the other blister agents. Instead, CX forms hard tissue masses like beesting wheals in which expelled CX may collect under scab materials, and may re-enter the body via adjacent tissue.

Initially, CX comes into contact with the skin and leaves a blanched area within 30 seconds where it is absorbed into the skin. A red, rash-like, ring immediately forms surrounding a forming wheal. Within a day the blanced area and rash will turn dark as broken down skin pigment pools near the surface. A scab will form over the whole in about a week, which may fall off after another three weeks. Depending on the total dosage recieved, total healing may take a week to about a year (severe cases).

Immediate death from systemic shock or trauma is possible. Effects from inhalation are little known in the west. This agent is readily water soluble (even though it precipitates), which might be an ameliorating factor.

This agent will dissolve in human sweat. A particularly insidious effect must be avoided through use of protective overclothing: if mixed in sweat, phosgene oxime would flow into the more tender parts of the body, to include the armpits, the hollows behind the elbows and knees, and to the area of the buttocks and crotch.

Phosgene oxime's effects are INSTANTANEOUS. Even immediate decontamination would do little to ease pain. Treatment may involve neuro blocking drugs.

Field behavior

Phosgene oxime in pure form is a colorless, crystalline solid which would probably be micropulverized into a fine powder or dust. It may also be encountered as a water based aerosol.

CX melts at about 40°C(104°F). Thus, below that temperature its pure compound would create no vapor pressure of its own. Contamination would be either by aerial or ground contamination.

CX would probably exist in the environment until fully diminished through rain, fog, or snow. In desert areas it would be expected to evaporate *where exposed to direct sunlight* when temperatures rise above 104°F.

Specific data

median lethal dosage (LCt_{50})

Unknown.

median incapacitating dosage (ICt_{50})

Minimal exposure causes accute discomfort.

skin toxicity

See Pathology.

eye toxicity

Highly toxic. Severe injury possible.

rate of action

Immediate. See Pathology.

protection required

Protective mask/respirator and full protective overclothing.

rate of detoxification

Not fully studied. Many cases last from between two months and a year for full recovery. Reoccurances can be as painful as initial contact.

decontaminants

Warm water effectively dissolves CX. Bleaches and strong oxidizers will break down the compound. Strong alkalai solutions (such as sodium hydroxide, NaOH) with live steam should be used on large ground and structural areas of contamination.

vapor density

None below 40°C(104°F). CX is normally a solid.

vapor pressure

None below 40°C(104°F). Temperature/pressure curve not fully studied.

solid density

Probably between 1.40 and 1.50 g/cc at 20°C(68°F).

persistency

See Field Behavior.

volatility

None below 40°C(104°F). See Vapor Pressure, above.

latent heat of vaporization

Indeterminate.

melting point

About 40°C(104°F)

boiling point

About 54°C(129.2°F), with decomposition.

decomposition point

At boiling point.

flash point

None.

rate of hydrolysis

Data not available.

hydrolysis products

Data not available.

stability in storage

Stable in steel containers when dry.

action on metals and other materials

Slightly acidic and corrosive when mixed with water.

molecular weight

113.92

Mixes

mustard-lewisite mix

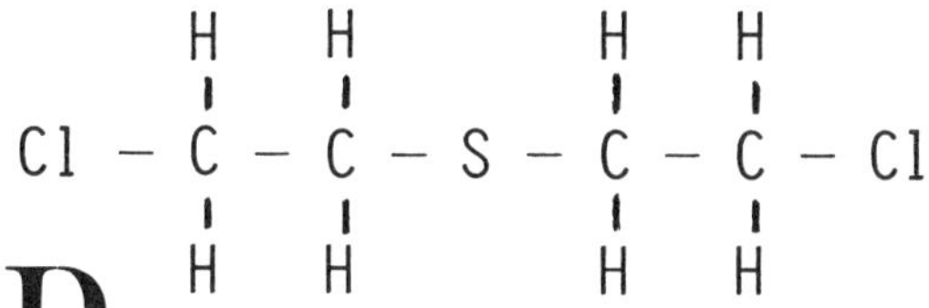

HD

37-50% by volume

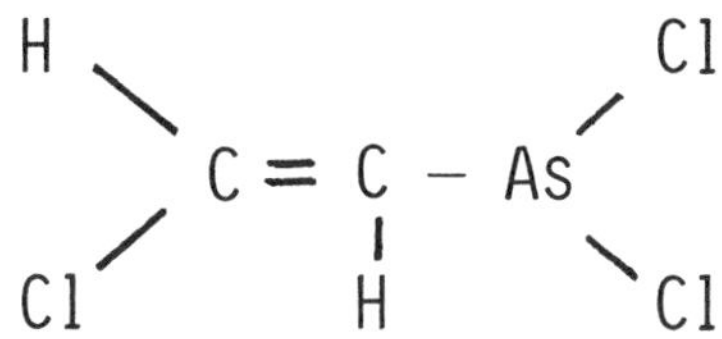

L

50-63% by volume

HL

Standard NATO agreement (STANAG) code: HL

Chemical name: (none)
Common name: ML mix
Formula: (as per components)

Family: casualty agent
Type: blister agent (mustard-arsenical mix)

A deep amber to dark brown oily liquid with a strong, musky, garlicly odor. Composed of off-the-shelf agents. Devised as a low-freezing mixture for use in cold weather operation and high altitude aerial sprays.

Specific data (HL)

median lethal dosage (*LCt_{50}*)

1500 mg-min/m^3 (inhalation); above 10,000 mg-min/m^3 (skin absorption).

median incapacitating dosage (*ICt_{50}*)

200 mg-min/m^3 (eye injury); 1500-2000 mg-min/m^3 (skin absorption).

skin toxicity

Highly toxic. Subcutaneous damage. Rash will form within an hour with blistering of entire reddened area within 13 hours. Dosages are accumulative and not detoxified.

eye toxicity

Highly toxic. Permanent damge to corneas with concentrations approaching 200 mg-min/m^3. Blindness would be expected. Dosages are accumulated and not detoxified.

systemic pathology

Dry-land drowning syndrome likely and permanent damage to lungs and endocrine system. Destruction of bone marrow and blood cells.

rate of action

Rapid. Immediate eye irritation. See above.

protection required

Protective mask/respirator and full protective clothing.

rate of detoxification

Not naturally detoxified within the human body.

decontaminants

Bleaches and oxidizers; strong alkalies, such as sodium hydroxide (NaOH). Closed areas and confined spaces should be cleaned out with strong alkalai solutions with live steam.

vapor density

6.5 times as heavy as air.

vapor pressure

0.02 mm Hg at -10°C(14°F); 0.248 mm Hg at 20°C(68°F); 1.03 mm Hg at 40°C(104°C).

liquid density

Average of 1.66 g/cc at 20°C(68°F).

persistency

Lasts about 1 to 1½ days under temperate weather conditions. About a week under extreme winter conditions.

volatility

240 mg/m^3 at -11°C(12.2°F); 2730 mg/m^3 at 20°C(68°F); 10,270 mg/m^3 at 40°C(104°F). Calculated from components.

latent heat of vaporization

Aprox 70 calories per gram. Average of components (see HD and L, then calculate by proportion).

freezing point

Between -24.5°C(-12.1°F) and -42°C(-43.6°F). Designed for cold weather use.

boiling point

About 190°C(374°F). Decomposes before boiling.

decomposition point

Above 100°C(212°F).

flash point

No immediate danger of explosion or fire.

rate of hydrolysis

Lewisite component hydrolyses as a vapor (see L), whereas distilled mustard hydroylses slowly (see HD).

hydrolysis products

Hydrochloric acid, thiodiglycol, chlorovinylarsenious oxide. Hydrolysis under alkaline conditions will destroy the blistering abilities of L and HD.

stability in storage

Best stored in laquered steel containers. No hazardous chemical reactions between components.

actions on metals or other materials

None of significance.

molecular weight

186.4 (based on 63% L and 37% HD composition)

mustard-T mixture

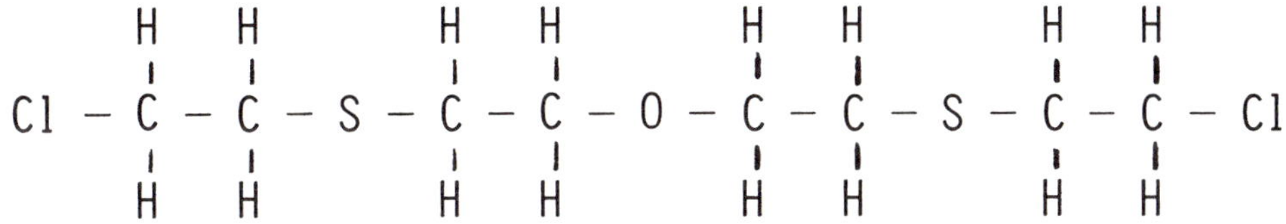

T

40% by volume

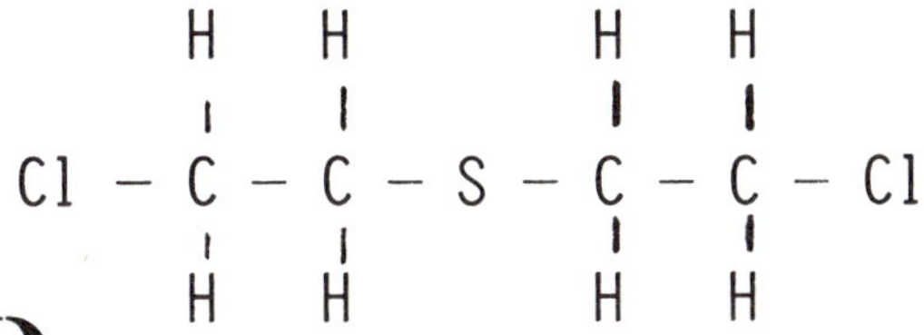

HD

60% by volume

HT

Standard NATO agreement (STANAG) code: HT

Chemical name: (none)
Common name: HT mix
Formula: (as per components, qv)

Family: casualty agent
Type: blister agent (mustard)

A clear yellow to pale amber liquid with about twice the persistency of HD alone. T has a low volatility, being designed for absorption rather than inhalation. Intended when first produced in the late 1930s for use in aircraft aerosols. Same pathology as HD. Superseded more by doctorine than by anything else, with the advent of persistent nerve agents. Semi-obsolete.

Code-designated blister agents not found in production

- Q
- T

Both these agents date from the years immediately prior to the second world war. T, an "extended" molecular version of HD, saw production as part of the mix HT (qv).

4, bis (methylchloroethyl sulfide)

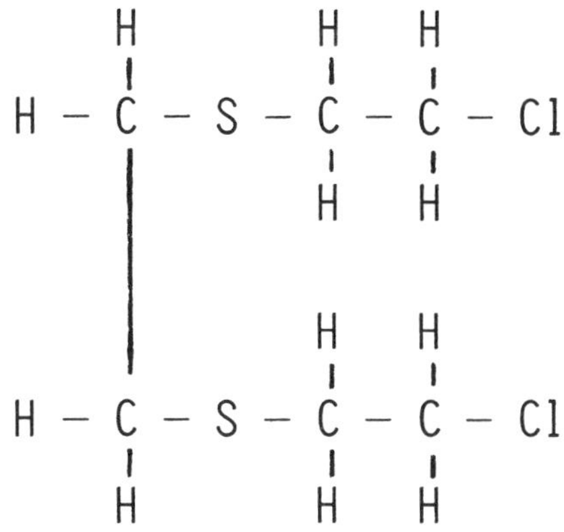

Q

$ICt_{50} = 300$ mg-min/m^3

Standard NATO agreement (STANAG) code: Q

Chemical name: 4, bis (methylchloroethyl sulfide)
Common name: Q
Formula: $(CH_2SC_2H_4Cl)_2$

Family: casualty agent
Type: blister agent (mustard)

In pure form a pale amber solid with little or no odor. Created in the mid 1930s at the British Porton Down facilities as a quick acting casualty agent with the asphyxiating qualities of phosgene, CG (qv), and the delayed blistering/systemic damage of distilled mustard. Compare with structure of HD.

Obsolete but easily synthesized. Used in solution with any of several organic solvents, as an aerosol.

bis(2-chloroethyl sulfide) monoxide

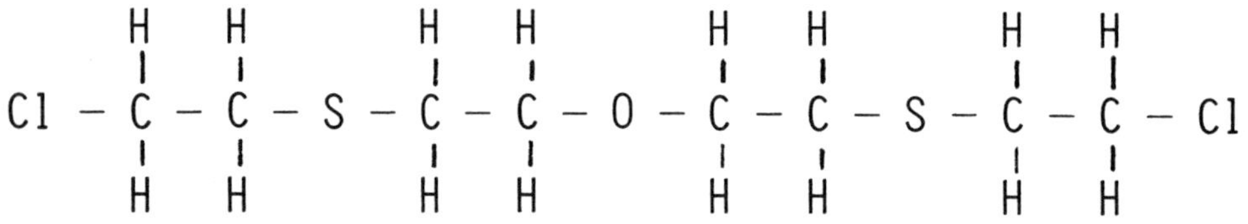

T

$ICt_{50} = 400\ mg\text{-}min/m^3$

Standard NATO agreement (STANAG) code: T

Chemical name: bis(2-chloroethyl sulfide) monoxide
Common name: T
Formula: $(ClC_2H_4SC_2H_4)O(C_2H_4SC_2H_4Cl)$; $O(C_2H_4SC_2H_4Cl)_2$

Family: casualty agent
Type: blister agent (mustard)

A dark oily liquid with little or no odor. Created in the mid 1930s at the British Porton Down facilities as a distilled mustard thickener (used in HT) for use in aerial sprays, or by itself in warm climates. As a pure agent it is obsolete. As a mixer it is semi-obsolete.

Structurally, T consisits of two HD groups tied together with an oxygen (ether) bond.

Comparative
Tables

comparative data

agent	*rate of action*	*state at 68°F*	*odor*	*volatility (mg/m³)*	*LCt_{50} (mg-min/m³)*	*ICt_{50} (mg-min/m³)*	*vapor density (x air)*	*vapor pressure (mm Hg)*
HD	delayed, hours to days	colorless to pale yellow liquid	raw garlic	610 at 68°F	1500 inhal; 10,000 skin	200 eye; 2000 skin	5.4	0.072 at 68°F
MD	rapid	colorless liquid	none when pure	74,900 at 68°F	3,000	25 inhal	5.5	7.76 at 68°F
PD	immediate eye; to 1 hr skin	colorless liquid	none when pure	390 at 77°F	2600 inhal	16 vomit; 1800 blist	7.7	0.033 at 77°F
ED	immediate irritation; blistering delayed	colorless liquid	none when pure	20,000 at 68°F	3000 inhal	5-10 inhal	6.0	2.09 at 68°F
L	rapid	dark oily liquid	may resemble geraniums	4480 at 68°F	1200 inhal 100,000 skin	300 eye; 1500 skin	7.1	0.394 at 68°F
HN1	delayed: 12 or more hours (blistering)	dark liquid	fishy or musty	1520 at 68°F	1500 inhal; 20,000 skin	200 eye 9000 skin	5.9	0.24 at 77°F
HN2	delayed: 12 or more hours (blistering)	dark liquid	soapy to fruity	3580 at 77°F	3000 inhal	100 eye	5.4	0.29 at 68°F
HN3	delayed, hours to days	dark liquid	none when pure	121 at 77°F	1500 inhal; 10,000 skin	200 eye; 10,000 skin	7.1	0.0109 at 77°F
CX	instantaneous	colorless solid if pure	like tear gas	none	unknown	any expos	none	none

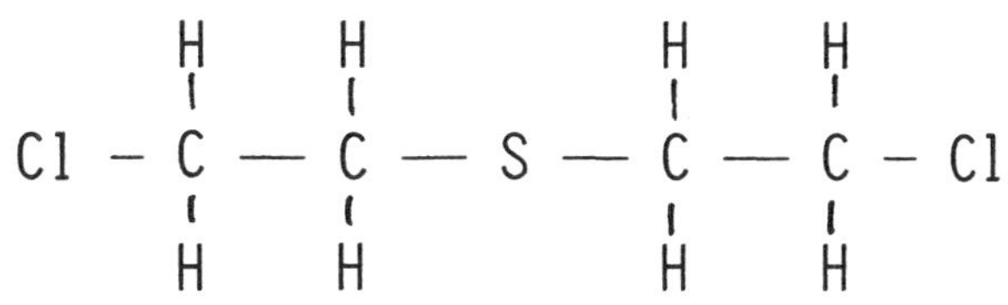

Distilled Mustard (HD)

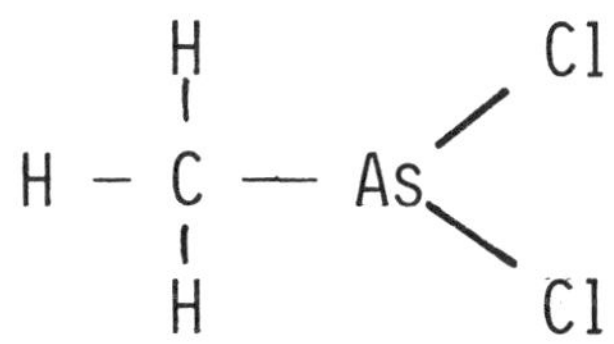

Methyldichloroarsine (MD)

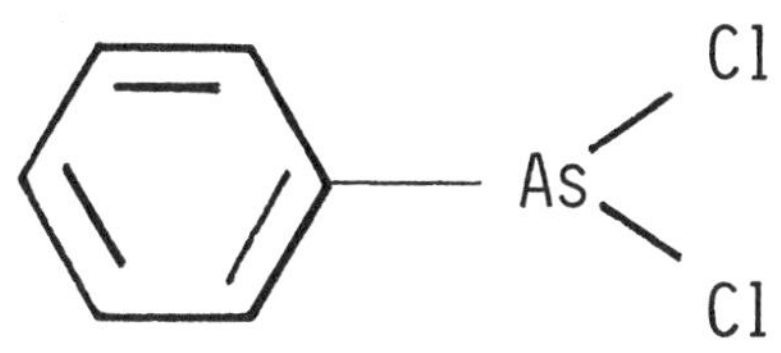

Phenyldichloroarsine (PD)

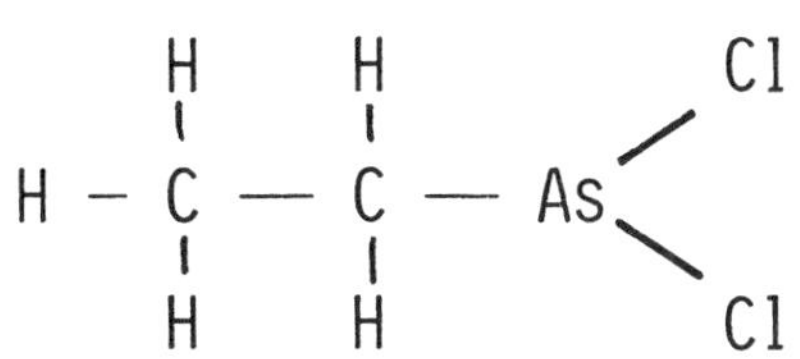

Ethyldichloroarsine (ED)

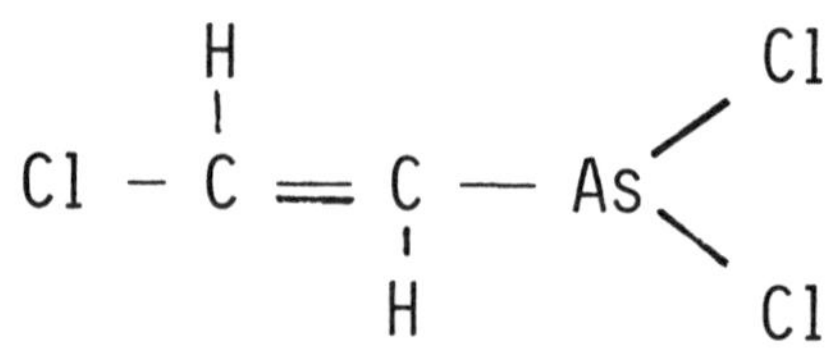

Lewisite (L)

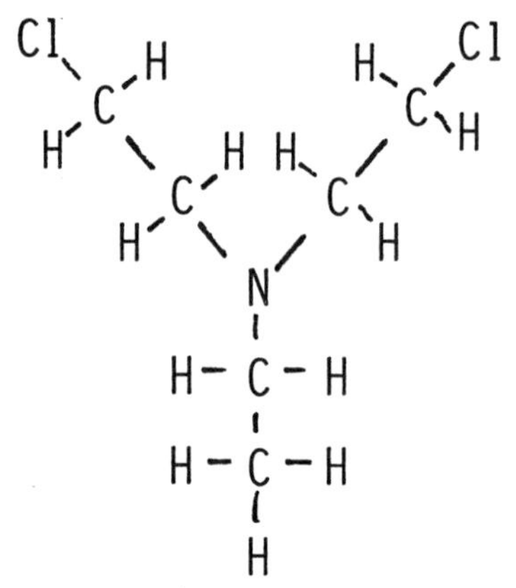

Nitrogen mustard One (HN-1)

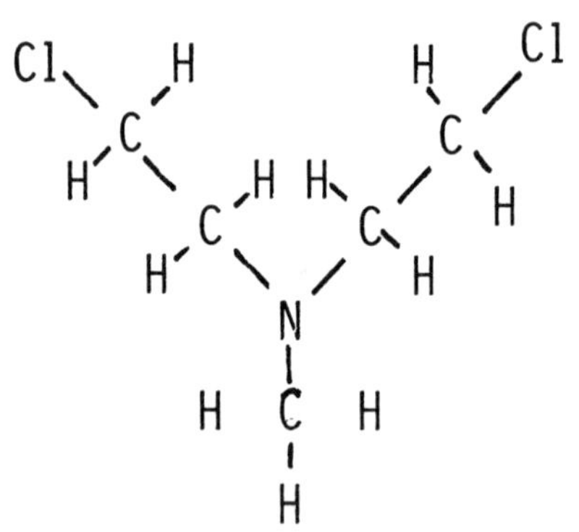

Nitrogen mustard Two (HN-2)

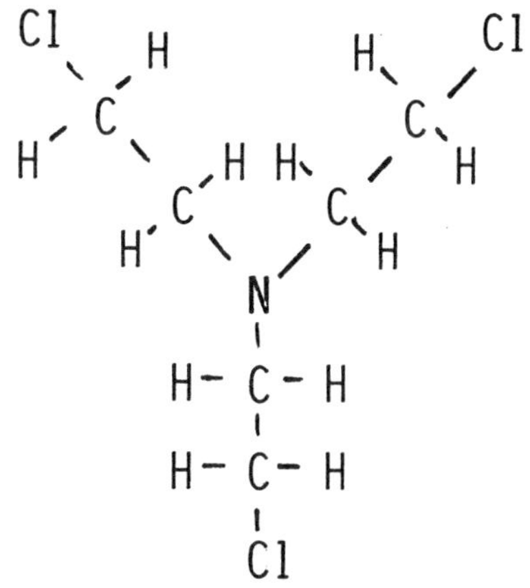

Nitrogen mustard three (HN-3)

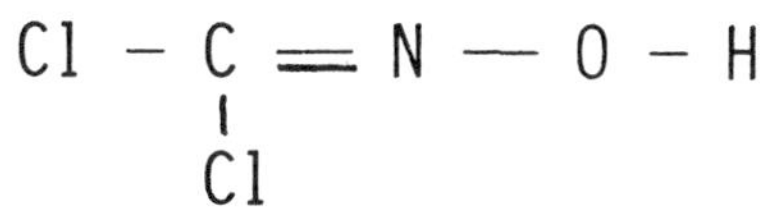

Phosgene oxime (CX)

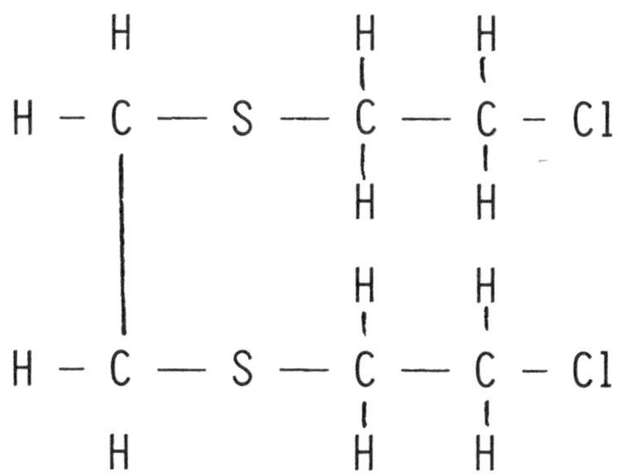

4,bis(methylchloroethyl sulfide)
(Q) *obsolete*

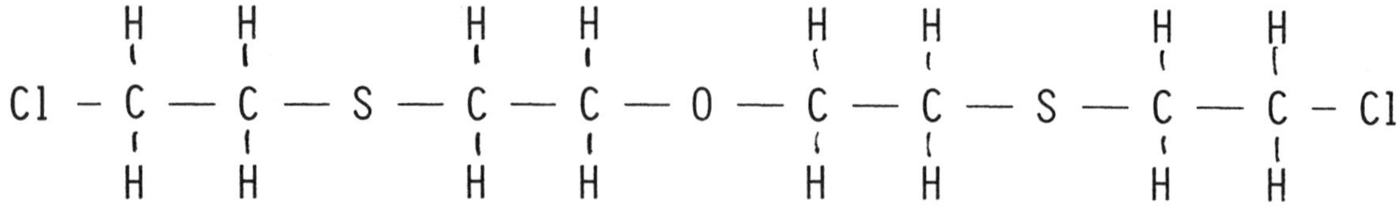

bis(2-chloroethyl sulfide) monoxide
(T) *obsolete*

RECOMMENDED READING

Clayton, George D and Clayton, Florence E, eds. *Patty's industrial hygiene and toxicology, third revised edition.* New York. John Wiley & Sons. 1978.

Crone, Hugh D. *Chemicals and Society, a guide to the new chemical age.* London. Cambridge University Press. 1986.

Daintith, John, ed. *Dictionary of chemistry, derived from the Oxford University Press concise science dictionary.* New York. Warner Books. 1986.

Douglass , Joseph D. and Livingstone, Neil C. *America the vulnerable, the threat of chemical and biological warfare.* Lexington, MA. Lexington Books. 1987.

Gad, Shayne C. *Evaluating irritation and corrosion hazards, chpater in Handbook of product safety evaluation, Shayne C. Gad, ed.* New York. Marcel Dekker. 1987.

Godman, Arthur and Denney, Ronald. *Barnes & Noble thesaurus of chemistry.* New York. Barnes & Noble. 1985.

Giese, Friedo. *Beilstein's index, trivial names in systemic nomenclature of organic chemistry.* Berlin. Springer-Verlag. 1986.

Harris, Robert and Paxman, Jeremy. *A higher form of killing, the secret story of chemical and biological warfare.* New York. Wang and Hill. 1982.

Masterson, William, et al. *Chemical principles.* Philadelphia. Saunders College Publishing. 1981.

Meyer, Eugene. *Chemistry of hazardous materials.* Englewood Cliffs, NJ. Prentice-Hall. 1977.

NIOSH. Lewis, Richard and Sweet, Doris, eds. *Registry of toxic effects of chemical substances.* U.S. Department of Health and Human Services, Centers for Disease Control. National Institute for Occupational Safety and Health. 1985.

Parker, Sybil B., ed. *McGraw-Hill dictionary of chemical terms.* New York. McGraw-Hill. 1984.

Research and Education Association staff. *The organic chemistry problem solver.* Research and Education Association. 1986.

Sax, Irving N., ed. *Dangerous properties of industrial materials.* New York. Van Nostrand Reinhold. 1984

Sax, Irving N. and Lewis, Richard J., Sr. *Rapid guide to hazardous materials in the workplace.* New York. Van Nostrand Reinhold. 1986.

Wahl, Andre. *The manufacture of organic dyestuffs.* London. Bell and Sons. 1914.

Windholz, Martha, et al, eds. *The Merck index, an encyclopedia of chemicals and drugs, tenth edition.* Rahway, NJ. Merck & Co. 1983.

Chapter Two

Blood Agents

official definition

Blood agents are absorbed into the body primarily by breathing. They effect body functions through action on the enzyme *cytochrome oxidase*, thus preventing the normal utilization of oxygen by the cells and causing rapid damage to body tissues.

FM 3-9

The three basic blood agents are covered in this chapter. Two are cyanide compounds and the third is the hydrate of arsenic.

- AC hydrogen cyanide
- CK cyanogen chloride
- SA arsine

Metabolism of the blood agents

The cells which constitute the human body must be supplied with nutrients and have their waste products removed. This is the function of the circulatory system. No cell in the human body is more than one other cell away from the blood.

Oxygen is taken to, and carbon dioxide removed from, the cells by a chemical substance called *hemoglobin* which is contained within the red blood cells.

Hemoglobin has two principal components. The first, *heme*, is a fairly simple chemical substance which attaches to the other main component. Heme contains an iron (Fe) bond which holds oxygen (O_2) or carbon dioxide (CO_2) to the main blood protein. Several thousand heme molecules can be bound to a single protein molecule. That protein is *globin*, a complex protein molecule consisting of about 574 amino acids bound together in a chain.

A third substance, *cytochrome oxidase*, has the function of lifting oxygen atoms from the hemo-globin group and replacing them with carbon dioxide molecules.

Cyanide (-C≡N) readily bonds with oxygen. The cyanide-based blood agents strip the iron atom from the hemo molecule. When that occurs, cytochrome oxidase cannot metabolize oxygen from hemoglobin and replace it with carbon dioxide waste products for removal. Cytochrome oxidase, a peptide chain of about 104 amino acids, relies on the iron component of hemoglobin to perform its function.

Arsenic (As) attacks hemoglobin by stripping off hemo molecules and incorporating their iron-oxygen groups into new molecules the human body cannot use.

Hydrogen Cyanide

$H-C\equiv N$

AC

Standard NATO agreement (STANAG) code: AC

Chemical name: hydrogen cyanide, hydrocyanic acid
Common name: hydrogen cyanide, prussic acid (solution)
Formula: HCN

Family: casualty agent
Type: blood agent

In pure form, a colorless gas having an odor similar to bitter almonds.

History

Cyanides have been used as poisons long before modern chemistry came into being. Metal cyanides, commonly based on iron and potassium, are common to many regions. They have long been used in the form of inorganic salts for the extraction of gold and similar metals from ores. Pure cyanogen (CN_2) processes were developed in 19th century Germany and France in fixing nitrogen compounds, from fertilizers to explosives. One of the oldest known pesticides.

The French military first investigated cyanides for their military potentials in the first months of 1916 and the British followed suit. Hydrogen cyanide, from prussic acid, was not used in the first world war due to inadequacy of then-current munitions and tactics. Artillery-delivered canisters tended to explode either in flight or on impact, while gas-cylinder released concentrations diluted significantly in the wind. The return to the hydrocyanic (prussic) acid formulation (HCN dissolved in water or water and ether) proved that hydrogen cyanide was ideal for aerial sprays and rocket munitions not containing bursting charges.

As prussic acid, HCN is an assasin's weapon. On October 15th, 1959, Stefan Bandera, a prominent Ukranian exile was assassinated at his Munich, Germany home when prussic acid was sprayed in his face. Through eye absorption and inhalation the agent rapidly caused Bandera's death through the sudden contraction of his blood vessels, simulating a heart attack.

Structure

Hydrogen cyanide is a weak acid formed by the hydration

of cyanide (CN_2) gas. Commonly prepared through the Andrussow process involving the catalytic oxidation of ammonia-methane mixtures or acidifying sodium cyanide.

Hydrogen cyanide gas rapidly dissolves in water, dissolves easily in alcohol, and dissolves slightly in ether. This agent owes its toxicity entirely to its cyanide component, not to any qualities as an acid. Upon mixture with any other acid, hydrocyanic acid releases its HCN from solution

Pathology

Hydrogen cyanide, as a gas is either inhaled or absorbed through breaks in the skin. As hydrocyanic acid it may be injested, absorbed through the skin or eyes, or inhaled as a mist. It is irritating to the eyes and upper respiratory tract, especially in liquid forms.

Hydrogen cyanide inactivates certain enzyme systems, most notably cytochrome oxidase, preventing the normal utilization of oxygen by the cells. Skin may appear flushed.

Low levels of injection cause weakness, headache, disorientation, nausea and vomiting. Increasing dosage will result in loss of consciousness; an end to respiration followed by death within 15 minutes.

An immediate lethal dosage will commonly cause a violent contraction of the blood vessels accompanied by severe shock, which in of itself may cause death before asphyxiation occurs.

Field behavior

Pure gas is lighter than air. Hydrocyanic acid is not much heavy than water and will evaporate at a similar rate. NATO munitions commonly involve aerial sprays and Warsaw Pact munitions emphasize rocket munitions. The vapors present two critical hazards. The first ~~is~~ involves its toxicological properties, the second its explosive tendencies. Vaporizing liquid over troop positions can be ignited by gunfire or electrical spark.

Primary battlefield use is that of a non-persistent asphyxiating agent.

Specific data

median lethal dosage (LCt_{50})

Varies according to concentration.
Vapor: 2000 mg-min/m^3 at 200 mg/m^3 concentration, or 4500 mg-min/m^3 at 150 mg/m^3 concentration; an average of 300 ppm in enclosed areas.
Liquid: splashed liquid giving a 50 mg dose.

median incapacitating dosage (ICt_{50})

Varies according concentration.
Vapor: 150 ppm in enclosed spaces.

skin toxicity

In less than lethal dosages the liquid is slightly irritating to the skin. Absorbed through breaks in the skin.

eye toxicity

In less than lethal dosages both the vapor and the liquid are slightly irritating to the eyes. Absorbed through the occular membranes.

rate of action

Immediate. Vapor inhaled lethal dosage will cause death within 15 minutes. Hydrocyanic inhaled or ingested will cause death within 2-5 minutes, with unconsciousness.

protection required

Protective mask/respirator against vapors in open areas. When liquid is present and in closed or confined spaces protective overclothing should be worn.

rate of detoxification

Rapid. Non-lethal dosage is detoxified by the human body at an average of 0.017 mg/kg per minute.

decontaminants

None required in open terrain. Aeriation may be sufficient for closed or confined spaces due to the high volatility of the agent. If complete decontamination is required, caustic soda with steam would be sufficient.

vapor density

0.93 times the weight of air.

vapor pressure

742 mm Hg at 25°C (77°F).

liquid density

0.687g/cc.

persistency

Vapor persistency is short, as the vapor rapidly dissipates. Hydrocyanic acid evaporates at a rate roughly that of tap water.

volatility

37,000 mg/m^3 at -40°C (-40°F); 1,080,000 mg/m^3 at 25°C (77°F). Vapor is EXPLOSIVE!

latent heat of vaporization

233 calories per gram.

freezing point

-13.3°C (8.06°F) for hydrocyanic acid.

boiling point

25.7°C (78.26°F).

decomposition point

About 66°C (150.8°F).

flash point

0°C (32°F). AC is ignited about 50% of the time when delivered (fired to the target) in artillery munitions.

rate of hydrolysis

Low rate of hydrolysis.

hydrolysis products

Mainly (NH_3) and (NCOOH).

stability in storage

Fixed munitions of HCN must not be stored for any extended period of time (in years) lest an explosive polymer form within the canisters. Impurities of phosphoric acid or sulfur dioxide (present in some ferrous alloys) will contribute towards instability.

action on metals or other materials

Little or none when pure. But see above.

molecular weight

27.02

Warning

The above specific data refer to hydrogen cyanide/hydrocyanic acid in its traditional form of a pure chemical. Microencapsulation techniques could make this into a moderately persistent poison presenting a profoundly greater hazard.

Cyanogen Chloride

$Cl-C\equiv N$

CK

Standard NATO agreement (STANAG) code: CK

Chemical name: cyanogen chloride
Common name: chlorocyanogen, chlorine cyanide
Formula: CNCl

Family: casualty agent
Type: blood agent

A colorless gas with a sharp, pepperish odor similar to that of most tear gasses. A liquid at temperatures below 55°F. May be delivered as an aerosol.

History

For a brief history of cyanide compounds as poisons and as industrial catalysts, see *hydrogen cyanide* (AC).

Cyanogen chloride is a compound first seeing use in manufacturing processes where the hydrogen compound presented too great a fire or explosive hazard. First usage was in the refining of metal ores and the chemical synthesis of dyestuffs. Its poisonous qualities made it ideal as a fumigant. More recent usages include the production of synthetic rubber.

Less lethal as a military casualty agent than hydrogen cyanide (AC), but easier to deploy because of its non explosive qualities. Developed as a military agent immediately following the first world war when new munitions designs allowing wide dispersal were created. As it is a liquid between 20°F and 55°F, cyanogen chloride proved useful as an aircraft delivered aerosol before the development of the nerve agents in the late 1930s.

Structure

Cyanogen chloride is commonly formed by the action of chlorine gas (Cl_2) on cyanide gas (CN_2). It may be considered to have many of the charactoristics of a chlorine salt without meeting the full definition, ie the solid precipitate of an acid-base reaction.

$$\text{Cl–Cl} + \text{N≡C–C≡N} \rightarrow \begin{matrix}\text{Cl–C≡N}\\ \text{Cl–C≡N}\end{matrix}$$

Pathology

Cyanogen chloride, both as a liquid and as a gas is either inhaled or absorbed through breaks in the skin. In both forms it is highly irritating to the eyes and upper respiratory tract.

Once inside the body, cyanogen chloride converts to hydrogen cyanide. It inactivates certain enzyme systems, most notably cytochrome oxidase, preventing the utilization of oxygen by the cells. Skin may appear flushed.

Low levels of injestion cause weakness, headache, disorientation, nausea and vomiting. Increasing dosages will result in loss of consciousness, an end to respiration, and death within 15 minutes.

An immediate lethal dosage will commonly cause a violent contraction of blood vessels accompanied by severe shock, which in of itself may cause death.

Field behavior

Liquid cyanogen chloride will evaporate at a rate similar to tap water in temperatures above 55°F. Munitions will include aerial sprays and rocket munitions, the latter being emphasized by Warsaw Pact nations in their delivery of blood agents. The vapors are not as toxic as those of hydrogen cyanide (AC) and do not involve any explosive hazard.

Primary battlefield use is that of a non-persistent asphyxiating agent.

Specific data

median lethal dosage (LCt_{50})
11,000 mg-min/m^3.

median incapacitating dosage (ICt_{50})

7,000 mg-min/m^3.

skin toxicity

The liquid is irritating to the skin.

eye toxicity

Both the liquid and gas are highly irritating to the eyes.

rate of action

Immediate. The liquid, if ingested, may cause death within 2 to 5 minutes.

protection required

Protective mask/respirator against vapors in open areas. When liquid is present and in closed or confined spaces protective overclothing should be worn.

rate of detoxification

Rapid. Non-lethal dosages are detoxified at a rate of between 0.02 to 0.1 mg/kg per minute.

decontaminants

None required in open terrain. Aeriation may be sufficient for closed or confined spaces. If complete decontamination is required against liquids, caustic soda with steam would be sufficient.

vapor density

2.1 times as heavy as air.

vapor pressure

1000 mg Hg at 25°C (77°F).

liquid density

1.18 g/cc at 20°C(68°F).

persistency

Short, although lethal concentrations may persist in jungle or forest terrain under temperature/pressure inversions

volatility

2,600,000 mg/m^3 at 12.8°C (55.04°F).

latent heat of vaporization

103 calories per gram.

melting point

-6.9°C(19.58°F).

boiling point

12.8°C(55.04°F).

decomposition point

Above 100°C (212°F).

flash point

None. Non flammable.

rate of hydrolysis

Very low.

hydrolysis products

HCl and CNOH

stability in storage

Stable for less than one month in canister munitions. May polymerize to form explosive compound (2,4,6 trinitrochloro-s-trizine $C_3N_3\ Cl_3$ -cyclic).

action on metals and other materials

None when pure.

molecular weight

61.48.

Warning

The above specific data refer to cyanogen chloride in it traditional form of a pure chemical. Microencapsulation techniques could make this into a mildly persistent poison presenting a profoundly greater hazard.

Arsine

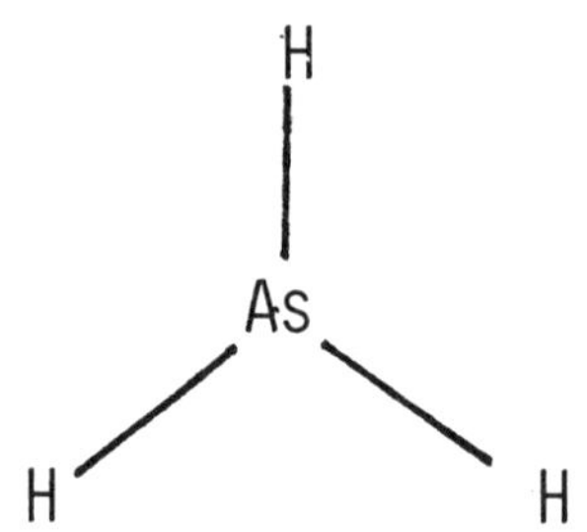

SA

Standard NATO agreement (STANAG) code: SA

Chemical name: arsenic trihydride
Common name: arsine
Formula: AsH_3

Family: casualty agent
Type: blood agent

A colorless gas having an odor similar to that of powdered garlic.

History

Albertus Magnus first isolated metalic arsenic (element Number 33 on the Periodic Table of the Elements) in the year 1250 by heat reducing the minerals orpiment (As_2S_3) and realgar (As_4S_4). Both these compounds had been used as poisons (animal, insect, and human) for millennia. White arsenic (As_2O_3), a chalky white powder, is one of the oldest known general pesticides. All three compounds have a long history in assassinations and homicides. Until the early years of this century cupric arsenite was commonly used as a paint pigment and universally used as a green fabric dye.

Arsenic hydride, or arsine, has long been used in the preparation of arsenic-based insecticides and in the manufacture of certain glass dyes. Recently it has become vital to the manufacture of microelectronic components. Its ready heat decomposition enables growing crystals to be doped with minute traces of arsenic to produce *n*-type semiconductors.

Arsine's history as a military casualty agent has fluxuated between the hypothetical and the experimental. It was first considered in the 1920s and found unacceptable due to its high volatility and low flash point. Its use would be limited to mines and other munitions which do not require bursting charges or impact-opening canisters. Arsine doubles as an explosive and has been known to ignite on contact with dry, warm air.

Structure

Arsine is a colorless gas produced commercially by the reduction of mineral acids with arsenic compounds of electropositive metals. It is also produced by the reduction of some arsenic compounds with free hydrogen ions.

Pathology

Arsenic compounds, including arsine, are known to accumulate in the body, displacing calcium in bone matter in the form of calcium arsenate. Production of new blood cells in the bone marrow is toxicically effected as such.

Arsine enters the bloodstream through the respiratory system or through cuts or breaks in the skin. It oxidizes cytochrome oxidase, rendering that enzyme useless and in addition damages the liver and the kidneys and may cause harm to the urinary tract. The skin may appear flushed.

Slight exposure causes headache and irritability. Increasing exposure results in chills, nausea and vomiting. Lethal dosages may cause blood vessel contraction and shock prior to any asphyxiating effects. Death from shock may occur within 2 minutes. Death from asphyxiation may be within ten to fifteen minutes. Death from kidney or liver damage may occur within as long as 11 days.

Field behavior

Heavier than air, arsine will seek the lowest elevations as it vaporizes. Highly explosive, it must not be used in artillery munitions but rather in mines and booby-traps. Both the explosive and toxic effects might be of military significance depending upon tactical considerations. Disperses rapidly.

Specific data

median lethal dosage *(LCt_{50})*

5,000 mg-min/m^3 or an average of 0.1 gram. Also in a ratio of 2 mg per kilogram (about 2 lbs) of body weight.

median incapacitating dosage *(ICt_{50})*

2500 mg-min/m^3 or about 0.5 ppm.

skin toxicity

None to bare skin, although arsine will enter the body through any breaks or cuts.

eye toxicity

None to the eyes themselves although arsine may penetrate through the tissues within the eyelids.

rate of action

Delayed for other than massive dosages. Principal ef-ects are through systemic poisoning (see Pathology).

protection required

Protective mask/respirator.

rate of detoxification

Slow. Principal effects are through systemic poisoning.

decontaminants

None are required in open areas. Aeriation of closed or confined spaces is hazardous because of explosive factor. Arsenic traces may be removed from walls, etc, by a solution of potassium permanganate and water.

vapor density

2.69 times as heavy as air.

vapor pressure

11,100 mm Hg at 20°C(68°F).

liquid density

1.34 g/cc at 20°C(68°F).

persistency

Very short. Vaporizes extremely fast and disperses rapidly.

volatility

30,900,000 mg-min/m^3 at 0°C (32°F).

latent heat of vaporization

53.7 calories per gram at -62.5°C(-80.5°F).

melting point

-116°C(-176.8°F).

boiling point

-62.5°C(-80.5°F).

decomposition point

280°C(536°F).

flash point

-116°C(-176.8) (melting point). Cannot be used in artillery munitions. Has been known to explode on contact with warm air.

rate of hydrolysis

Very rapid.

hydrolysis products

Arsenic acids and hydrides.

stability in storage

Must be stored in glass-lined cannisters. Will rapidly decompose if stored in simple steel canisters.

action on metals and other materials

Metals will cataylse decomposition, with the formation of acids and hydrides.

molecular weight

77.93

Warning

The above specific data refer to arsine in its traditional form as a pure chemical. Microencapsulation of arsenic compounds could make these into highly persistent poisons presenting a profoundly greater hazard.

Field treatment for blood
agent poisoning

amyl chloride

amyl chloride

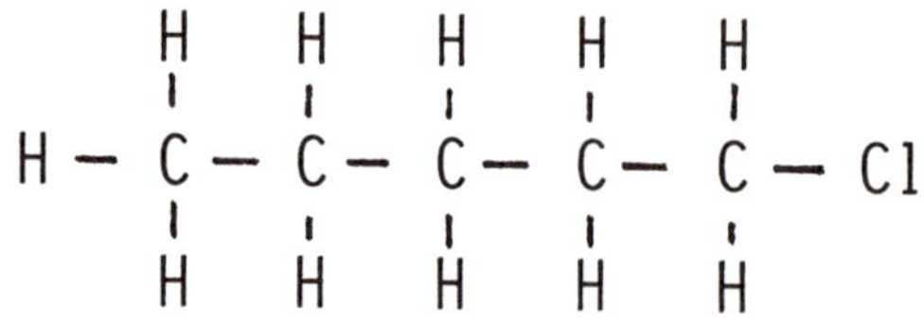

Chemical name: 1-chloropentane; n-amyl chloride; n-butylcarbonyl chloride

Warning: of limited use against the effects of arsine.

Used in the form of an inhalant to restore the effects of *cytochrome oxidase* within the human body.

Military issue field antidote takes the form of an inhaler similar to that used for ammonia sniffers, i.e. a fabric-wrapped glass or frangible plastic tube to be broken between the fingers. Most military preparations may contain an admixture of 2- and 3-chloropentanes to act as a buffer to amyl chloride's slow, but profound, anesthetic effects.

In normal procedures, two capsules are to be broken and stuffed inside the victim's mask under each eye or on the ledge of each eyepiece, presuming the victim has a protective mask.

Placing an opened capsule directly into the victim's mouth would not be recommended as it might render the victim comatose or into shock under many conditions.

The final effect of the amyl chloride is that of prolonging the victim's life long enough for the body's natural process of detoxicification to proceed. Further medical observation and treatment should follow.

Comparative
Tables

blood agents comparative data

agent	rate of action	state at 68°F	odor	volatility (mg/m^3)	LCt_{50} ($mg\text{-}min/m^3$)	ICt_{50} ($mg\text{-}min/m^3$)	vapor density (x air)	vapor pressure (mm Hg)
AC	rapid	colorless gas or liquid	bitter almonds	1,080,000 at 77°F	2000 to 4500 in open; 300 ppm inclosed areas	150 ppm	0.93	742 at 77°F
CK	rapid	colorless gas	very faint odor of bitter almonds	2,600,000 at 55°F	11,000	7000	2.1	1000 at 77°F
SA	delayed: 2 hours to 11 days	colorless gas	mild garlic	30,900,000 at 32°F	5000	2500	2.69	11,100 at 68°F

blood agents   comparative structures

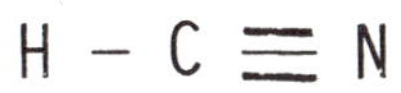

Hydrogen cyanide (AC)

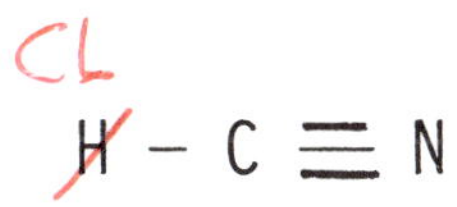

Cyanogen chloride (CK)

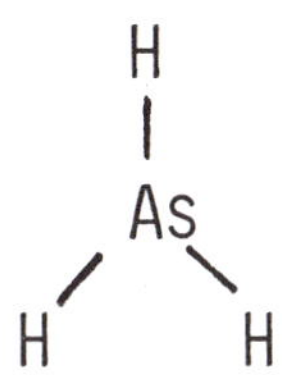

Arsine (SA)

REFERENCES

Clayton, George D and Clayton, Florence E, eds. *Patty's industrial hygiene and toxicology, third revised edition.* New York. John Wiley & Sons. 1978.

Daintith, John, ed. *Dictionary of Chemistry, derived from the Oxford University Press concise science dictionary.* New York. Warner Books. 1986.

Douglass, Joseph D. Jr. *Biochem warfare: new dimensions and implications, in Defense and Foreign Affairs, p.41.* April, 1987.

Douglass, Joseph D. Jr and Livingstone, Neil C. *America the vulnerable: the threat of chemical and biological warfare.* Lexington, MA. Lexington Books. 1987.

Gad, Shayne C. *Evaluating irritation and corrosion hazards, chapter in Handbook of product safety evaluation, Shayne C. Gad, ed.* New York. Marcel Dekker. 1987.

Harris, Robert and Paxman, Jeremy. *A higher form of killing, the secret story of chemical and biological warfare.* New York. Wang and Hill. 1982.

McGeorge, Harvey J. II. *Chemical warfare: seeking an East/West balance, in Defense and Foreign Affairs, p.29.* April, 1987.

Masterson, William, et al. *Chemical principles.* Phildelphia. Saunders College Publishing. 1981.

Mehlman, A.A., ed. *Safety evaluation.* Princeton, NJ. Princeton Scientific Press. 1987.

Meyer, Eugene. *Chemistry of hazardous materials.* Englewood Cliffs, NJ. Prentice-Hall. 1977.

NIOSH. Lewis, Richard, and Sweet, Doris, eds. *Registry of toxic effects of chemical substances.* U.S. Department of Health and Social Services, Centers for Disease Control. National Institute for Occupational Safety and Health. 1985.

Research and Education Association staff. *The organic chemistry problem solver.* New York. Research and Education Association. 1986.

Windholz, Martha, et al, eds. *The Merck index, an encyclopedia of chemicals and drugs, ninth edition.* Rahway, NJ. Merck & Co. 1976.

Sax, Irving N., ed. *Dangerous properties of industrial materials.* New York. Van Nostrand Reinhold Co. 1984.

Chapter Three

Choking Agents

official definition

Choking agents injure an unprotected man chiefly in the respiratory tract - that is, in the nose, throat, and, particularly, the lungs. In extreme cases membranes swell, lungs become filled with liquid, and death results from lack of oxygen; thus, these agents "choke" an unprotected man. Fatalities of this type are referred to as "dry-land drownings."

FM 3-9

The two standard choking agents, phosgene and diphosgene are based around a ClC:O bond:

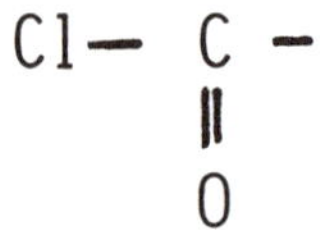

Phosgene was the more often used of the chemical agents deployed during the first world war. Warfare in that conflict was mainly an affair of static battles fought from trenches. Mechanized warfare demanded the development of lethal compounds which were effective within minutes, not hours. As the choking agents are gaseous, not liquid, their persistency is erratic at best and their ability to contaminate equipment and stores never matched that of the blister, and later the liquified nerve agents. For these reasons the catagory was not developed further, and was superceded for the most part by the nerve agents. However, phosgene is often used as a chlorinating agent in organic chemical manufacturing processes, and due to its availablity should not be written off. The phosgenes are no less lethal today than they were in 1915.

The common choking agents are:

- CG phosgene (carbonyl chloride)
- DP diphosgene (trichloromethyl chloroformate)

Chlorine

Cl – Cl

Standard NATO agreement (STANAG) code: none

Chemical name: chlorine

Formula: Cl_2

Family: casualty agent

Type: choking agent

Foglike in its initial concentrations, it becomes a dense yellow-green gas. Has an odor like concentrated bleach.

History

Chlorine was the first chemical battlefield agent used in the first world war. First used on the 22nd of April, 1915 against French reserve and colonial troops in their positions around the village of Langemarck, near Ypres. German engineers of the 23rd and 26th Army Corps released the contents of 6,000 cylinders along a four mile front. The vapor mass rolled westwards in a dense cloud to inundate the French troops and nearby British elements. Five thousand fatalities occured within minutes and mass panic ensued among troops escaping their trenches. Everything made of metal (brass, copper, silver, steel, aluminum, etc.) was etched and corroded within fifteen minutes, even artillery breech blocks rusting shut. Ten thousand French and British troops became chemical casualties, most of whom were no longer fit for military service. If the German army had forseen the consequences of what was initially viewed as a hare-brained experiment, they might have massed troops enough to push through to the sea that very day and the war might have ended. As it was, that day was to see the birth of modern chemical warfare.

Chlorine was too tricky to use. It quickly gave way to things just as nasty but more practical in the field.

Structure

Chlorine is a pure element rather than a chemical compound or mixture. It is Number 17 on the Periodic Table of Elements, a member of the *halogen* family (which also includes flourine, bromine, iodine, and astatine). Like all of them, chlorine is an extremely reactive element.

Chlorine is normally a gas, but it liquifies under pressure. It is stored as a liquid within pressure cylinders. Liquid or gaseous, chlorine atoms (like those of hydrogen) bond together in pairs:

$$Cl - Cl$$

Pathology

Chlorine reacts with organic tissue as it tries to replace hydrogen bonding in hydrocarbon compounds with its own bondings, freeing up carbon and oxygen bonding patterns. In short, it destroys tissue. Inhaled, it strips the lining from broncial tubes and lungs. Inflammation is instant and massive amounts of phlem are formed along with hemorrhaging. Dead tissue and liquids fill up the lungs. Remaining within a cloud of chlorine in and of itself is asphyxiating. Vomiting and diarrhoea are common side effects of the nausea caused by light inhalation.

Surviving casualties typically cough up lung detritus for extended periods. Lung damage is permament and for all practical purposes is accumulative. Casualties require extensive medical treatment.

Field behavior

Chlorine must be used in heavy concentration to be tactically useful. This cannot be done with conventional munitions unless tremendous quantities are utilized. The other alternative is to release the agent from massed cylinders, relying on often fickle winds to carry it to a target area.

Specific data

median lethal dosage (LCt_{50})

19,000 mg-min/m^3.

median incapacitating dosage (ICt_{50})

1,800 mg-min/m^3

skin toxicity

Little or no irritation to the skin. Irritating to open wounds or cuts.

eye toxicity

Irritating to the eyes.

rate of action

Immediate.

protection required

Protective mask/respirator.

rate of detoxification

Rapid for amounts below incapacitating amounts, above which tissue damage may occur.

decontaminants

None required. All concentrations dissipate.

vapor density

2.4 times heavier than air.

vapor pressure

4,992 mm Hg at 20°C(68°F).

liquid density

1.41 g/cc at 20°C(68°F).

persistency

Short. Rapid dissipation.

volatility

19,369,000 mg/m^3 at 20°C(68°F).

latent heat of vaporization

68.8 calories per gram.

melting point

-101°C(-149°F).

boiling point

-34.5°C(-30.1°F).

decomposition point

Greater than 1,000°C(1832°F).

flash point

None. Does not ignite.

rate of hydrolysis

Slow.

hydrolysis products

HCl and HOCl.

stability in storage

Stable when stored in liquid form (pressure canister).

action on metals & other materials

Highly corrosive to all metals in the presence of any hunidity factor.

molecular weight

70.91

Phosgene

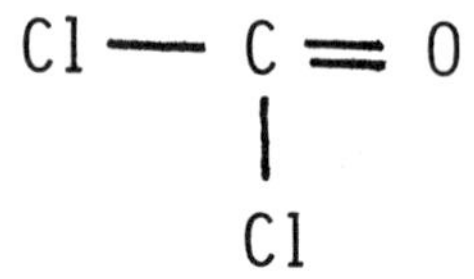

CG

Standard NATO agreement (STANAG) code: CG

Chemical name: carbonyl chloride
Common name: phosgene, collognite, D-Stoff
Formula: $COCl_2$

Family: casualty agent
Type: choking agent

Foglike in its initial concentrations, it becomes colorless as it spreads. Has an odor like new-mown hay.

History

Phosgene was first used in the dye industry in the late 19th century to process colorfast materials. About the turn of the century it began to see some limited use as a pesticide after it was noticed it effectively killed insects and vermin exposed to its effects in dye processing plants.

IG. Farbin, the German dye and chemical works donated their research to the Kaiser Wilhelm Institute in the late spring of 1915, and the latter began production studies. The Allies had just begun their own use of chlorine and the Central Powers felt they needed a new casualty agent in reply. It was first used against the British at Ypres on December 19th of that year. In its battlefield concentrations it was viewed mainly as a nuisance, an impurity in the chlorine gas released at the same time. Two days later mass casualties occured from pulmonary edema. British production began at the newly-founded laboratories at Porton Down and it was first used as an artillery munition by the British at the second battle of the Somme in June 1916. American production began at the newly-founded Edgewood Arsenal in mid-1918. By some estimates, more than 80% of all chemical agent fatalities in the first world war were from phosgene.

In the 1920s phosgene was manufactured as a military agent by all the major powers and several minor powers. It has remained in the chemical arsenals ever since.

Structure

Phosgene is deceptively easy to manufacture. It is prepared from chlorine and carbon dioxide under pressure.

It may ~~be~~ similarly be prepared from carbon monoxide and nitrosyl chloride. In either case it involves taking a single or double carbon-oxygen bond:

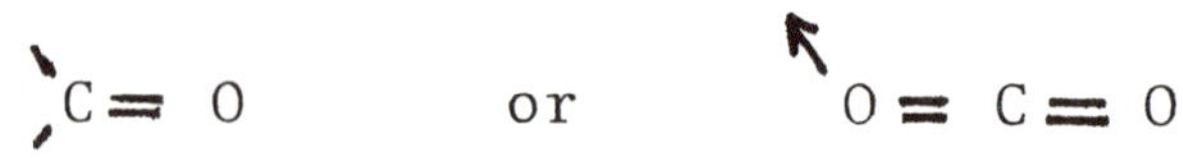

carbon monoxide *carbon dioxide*

and making a dual chlorine bond:

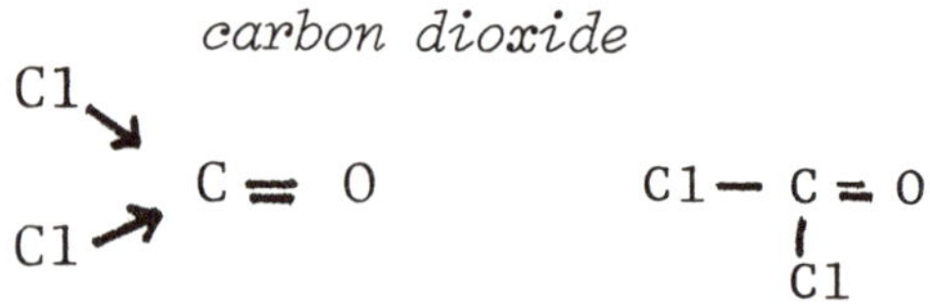

A du Pont process involves adding an oxygen bond to the Carbon ion while breaking down a carbon tetrachloride molecule:

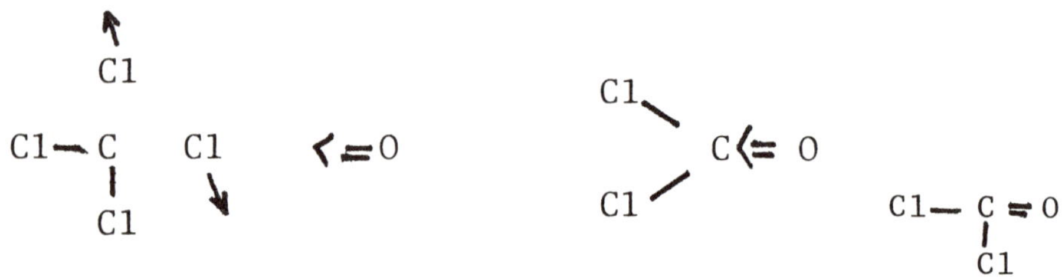

Phosgene, like arsine, serves many legitimate uses. It is an important catalyst in the preparation of a number of organically-based chemicals.

Phosgene is only slightly soluble in water and freely soluble in benzene, toulene, acetic acid, and most other liquid hydrocarbons.

Pathology in animals and plants

Evidence dating from world war one usage has shown phosgene to be fatal to most insects, reptiles, and mammals when used in concentrations. The same evidence further suggests it is toxic to many broad-leaf plants and trees. Phosgene, as a basic carbonyl, is used in the manufacture of many pesticides and herbicides.

Pathology in humans

Phosgene is immediately although mildly irritating to the eyes. In this regard it may be mistaken for any number of chemical agents, non-toxic as well as toxic. In concentrations approaching 1600 mg-min/m^3 it may be mistaken for tear gas.

Lethal effects are not immediately manifest. The body does not detoxify this agent, which accumulates within the system. First attacked are the lung capillaries and then the membranes of the lung sacs where phosgene is directly exchanged into the blood, causing the lungs to flood with watery fluids. The full effect of lethal dosages may not be apparent until about 4 hours after exposure. Victims of accumulating dosages might go for up to a day before manifesting traumatic symptoms or sudden death.

Field behavior

Phosgene vapors are heavier than air and are non explosive. They will seek the lower levels of terrain and man-made structures. They will dissipate within 20 minutes in open terrain but may persist upwards of almost 10 hours in shady areas, low terrain, and in moderate temperatures (below 68°F) under inversion conditions. In confined spaces it may persist for days. Under arid conditions in full sun it may dissipate within 5 minutes.

The further phosgene dilutes the greater its ability to hydrolyse. Under humid conditions, as in a forest or jungle following rain, or near large bodies of water, phosgene readily hydrolyses.

Specific data

median lethal dosage (LCt$_{50}$)

3200 mg-min/m^3.

median incapacitating dosage (ICt$_{50}$)

1600 mg-min/m^3.

skin toxicity

None in open terrain or short exposure.

eye toxicity

Irritating in concentration. No permament damage in open terrain or from short exposure.

rate of action

Immediate attack on the body. Delayed for several hours in showing symptoms. Many low dosages may add up to one large dosage due to accumulative effect.

protection required

Protective mask/respirator in open areas.

rate of detoxification

Not detoxified naturally within the body. Dosage is accumulative.

decontamination

None required in open areas. Aeration and water are sufficient for closed or confined spaces.

vapor density

3.4 times as heavy as air.

vapor pressure

365 mm Hg at -10°C (14°F), 555 mm Hg at 0°C (32°F), 1173 mm Hg at 20°C (68°F).

liquid density

1.373 g/cc at 20°C (68°F).

persistency

Short duration. Very volatile. May persist in sheltered areas and in structures for up to several days in diminishing concentrations.

volatility

528,000 mg/m^3 at -40°C (-40°F), 2,200,000 mg/m^3 at -10°C (14°F), 4,300,000 mg/m^3 at 7.6°C (45.7°F).

latent heat of vaporization

59 calories per gram.

freezing point

-128°C (-198°F).

boiling point

7.6°C (45.7°F).

decomposition point

800°C (1472°F).

flash point

None. Non flammable.

rate of hydrolysis

Rapid, especially in wet jungle or forest conditions.

hydrolysis products

Hydrochloric acid and carbon dioxide.

stability in storage

Stable in steel containers.

action on metals and other materials

None in pure form. When hydrolysing it becomes slightly corrosive with buildup of HCl.

molecular weight

98.92.

Warning

The above specific data refer to phosgene in its tradit-ional form of a pure chemical. Microencapsulation techniques could make this into a highly persistent poison presenting a profoundly greater hazard.

Diphosgene

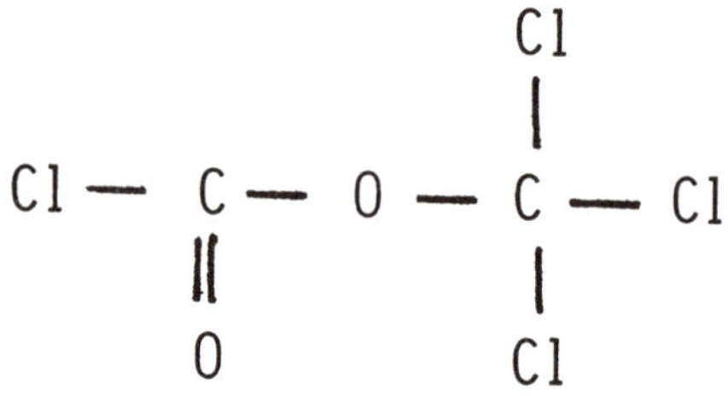

DP

Standard NATO agreement (STANAG) code: DP

Chemical name: trichloromethyl chloroformate
Common name: diphosgene
Formula: $ClCOOCCl_3$

Family: casualty agent
Type: choking agent

Foglike in its initial concentrations, it becomes colorless as it spreads. Has an odor like new-mown hay or green corn. Diphosgene may cause a stinging sensation to the eyes and upper respiratory tract. A rapidly vaporizing liquid.

History

Diphosgene was created in, or shortly after (according to different sources) the first world war as an improved version of phosgene (CG). Like phosgene, it was an agent suited for the static warfare of the western front.

Diphosgene typifies the phenomenon of the second-generation chemical agent. The chemical filters of the day were developed to screen out phosgene. On the other hand, they could be penetrated by chloroform. Diphosgene is basically phosgene with chloroform grafted onto it. The latter will destroy the filter allowing the former to seep through.

Like phosgene, diphosgene fell out of favor by the 1930s and was superceded by the nerve catagory of agents.

Diphosgene with its chlorine atoms replaced by hydrogen (methyl formate) is a common fumigant (see below).

Structure

The manufacture of diphosgene takes the manufacture of phosgene one further by combining both the carbon *di*oxide/nitrosyl chloride and du Pont processes. Keeping the second oxygen-carbon bond, a third carbon-oxygen bond is form with the loss of a chlorine atom from a carbon tetrachloride group:

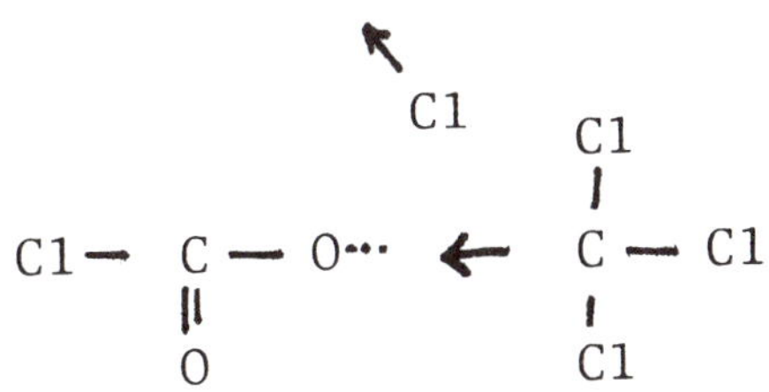

Chlorine is highly reactive. The resulting compound (diphosgene) tends to break down in the presence of any suitable catalyst. Diphosgene must be in as pure a form as possible and in glass canisters. In a metal canister it would oxidize in short order to chloroform ($CHCl_3$), phosgene, and water:

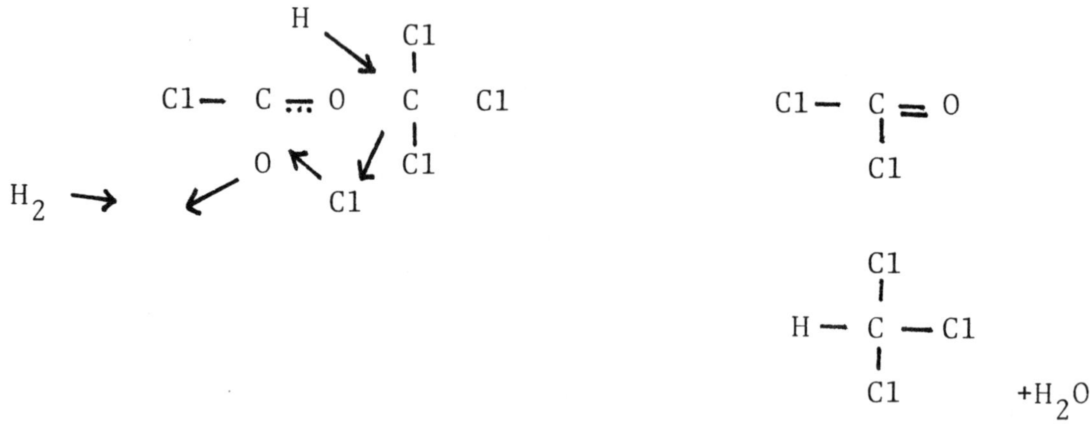

A similar looking compound, mentioned above, is methyl formate ($C_2H_4O_2$):

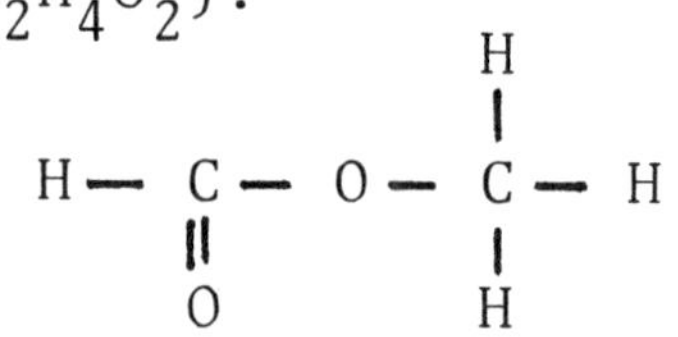

which is commonly used as a fumigant and larvacide with tobbacco, dried fruits, and cereals. While capable of causing narcosis and death from pulmonary irritation from overdose as does diphosgene, methyl formate lacks the same degree of lethality. It is a derivative of formic (methanoic) acid (HCOOH)and its configuration is derived from a different process than does diphosgene. It is not a military agent and is mentioned here only to make the distinction.

Pathology

The effects of diphosgene are identical to those of

phosgene in the simple fact that diphosgene oxidizes and converts to phosgene, chloroform, and water in the same manner as mentioned above. It attacks the lung capilaries and then the membranes of the lung sacs, causing severe irritation (and later scarring the tissue) as the agent enters directly into the bloodstream to cause further systemic damage, in particular to the liver and kidneys. The effects of a lethal dosage may not be apparent for several hours. Effects, as with dosages of phosgene, are accumulative. Victims might suffer trauma or sudden death up to a day after the last dosage, or they may suffer effects years later.

Diphosgene differs from phosgene in the field in being slightly irritating to the nose and eyes because of its high chlorine content.

Field behavior

Diphosgene vapors are heavier than air and they are non explosive. Diphosgene, being more volatile than phosgene, tends to dissipate at a quicker rate than phosgene. This limits its capacity to be used in "surprise" concentrations for the unwary. Its practical persistency may tend to be about half that of phosgene in temperate climates (under 20°C or 68°F), or about 5 hours in dry, shady areas in low-laying terrain and building substructures. It will break down quickly in direct sunlight. As it dissipates diphosgene will break down both into phosgene and hydrolysis products. Under humid conditions, as in a forest or jungle following rain, or near a large body of water, diphosgene would quickly break down.

Diphosgene would be damaging to some air and water filtration equipment due to its chlorine components.

Specific data

median lethal dosage (LCt_{50})

3200 mg-min/m^3.

median incapacitating dosage (ICt_{50})

1600 mg-min/m^3.

skin toxicity

None in open terrain or in short exposures.

eye toxicity

None in open terrain or in short exposures. Slight lacrimatory effect (see text).

rate of action

Immediate attack on the body. Delayed for several hours in manifesting symptoms. Many low dosages add up to one large dosage due to accumulative effect.

protection required

Protective mask/respirator in open areas.

rate of detoxification

Not detoxified naturally within the body. Dosage is accumulative.

decontaminants

None required in open areas. Aeration and water are sufficient for closed or confined spaces.

vapor density

6.8 times as heavy as air (twice as heavy as phosgene).

vapor pressure

1 mm Hg at 0°C (32°F), 4.2 mm Hg at 20°C (68°F).

liquid density

1.653 g/cc at 20°F (68°F).

persistency

Short duration. More volatile than phosgene. May per sist in sheltered areas and in structures for up to a day or so at the most in diminishing concentrations.

volatility

12,000 mg/m^3 at 0°C (32°F), 45,000 mg/m^3 at 20°C (68°F), 270,000 mg/m^3 at 51.7°C (125°F).

latent heat of vaporization

57.4 calories per gram.

melting point

-57°C (-70.6°F).

boiling point

127°C (260°F).

decomposition point

Above 300°C (572°F) diphosgene will break down into CG (assuming in pure form, no catalysts), with a further complete breakdown at 800°C (1472°F).

flash point

None. Non flammable.

rate of hydrolysis

Slow hydrolysis. Must first break down into phosgene, which depends on catalyst actions. Then, hydrolysation is as at the rate of phosgene. (see text)

hydrolysis products

Hydrochloric acid and CO_2, following breakdown into Phosgene.

stability in storage

Unstable in anything but glass. Eventually will convert to phosgene if any cataylst is present. (see text)

hydrolysis products

Most metals catalyse diphosgene to phosgene. Then, if hydrolysed it becomes slightly corrosive with buildup of HCl.

molecular weight

197.85

Warning

The above specific data refer to diphosgene in its traditional form of a pure chemical. Microencapsulation techniques could make this into a highly persistent poison presenting a profoundly greater hazard.

Comparative Tables

choking agents — comparative data

agent	*rate of action*	*state at 68°F*	*odor*	*volatility (mg/m^3)*	*LCt_{50} ($mg\text{-}min/m^3$)*	*ICT_{50} ($mg\text{-}min/m^3$)*	*vapor density (x air)*	*vapor pressure (mm Hg)*
chlorine	immediate	yellow gas	like bleach	19,369,000 at 68°F	19,000	1800	2.4	4992 at 68°F
GG	immediate to 3 hours, depending on concentration	colorless gas	new-mown hay; green corn	4,300,000 at 45°F	3200	1600	3.4	1.173 at 68°F
DP	immediate to 3 hours, depending on concentration	colorless gas	new-mown hay; green corn	45,000 at 68°F	3200	1600	6.8	4.2 at 68°F

choking agents — comparative structures

Cl - Cl

Chlorine

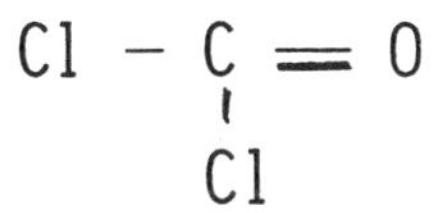

Phosgene (CG)

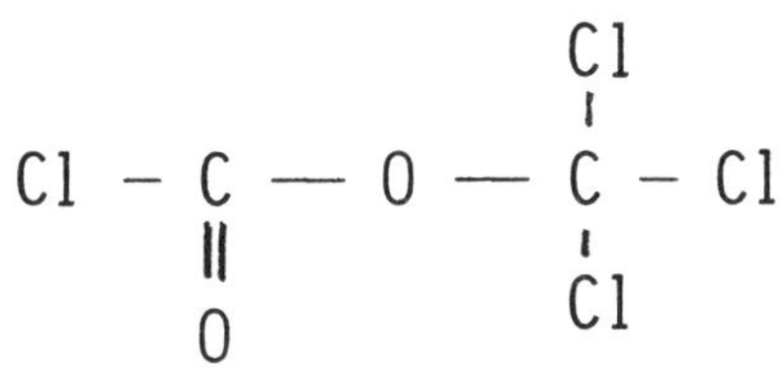

Diphosgene (DP)

REFERENCES

Dainith, John, ed. *Dictionary of chemistry, derived from the Oxford University Press concise science dictionary.* New York. Warner Books. 1986

Douglass, Joseph D. Jr and Livingstone, Neil C. *America the vulnerable, the threat of chemical and biological warfare.* Lexington Books. 1987.

Gad, Shayne C. *Accute toxicology testing.* Caldwell, NJ. Telford Press. 1987.

______________, ed. *Evaluating irritation and corrosion hazards, in Handbook of Product Safety Evaluation.* New York. Marcel Dekker. 1987.

Harris, Robert & Paxman, Jeremy. *A higher form of killing, the secret story of chemical and biological warfare.* New York. Hill and Wang. 1982.

Hayes, A.W., ed. *Principles and methods in toxicology.* New York. Raven Press. 1987.

Masterton, William, et al. *Chemical principles.* Philadelphia. Saunders College Publishing. 1981.

Meyer, Eugene. *Chemistry of hazardous materials.* Englewood Cliffs, NJ. Prentice-Hall. 1977.

NIOSH. Lewis, Richard and Sweet, Doris, eds. *Registry of toxic effects of chemical substances.* U.S. Department of Health and Social Services, Centers for Disease Control. National Institute for Occupational Safety and Health. 1985.

Research and Education Association staff. *The organic chemistry problem solver.* New York. Research and Education Association. 1986.

Windholz, Martha, et al. *The MERCK Index, an encyclopedia of chemicals and drugs, 10th edition.* Rahway, NJ. Merck & Co. 1983.

HISTORICAL REFERENCE

Wahl, Andre. *The manufacture of organic dyestuffs,* translated by F.W. Atak. London. G. Bell and Sons. 1914.

Chapter Four

Nerve Agents

official definition

While the individual nerve agents differ in molecular structure, all of these agents have the same physiological action on man in that they cause an increase in acetylcholine throughout the body by their interference with the vital enzyme called *cholinesterase.*

In general, the peripheral nervous system of the human body makes use of either of two chemical neurotransmitters. The neurons of the sympathetic nervous system release *norepinephrine* to carry the final impulse to the end organs. Those of the parasympathetic nervous system release *acetylcholine.* Acetylcholine also plays a vital role in the innervation (control) of skeletal muscles, autonomic ganglia, and many structures within the central nervous system.

Normally, the enzyme *cholinesterase* prevents the accumulation of acetylcholine after its release in the nervous system.

Nerve agents (*cholinesterase inhibitors*) permit acetylcholine to persist at the above sites, mimicking the effects of a massive release of acetylcholine.

Thus, the major effects will be in skeletal muscles, parasympathetic end organs, and the central nervous system.

The four cardinal principles of therapy for nerve agent intoxication are assisted ventilation, parasympathetic blockage (*atropine*), decontamination, and enzyme reactivation with an oxime such as *2-PAM-chloride*.

FM 3-9

The current common nerve agents are organophos-~~phos~~phates owing their ancestry to the insecticide industries of Germany and Czechoslovakia. As the first three, tabun, sarin, and soman were developed by the German army after tabun's accidental discovery in 1937, this author shall refer to them as the Wehrmacht Agents rather than as the "G" series. In fairness to the British, this German series is based on aconitine, a test agent from Porton Down. In fairness to the Wehrmacht, although they developed tabun, sarin, and soman, they never used them in battle. In 1952 the Tripartite countries of Britain, the United States, and Canada invented the fourth agent, VX, whose formula mysteriously appeared in Soviet sources as VR-55.[1]

Nerve agents were supposed to replace the choking agents in tactical theory. After 1918 nobody ever fought a major war with chemicals so the idea was moot.

1. Not identical but similar. See VX: history.

Of the Wehrmacht series only two, tabun and sarin, were fully developed. The third, soman was developed from German specifications by the USSR. In their basic formulations all three are gaseous and non-persistent.

VX (VR-55) was designed for small vapor mass and consequent high persistency.

The classical textbook symptoms of nerve gas poisoning includes:

- difficulty in breathing;
- drooling and excessive sweating;
- vomiting, cramps, involuntary defecication, urination;
- twitching, jerking, and staggering;
- headache, confusion, drowsiness, convulsion, and coma;
- dimness of vision and pinpointing of the pupils (from direct eye exposure).

These are the major nerve agents:

- GA (tabun) (semi-obsolete)
- GB (sarin)
- GD (soman)

- VX

These are code-designated nerve agents which were not adopted for production:

- GF (British variation of sarin)
- VE (precursor to VX)

Summary of the human nervous system, neurotransmitters, and organophosphorus compound interference

All of the functions of the human body are coordinated by its nervous system. Physically, the nervous system is an extension of the brain, down through the spine and major ganglia (*central* nervous system) to the organs and various glands, to the fine network of sensory and activator nerves (often called the *peripheral* nervous system).

There is a second way of dividing the human nervous system, based on function rather than structure. To put it in extremely simple terms, the functioning of the entire human body consists of a series of two-part commands originating in the brain. The first, the *sympathetic* nerve chain, produces epinephrine (adrenaline) and a similar substance called sympathin. In general terms, this system of nerves initiates enzyme action and muscle/tissue movements. The sympathetic nerves work in conjunction, and are intertwined with the *parasympathetic* nerve chain whose function is to contain or reverse the same functions that the sympathetic nervous system initiates. Thus the sympathetic nervous system will accelerate heartbeat and the parasympathetic nervous system will slow down the heartbeat when increased blood flow is no longer deemed neccessary by the brain. A similar action occurs throughout the entire body with all its functions.

The human body works like an electro-chemical computer, with the nervous system(s) the wiring that carries its messages and commands.

The nerve cells do not directly connect with each other, but rather they meet at coupling points called *synapses*. The impulses pass from one cell to another at these points. These consist of electro-chemical signals instantaneously jumping from one cell to another through chemical "bridges" known as *neurotransmitters*. These chemicals break down, are re-absorbed, and re-released as instantaneously as the neural impulses they carry.

There are four principal neurotransmitters dealt with in this book. The first four:

- norepinephrine (noradrenaline)
- serotonin
- dopamine

work almost exclusively within the brain or the higher portion of the spinal cord. See the INCAPACITATING AGENTS for substances effecting these three.

There is a principal neurotransmitter directly effecting the body muscles and the other structures within the parasympathetic nervous system:

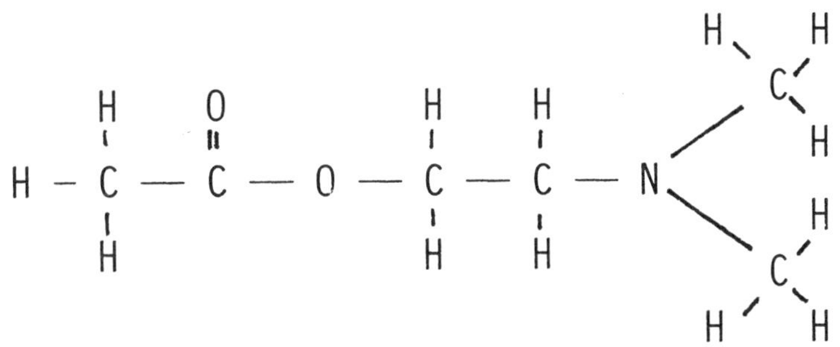

- acetycholine

mol wt 163.2 *parasympathomimetic*

All of the neurotransmitters do not break down of their own accord. Thus, the body supplies its own enzymes, called the *-erase(s)* which break them down into components which will a) break down them far enough so as not to transmit an impulse, but b) are not broken down so far that the body can not immpediately re-cycle them to make more of the origional neurotransmitter.

The -esterase for acetycholine is called

acetycholin<u>esterase</u>.

It breaks acetycholine down into *choline*

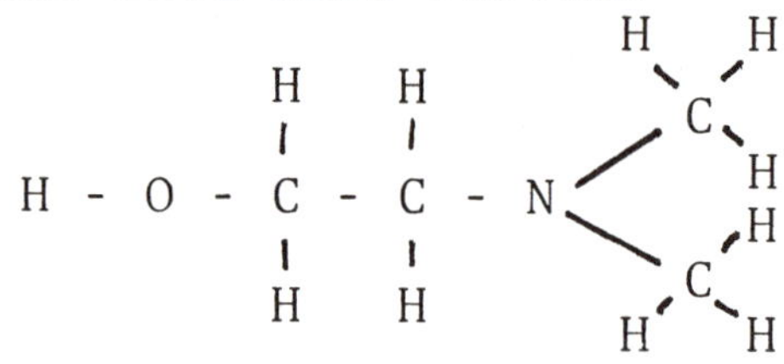

and *acetic acid*

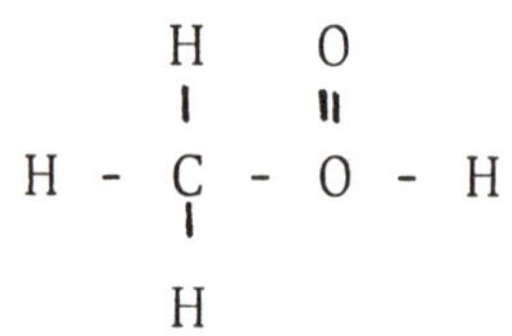

If acetycholinesterase is not allowed to function, acetycholine remains in the billions of effected neural synapses in the body. The result can be compared to a massive electrical short circuit.

The nerve agents do not allow acetycholinesterase to function.

Relationship of the nerve agents to the Incapacitating Agents

The six organophosphate nerve agents discussed in this chapter could be properly classed as acetycholine psychedelics.

Only the immediate lethality of the nerve agents prevent their use (and abuse) as psychoactive substances. It is not known whether nerve agent victims hallucinate before they die.

In this regard, these nerve agents fall into a catagory which includes physostigmine, scopolamine, muscarine, and atropine.

Atropine is the principal, and to date, the most effective antidote to these nerve agents.

The Wehrmacht nerve agents

- GA
- GB
- GD

Code names standardized by the Tripartite pact, the precursor of NATO. Tabun, Sarin, and Soman are the origional German code names.

There is *not*, nor has there ever been, a nerve agent of this series coded "GC." GC was the old medical code for gonorrhea. These three agents were too serious a matter to make bad jokes about.

The *G* stands for *German*, as in *German*-A, *German*-B, etc.

dimethylphosphoramidocyanidate acid, ethyl ester

Tabun

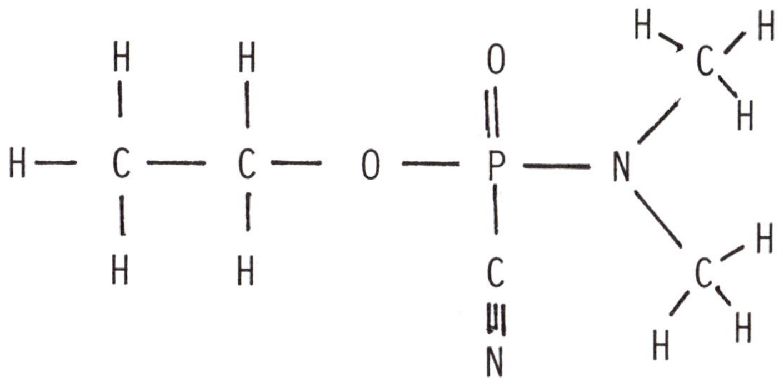

GA

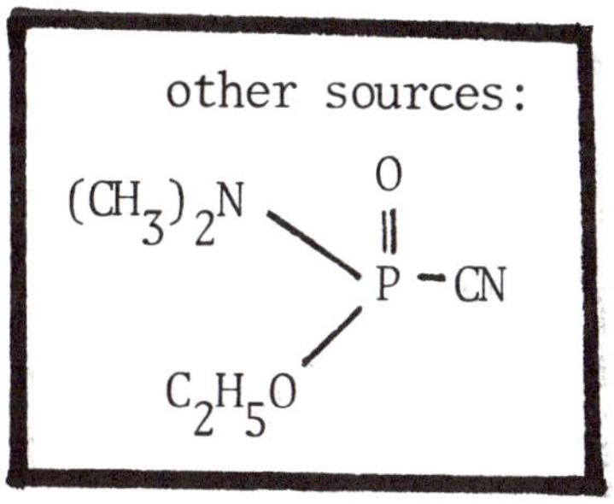

Standard NATO agreement (STANAG) code: GA

Chemical name: ethyl N,N-dimethyl phosphoramidocyanidate
Common name: tabun, GA
Formula: $C_2H_5OP(O)(CN)N(CH_3)_2$

Family: casualty agent
Type: nerve agent

A pale to dark amber liquid giving off a colorless vapor. Little odor in pure state, gives off a smell like rotting fruit as it oxidizes.

History

Working on formulations dating back to 1902 based upon (O)P:O(CN)(N) bondings, a Dr Gerhard Schrader came across the compound which came to be known as tabun. Schrader, a researcher at IG Farben, had been conducting a search for effective pesticides based upon organophosphorus bondings.

During initial testing in January 1937, a drop of tabun was spilled onto a lab bench. Within minutes Dr Schrader and his assistants suffered from contracted pupils, dizziness, and an accute difficulty in breathing. It took the lab staff three weeks to recover. More cautious testing in March showed that all test animals exposed to vapors died within twenty minutes of exposure. Tabun was abandoned as a pesticide. The matter might have ended there had not a Reichs Ordinance of 1935 mandated that studies of toxic substances (and anything else of military significance) be under government report. The law further specified that all such research be classified as Secret.

Dr Schrader was summoned to the Wehrmacht chemical lab at Berlin-Spandau. Tests of tabun were conducted under the facility director, a Dr. colonel Rüdriger. In the fall of that year tabun was adopted as the world's first nerve agent and a production facility was established at Elberfeld in the Ruhr. In 1940, production was transferred to a secret facility at Dyhernfurth-am-Oder near Breslau in Silesia.

In all, about 12,000 tons of tabun was produced, never to be used in combat. In 1944-1945 most of this stock was broken down with alkalies and dumped into the Oder river to prevent capture.

The German production code names were, in order: Le100, Gelan, Stoff-83, then Trilon-83 (Trilon was the name of a popular detergent).

In the west, Allied postwar testing was conducted at Porton Down (UK) and Edgewood Arsenal (US). Tentative adoption for use by Great Britain, Canada and the United States was shelved by the early 1950s in favor of tabun's successor, sarin (GB), which became the NATO standard.

Structure

The basic structure of tabun is formed by the interaction of dimethylamidophosphoryl dichloride and sodium cyanide in the presence of ethanol. Manufacture must be done under highly controlled conditions involving high-speed ventilation and atmospheric filtration.

Tabun is an organophosphate containing a cyanide (CN) bond. Its central structure is thus:

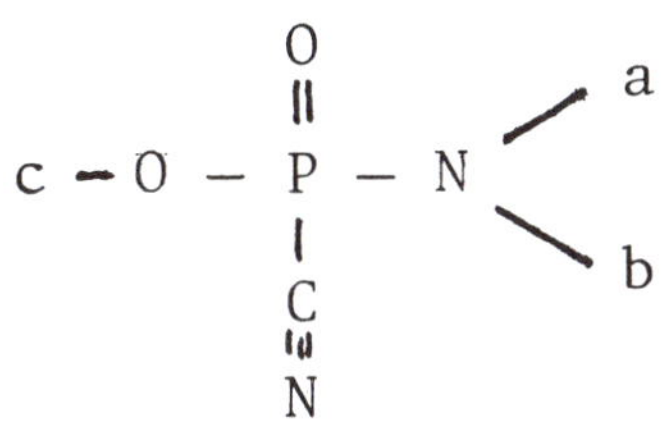

Points (a) and (b) contain methyl (CH_3)- nitrogen bonds and point (c) contains an ethyl ($C_2H_{(4)}$) group. Phosphorus is the key to the whole structure. An ether bond (-O-) next to a keytone bond (:O) would indicate a structure very likely to react with enzyme strings, given the phosphorus-nitrogen chain which would behave like a molecular chainsaw. GB and GD rely on an OP:OF pattern in which a propyl group replaces a nitrogen bond, but which is more reactive in the presence of a fluorine ion. The V-series return to the nitrogen bond. The cyanide group bespeaks of pre-peptide insecticide technology and on the whole is superfluous. What use is hemo-glauben poisoning in a victim already dead?

Readily soluble in all organic solvents. Rapid hydrolysis in presence of strong acid or alkalai bias.

Pathology

Tabun is either absorbed through the skin as a liquid or inhaled as a vapor. Skin absorbsion presents the greater hazard, in that between 1.0 and 1.5 grams of liquid solution (representing an average of 0.01 mg/kg concentration) will cause death within two minutes. Inhalation of vapors will require about 400 mg-min/m^3. Precaution as to vapor concentrations should be heeded, especially in the area where munitions have detonated: concentrations above 20,000 mg-min/m^3 will readily penetrate the skin and the membranes of and around the eyes will begin absorbsion at any level of concentration. Gradual dosages, as opposed to immediate lethal dosages, typically take between ten and twenty minutes before death occurs. Body detoxification proceeds very slowly.

Tabun interferes with the formation of cholinesterase in the neural synapses. In very simple terms, the peripheral and central nervous system proceeds to stimulate itself to its own destruction. Over-stimulation of the nervous system causes over-reactivity in the muscles and malfunctioning of the various body organs. Autopsies of victims typically show a massive congestion of various body enzymes and fluids in all the major organs, throughout the nervous system, and most notably in the brain. Survivors, most notably those who did not recieve prompt medical treatment, may be suffer permanent neurological damage. See Nerve Agents, official definition.

Field behavior

Tabun presents the least vapor hazard (in terms of vapor spread, not lethality) of the three Wehrmacht-created agents, about 1/36th that of sarin (the most vaporous) at 77°F. On the other hand, the liquid may remain in shaded areas for about two days under temperate climatic conditions. As the vapor density of tabun is about 5½ times that of air, these will be expected to seek lower elevations in the terrain and will flow into the substructures of buildings, utility conduits, sewers, and the like.

Tabun is a liquid, origionally designed to be delivered by artillery munitions or aerial spray. Its flash point of 172°F precludes any explosive hazard. Although it develops a fruity to bitter almond smell (courtesy of its CN component) upon vaporization, the pure compound has very little odor.

Specific data

median lethal dosage (LCt_{50})

400 mg-min/m^3 (inhalation or eye). 1.0-1.5 g at 0.01 mg/kg liquid (skin).

median incapacitating dosage (ICt_{50})

300 mg-min/m^3 (inhalation).

skin toxicity

Extremely toxic. Vapor concentrations above 20,000 mg-min/m^3 will penetrate the skin. Liquid agent will always penetrate the skin.

eye toxicity

Extreme hazard. Eye membranes form an efficient entry point for tabun. Dimness of vision and pinpointing of the iris occurs when exposure is from this source.

rate of action

Immediate. Lethal skin dosage will cause death within two minutes. Vapor inhalation may be within ten minutes.

protection required

Protective mask/respirator and full protective overclothing at all times in all concentrations. Normal cloth absorbs.

rate of detoxification

Slight, allowing cumulation of dosage. Medical treatment is manditory.

decontaminants

Bleach slurry, alkalai solutions, caustic soda (sodium hydroxide), or alcohol. Closed or confined spaces should be further flushed with ammonia and live steam. Note: chlorine-based decontaminants will create HCN as a by-product, so flushing is mandated with their use.

vapor density

5.63 times as heavy as air.

vapor pressure

0.070 mm Hg at 25°C(77°F) (low).

liquid density

1.073 g/cc at 25°C(77°F).

persistency

Splashed liquid may remain in the immediate vicinity for several days in temperatures not exceeding 77°F. Evaporates quickly in daytime desert temperatures. May remain for indeterminate periods in cold weather although hydrolysing with snow.

volatility

0°C(32°F), 90 mg/m^3; 25°C(77°F) 610 mg/m^3; 30°C(86°F) 856 mg/m^3.

latent heat of vaporization

79.56 caloroes per gram.

freezing point

-50°C(158°F).

boiling point

120°C(248°F).

decomposition point

150°C(302°F) - for 3 hours.

flash point

78°C(172.4°F).

rate of hydrolysis

Slow with distilled water at pH 7.0 but increasingly rapid with any acid or alkalai present. Phosphates readily catalyse hysrolysis by destruction of tabun's OP:O central bonding pattern.

hydrolysis products

Various ammoniuim-based compounds and HCN.

stability in storage

Stable in munitions where no water vapor is present.

action on metals and other materials

No significant reactions

molecular weight

162.3

Warning

The above specific data refer to tabun in its traditional form as a pure compound. Microencapsulation techniques could make this into a highly persistent poison presenting profoundly different types of hazards.

methylphosphonofluoridic acid
1-methylethyl ester

Sarin

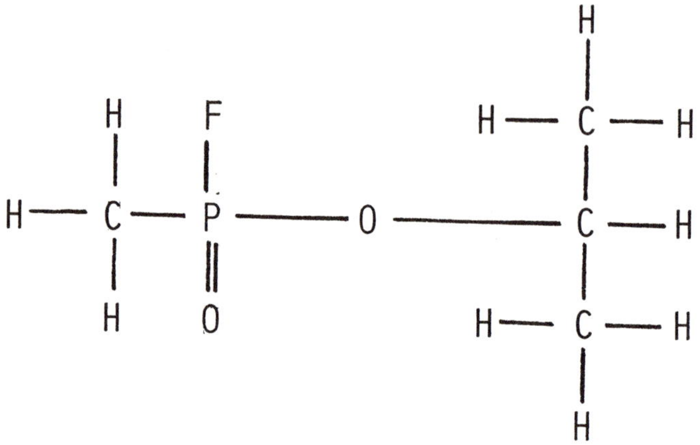

other sources:

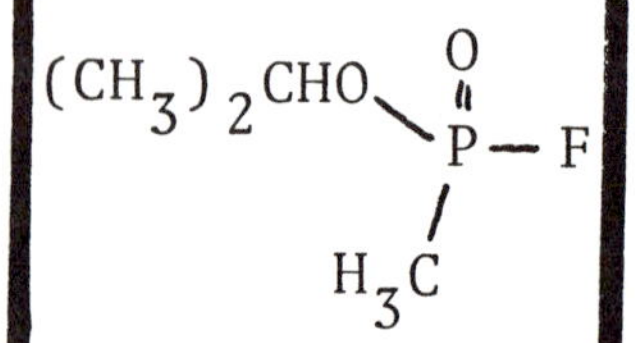

GB

Standard NATO agreement (STANAG) code: GB

Chemical name: isopropyl methyl phosphonofluoridate
Common name: sarin
Formula: $CH_3P(O)(F)OCH(CH_3)_2$

Family: casualty agent
Type: nerve agent

A colorless liquid which gives off a colorless vapor. Almost no odor in its pure state, in impure solutions it will have a slight odor like rotting fruit.

History

Sarin was the second in a series of organophosphorus based nerve agents (the first being tabun) developed by Dr Gerhard Schrader, origionally of IG Farben. Now an employee of the German army working at a new facility at Elberfeld in the Ruhr, in 1938 he developed a compound related to tabun which he felt had a greater potential as a war agent. As the formulation and manufacturing process were completed by fall of that year, Dr Schrader named the substance after the individuals involved in its creation: Schrader, Ambrose, Rüdriger, and van der Linde. Tests on lab animals at the Wehrmacht chemical laboratories at Berlin-Spandau in June of 1939 showed sarin to work ten times as fast as tabun in absorbed dosages.

Plans for the production of sarin were put on the back burner by the advent of the war in 1939, as plans for the development of the tabun plant at Dyhernfurth-am-Oder, Silesia went into execution. Small-scale sarin production began there at a small complex known as "Building 144." Construction of a seperate sarin production facility at Falkenhagen, southeast of Berlin, had almost been completed in 1945 before being captured by the Soviet forces.

Sarin, like tabun, had only come to the attention of the western allies when some prototype munitions were captured in the Ruhr. Their analysis at Porton Down and Edgewood Arsenal opened a lot of eyes, as the Allies had not even suspected the existence of nerve agents beyond a theoretical basis. Being the most potent of the known nerve agents (the Soviets were keeping soman to themselves, and had carted off the Dyhernfurth and Falkenhagen facilities back home), soman (recoded as GB by the British) was developed by the Tripartite nations of Britain, the United States, and Canada as a standard war agent. The earlier tabun was out of the running by 1952. With sarin's mLd of 70 mg-min/m^3 to tabuns 400 mg-min/m^3 there was simply no contest. At the formation of NATO, sarin was adopted as standard and so remains.

Structure

Sarin is an organophosphate containing a fluorine (F) bond. Its central structure

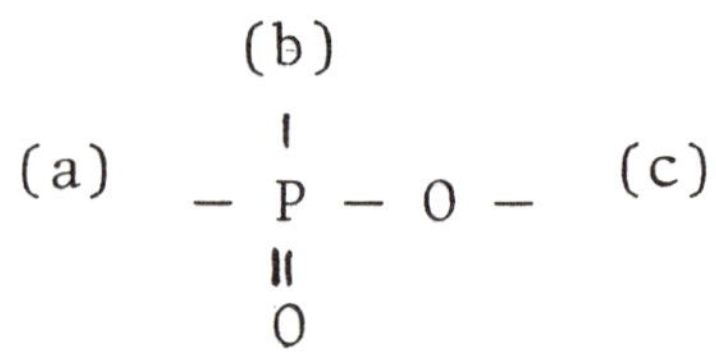

is identical to that of tabun. Differences: at (a) tabun's $N(CH_3)_2$ is replaced by a simple methane (CH_3); at (b) tabun's mostly superfluous cyanide (CN) is replaced by a more reactive fluorine (F) bond; and at (c) tabun's ethyl ($C_2H_{(5)}$) group is replaced with a more readily oxidized propyl ($C_3H_{(7)}$) group. The result is an agent which is more rapidly absorbed than the parent compound.

A disadvantage is that the fluorine ion reacts quickly with water, especially in the presence of alkalai solutions. While of benefit to internal assimilation, this permits environmental dissipation. While highly toxic, sarin in its pure form is not very persistent, evaporating at about the same rate as water as a result.

Origional decontaminants included bicarbonate of soda. Sodium carbonate and sodium hydroxide (caustic soda) work well. Hot soapy water works well as a field expedient, and warm water alone would eliminate an immediate threat from liquid sarin.

Pathology

Sarin is the most toxic of the three Wehrmacht agents. Either inhaled as a vapor or directly absorbed through the skin, death is rapid. Direct ingestion of liquid in concentraions of 0.01 mg/kg or more may cause death within one minute. Vapor concentrations above 8,000 mg-min/m^3 will immediately penetrate the skin. Eye membranes form an efficient entry point for sarin as well. The only moderating factor in sarin's lethality is its high volatility. Normal body detoxification is slow, allowing dosage to accumulate. Death from dosage accumulation takes about ten minutes.

Sarin interferes with the formation of cholinesterase in the neural synapses. In very simple terms, the peripheral and central nervous system proceeds to stimulate itself to its own destruction. Over-stimulation of the nervous system causes over-reactivity in the muscles and malfunctioning of the various body organs. Expected would be a massive congestion of various body enzymes and fluids in all the major organs, throughout the nervous system, and within the brain. Survivors, especially those who do not recieve prompt medical treatment, are likely to suffer permanent neurological damage. See Nerve Agents, official definition.

Field behavior

Sarin is the most volatile of the three Wehrmacht agents, forming a vapor mass about 36 times as quickly as tabun. However, high volatility can also mean swift evaporation with a liquid prone to rapid hydrolysis. This is not to understate the acute lethality of this agent, but to emphasize its lack of persistency in its normal liquid state.

At about five times the weight of air, sarin vapors may be expected to flow downwards into lower terrain and the substructures of buildings.

Sarin represents no fire or explosion hazard. Artillery or aerial spray delivered.

Specific data

median lethal dosage *(LCt_{50})*

70 mg-min/m^3 (inhalation); 12,000 mg-min/m^3 (vapor through skin; 0.01 mg/kg concentration (ingestion).

median incapacitating dosage *(ICt_{50})*

35 mg-min/m^3 (inhalation); 8,000 mg-min/m^3 (vapor through skin).

skin toxicity

Not toxic to skin tissue, however any liquid will immediately penetrate the skin, as will vapor in concentration above 8,000 mg-min/m^3.

eye toxicity

Causes neurological desensitivity. Eye membranes form an efficient pathway for sarin into the body.

rate of action

Immediate. Ingested liquid may cause death within one minute. Average vapor concentrations will cause lethal toxicity within ten minutes.

protection required

Protective mask/respirator and protective overclothing must be worn.

rate of detoxification

Natural detoxification within the body is slow. Lethal dosages may accumulate.

decontaminants

Caustic soda (sodium hydroxide) is most efficient, although any bleaching solution works well. Ammonia or alkalai solutions with live steam should be used to decontaminate closed or confined spaces.

vapor density

4.86 times as heavy as air.

vapor pressure

2.9 mm Hg at 25°C(77°F).

liquid density

1.09 g/cc at 25°C (77°F).

persistency

Essentially non-persistent, as sarin evaporates at about the same rate as water, with high volatility as a factor in vapor dispersion.

volatility

4100 mg/m^3 at 0°C(32°F); 22,000 mg/m^3 at 25°C(77°F); 29,000 mg/m^3 at 30°C(86°F).

latent heat of vaporization

80 calories per gram at 25°C(77°F).

melting point

-50°C(-68.8°F).

boiling point

158°C(316.4°F).

decomposition point

150°C(302°F) for 2½ hours.

flash point

None. Sarin does not burn.

rate of hydrolysis

Very rapidly hydrolysed in alkaline solutions. Acidic conditions will destroy sarin in the lab within fifteen hours. Munitions not airtight may completely hydrolyse within 30 hours.

hydrolysis products

In low pH (acidic), hydrogen fluoride (HF); in high pH (alkaline), isopropyl alcohol and various polymers.

stability in storage

Stable in steel canisters under normal temperature gradients.

action on metals and other materials

Slightly corrosive to ferrous alloys.

molecular weight

14.10

Warning

The above specific data refer to sarin in its traditional form as a pure compound. Microencapsulation techniques could make this into a highly persistent poison presenting profoundly different types of hazards.

Sarin is commonly thickened by admixture with certain oils and other petroleum products.

methylphosphonofluoridic acid 1,2,2-trimethylpropyl ester

Soman

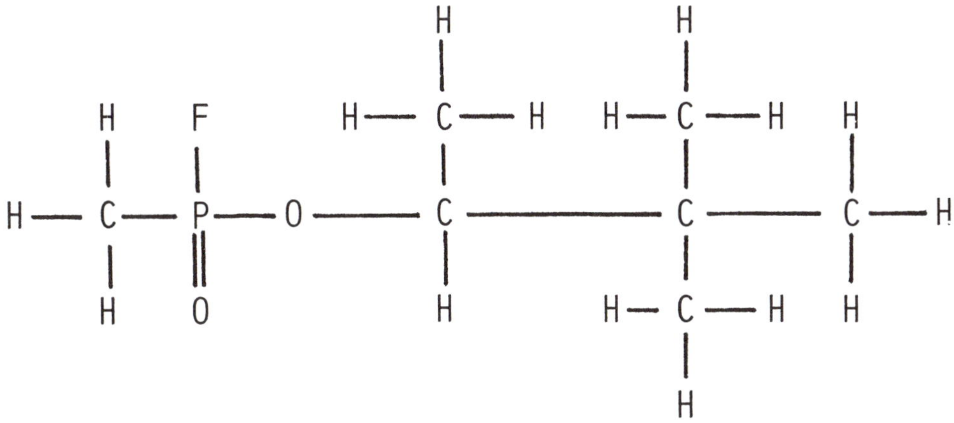

GD

other sources:

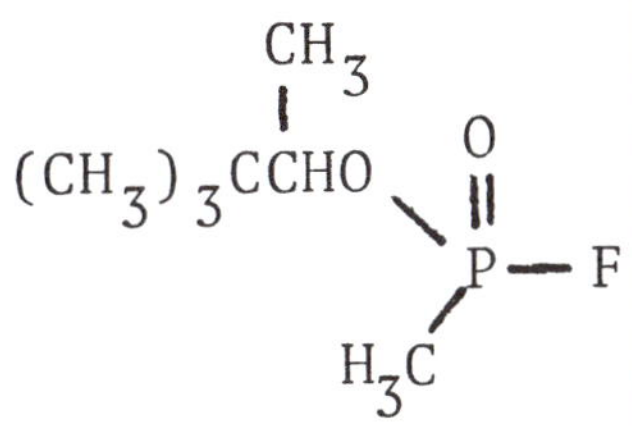

Standard NATO agreement (STANAG) code: GD

Chemical name: pinacolyl methyl phosphonefluoridate

Common name: soman

Formula: $CH_3P(O)(F)OCH(CH_3)C(CH_3)_3$

Family: casualty agent

Type: nerve agent

A colorless liquid which gives off a colorless vapor. Will have an odor similar to that of rotting fruit, and with impurities may have a camphorlike smell.

History

Soman was the last of the three major Wehrmacht-designed nerve agents. Tabun was relatively slow acting, but formed a stable cloud over a moderately persistent liquid. Sarin was extremely fast acting, but due to its volatility tended to evaporate at the same rate as water. Soman was a compromise. It had an evaporation rate sufficient to allow it to remain in an area for about a day while producing a dependable vapor mass which produced a significant downwind hazard. Although soman's median lethal dosage requires 30% more exposure than sarin, soman is considered more readily absorbed into the bloodstream and more immediately reactive with neural tissue, in particular that in the brain. So the tests in the Spring and Summer of 1944 seemed to show. Soman remain mostly theory.

Major investment had already been made in the tabun plant at Dyhrenfurth and the sarin factory at Falkenhagen, where preliminary soman testing occurred. By January of 1945 the Falkenhagen archives were kept in a converted mine-shaft complex about ten miles east of Berlin. Before they could be destroyed in March of that year the whole was captured by a soviet task force under GRU (Soviet military intelligence) direction. Investigation of the find was done by a chemical officer of the Soviet general staff, a Professor Colonel Kargin, who immediately ordered everything be shipped directly to the Karpov Institute in Moscow. By the end of 1946, Soviet production facilities for soman had been established.

There are sundry theories about the derivation of the name "soman." Probably the most convincing involves a double pun. In Greek derivation it may refer to *sleep*.[1] In many Latin based languages it refers to *bludgeon*. Both are appropriate.

1. although in direct translation *soma* means *body*, and in physiology the body tissues as distinguished from the germ cells.

Structure

Soman is an organophosphate containing a fluorine (F) bond. Its central structure

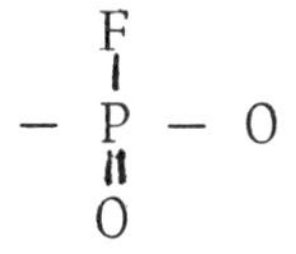

is identical to that of both tabun (GA) and sarin (GB). Soman is in fact based closely on sarin. The "left hand" portion:

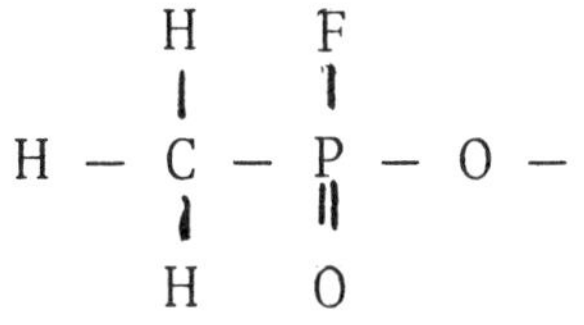

is identical. Sarins "right hand" propyl group, C_3H_7 , has been extended, the old C_3H_7 becoming a carbon bond with a methyl (CH_3) group filling the (top planar) structure, with an opposing single hydrogen (H) bond. Attached to the remaning orbital is a 2-methylpropane [CH_3C-$(CH_3)_2$] group. To compare:

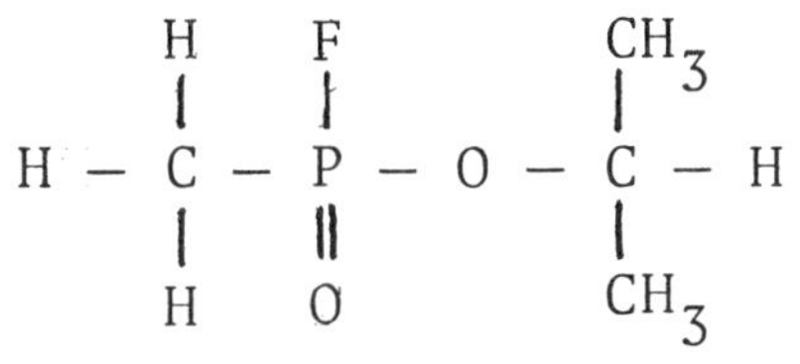

Sarin

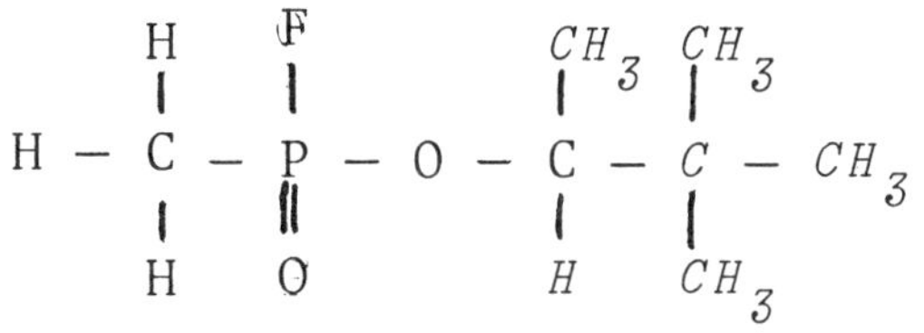

Soman

The effect of the 2-methylpropane group is to create a heavier liquid which by coincidence is slightly more interactive with certain proteins commonly found in the blood giving soman a slight edge over sarin in permeating certain neural membranes while preserving the cholesterase destroying qualities of the latter.

Pathology

Soman is the second most toxic of the Wehrmacht agents under field conditions. It is the most neurologically active. Dosages above 100 mg-min/m^3 (inhalation) or 0.01 mg/kg (ingestion or skin absorption) concentration liquid, may bring death within one minute. As body detoxification is very slow, dosage accumulation typically brings death within 15 minutes.

Skin *vapor* absorption represents a lesser hazard in open terrain due to soman's 5570 mg/m^3 volatility at 86°F, which is probably 30-40% of that required to penetrate the skin. Eye membrane absorption, on the other hand, is rapid.

Soman's one to two day persistency under moderate weather conditions increases the liklihood of mass casualties through dosage accumulation. Both vapor and liquid entering through open wounds will cause immediate spasmotic reactions with death following quickly.

Soman prevents the formation of cholinesterase in the neural synapses. The peripheral and central nervous systems stimulate themselves to their own destruction. This over stimulation causes violent muscle activity and malfunctioning of the various body organs. Most profoundly effected is the brain, which ceases to function before the body stops its *danse macabre*. Survivors will suffer permanent systemic damage.

Field behavior

Soman is a mildly persistent agent resembling clear a clear, heavy solvent or a very light machine oil. As this mixes with its environs its odor changes from something resembling overripe peaches to camphor. It will hydrolyse under most circumstances, most rapidly with alkalines and most slowly with acids.

Almost six and a half times as heavy as air, soman vapors

may be expected to flow downwards into lower terrain and into the substructures of buildings, tunnels, conduits, sewers and the like. Soman represents a much greater threat in enclosed or confined spaces than it does in open areas, especially where a stable vapor mass is permitted to accumulate.

To present a fire hazard, soamn must be heated to above 173°F. This is only possible in conflagrations or the most extreme of desert conditions where munitions might be exposed to direct sunlight.

Specific data

median lethal dosage (LCt_{50})

100 mg-min/m^3 (inhalation); 0.01 mg/kg (liquid concentration.

median incapacitating dosage (ICt_{50})

35 mg-min/m^3 (inhalation).

skin toxicity

Not toxic to skin tissue, however any liquid will penetrate the skin and there enter the blood.

eye toxicity

Causes neurological desensitivity. Eye membranes form an efficient entry path.

rate of action

Immediate. Ingested liquid may cause death within one minute. Inhaled vapor concentrations may cause death within ten to fifteen minutes. Harder to treat medically than either tabun or sarin.

protection required

Protective mask/respirator with protective overclothing at all times.

rate of detoxification

Slow. Effects are essentially accumulative and dosage builds up rapidly.

decontaminants

Caustic soda (sodium hydroxide) is most efficient, although any bleaching solution will work. Ammonia or alkalai solutions with live steam should be used to decontaminate closed or confined spaces.

vapor density

6.33 times as heavy as air.

vapor pressure

0.40 mm Hg at 25°C(77°F).

liquid density

1.022 g/cc at 25°C(77°F).

persistency

Mildly persistent. May last in shaded areas for about two days under moderate climatic conditions.

volatility

531 mg/m^3 at 0°C(32°F); 3900 mg/m^3 at 25°C(77°C); 5570 mg/m^3 at 30°C(86°F).

latent heat of vaporization

72.4 calories per gram at 25°C(77°F).

freezing point

-42°C(-43.6°F). Does not form a crystaline solid.

boiling point

198°C(388.4°F) with decomposition.

decomposition point

130°C(266°F) at four hours when exposed to air. Same temperature will degrade canistered munitions within 200 hours.

flash point

Above 78°C(172°F).

rate of hydrolysis

Varies according to pH. Complete hydrolysis in sodium hydroxide (NaOH) within 5 minutes. Will hydrolyse in almost neutral (pH 6.65) solutions within 45 hours.

hydrolysis products

Mainly hydrogen fluoride (hydrofluoric acic) (HF).

stability in storage

Less stable than tabun or sarin, in pure liquid form. Older conventional munitions might be suspect.

Action on metals and other materials

Slightly corrosive to most metals.

molecular weight

182.178

Warning

The above specific data refer to soman in its traditional form as a pure chemical. Microencapsulation techniques could make this into a very persistent poison presenting a profoundly greater hazard.

Soman is commonly thickened by admixture with certain oils and other petroleum products.

The V-series nerve agents

•VX

VX is the origional NATO version. VR-55 is a slight modification. Both appear to have been satisfactory for their mission, so further formula variations were not deemed necessary.

ethyl S-2-diisopropyl aminoethyl methylphosphoro-
thiolate

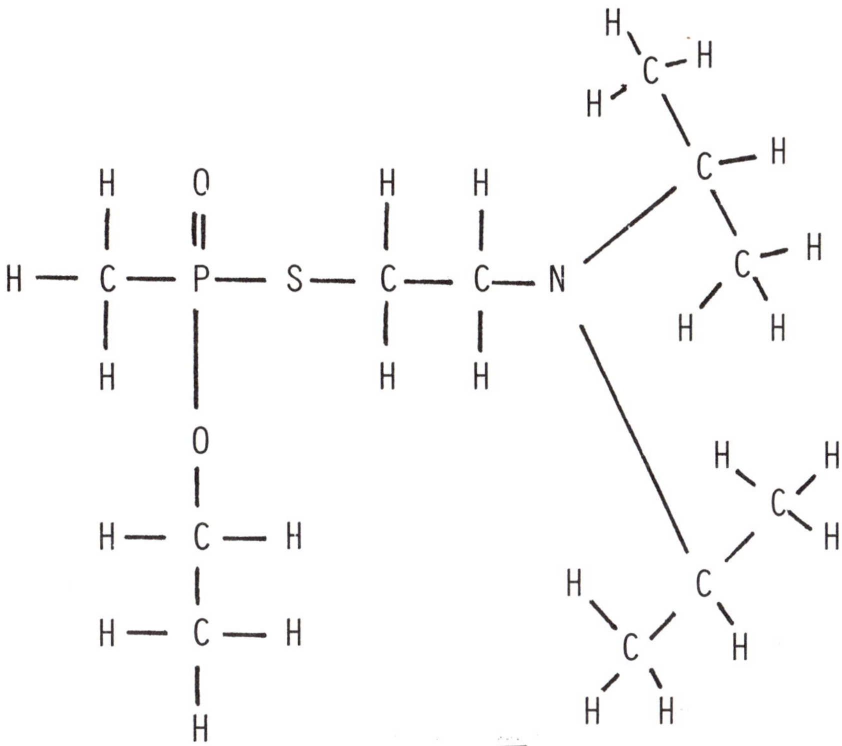

VX

Standard NATO agreement (STANAG) code: VX

Chemical name: ethyl S-2-diisopropyl aminoethyl methylphosphoro-thiolate
Common name: VX
Formula: $(C_2H_5O)(CH_3)(O):(P):SCH_2CH_2N[CH(CH_3)_2]_2$

Family casualty agent
Type: nerve agent

An odorless pale amber liquid similar in appearence to 20-weight motor oil. Gives off a colorless vapor.

History

In 1952 the Plant Protection Laboratory of Imperial Chemical Industries was conducting a search for new pesticides to replace DDT. A Dr. Ranajit Ghosh discovered an organophosphate/sulfur compound that was immediately toxic to mammals as well as to insects. The formula, along with samples was sent to the British military lab at Porton Down.

At this time, the British were commited to the adoption of either tabun or sarin and although intrigued by the new compound, decided to pass it on to Canada and the United States. Canada declined and the United States took the formula under study, refining the origional formula at its Edgewood Arsenal. This final version was coded VX.

Meanwhile, somewhere between ICI and Porton, Soviet military intelligence (the GRU) got ahold of the Dr Ghosh's formula and proceeded to develop their own version by 1955, which they call VR-55.

Porton Down developed the VX production technology at its Nancekuke, Cornwall, test station. Shortly thereafter the British cabinet ordered a halt to chemical weapons production. All work on VX was transferred to the United States.

By 1960 a small state-of-the-art plant was established at Newport, Indiana. About 1300 lbs a year (for a total of about 2½ tons) were produced until production was halted in 1968 following the Skull Valley Incident. In that incident about 20 lbs of VX leaked from an aerial spray tank (thought to be emptied) and drifted over the boundries of the Dugway, Utah, Proving Grounds, killing about 6000 sheep. An improperly stored canister of VX leaked on Okinawa in the summer of 1969. Following an inquiry, President Nixon issued an executive order in November 1969 halting U.S. production and development of chemical weapons.

Structure

Two bonding groups form the basis of a VX molecule:

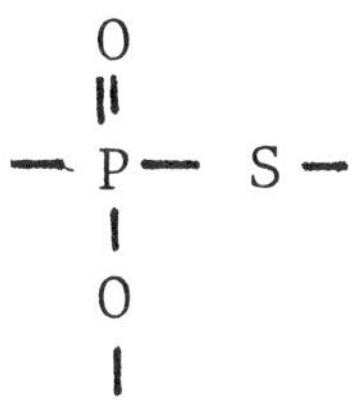

and

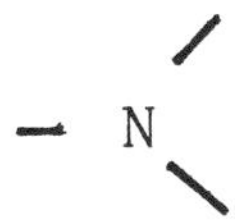

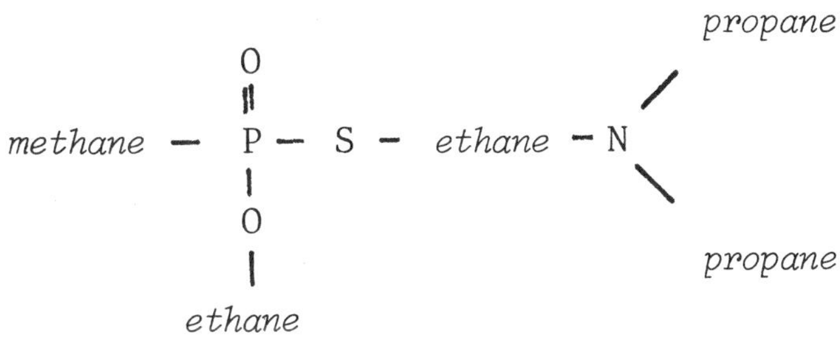

VX is a very heavy molecule which is highly reactive with animal enzymes, in part due to its eleven unsaturated hydrocarbon bonds in five major groups. All phosphorus bonds are reactive and, phosphorus being a crucial ingredient in neuroenzymes, organophosphorus groups catalyse ion substitution in those enzymes, thus destroying them. Nitrogen, especially as it releases heavy hydrocarbon bonds in the latter environment, promotes all the wrong types of oxidation for the health of the victim. The sulphur bond is crucial to the binding together of the reactive groups into a stable compound of noted longevity in all climatic conditions.

Pathology

Death from vapor inhalation (mLd 100 mg-min/m^3) would only be probable if the victim was in extreme proximity to a sizable puddle of the stuff. VX was designed to create its casualties through skin absorption or from mist formed by aerial sprays or air-bursting types of munitions (artillery round or rocket). Skin absorption requires perhaps 0.001 gram through a cut or scrape. Any quantity of liquid large enough to be seen with the unaided eye might easily penetrate unbroken skin. Slowly detoxified, all effects are cumulative.

VX destroys all neuroenzymes and is rapidly absorbed into the bloodstream. Cholesterase is only one of the neurotransmitters VX effects. Some victims with moderately lethal dosages may exhibit the spasmotic symptoms (jerking, urination, defecation, etc.) normally associated with nerve agents. But those who have recieved massive amounts of VX into their systems may simply go out like a candle, their nervous systems and involuntary muscles (heart, lungs, etc.), along with their brain functions, simply and immediately ceasing to function. Among survivors, systemic damages will be permanent.

Field behavior

VX is a thick liquid resembling 30-weight motor oil. With low volatility (10.5 mg/m^3) and vapor pressure (0.0007 mm Hg at 77°F), inhalation does not represent as great a threat as does absorption. For this reason, VX was designed to be a lethal contaminant, something that would cling to equipment, vehicles, clothing, and stores. Concentrations would prevent passage or occupation of terrain or structures.

VX (and its Soviet counterpart, VR-55) are most efficient when disseminated by aerial spray. Second most effective are artillery (cannon or missile/rocket) munitions fused to burst over a target. Low-explosive land mines were developed for the purpose of contaminating vehicles and cargo.

VX has the same viscosity as motor oil and would be expected to cling to whatever it splatters on. Decontamination must be immediate. VX may persist for up to several weeks in most climatic conditions, hydrolyzing slowest in acidic soils.

The vapors do present a unique type of hazard. In that

they are about nine times as heavy as air, VX deployed at higher levels of enclosed buildings would vapor contaminate lower levels. Similarly, conduits, tunnels, sewers, and caves could be made uninhabitable by the agent.

VX (and VR-55) presents the greater, and the most insidious threat among the nerve agents covered in this book.

Specific data

median lethal dosage (LCt_{50})

100 mg-min/m^3 (inhalation); 0.001 gr (ingested).

median incapacitating dosage (ICt_{50})

50 mg-min/m^3.

skin toxicity

Not toxic to skin tissue, but VX will penetrate the skin. Scrapes or cuts present an immediate entry point. This includes freshly shaved skin, vapor and liquid.

eye toxicity

May cause neuralinsensitivity. Eye membrane and tissues around the eyes are a point of immediate penetration, vapor of liquid.

rate of action

Immediate.

protection required

Protective mask/respirator and full protective clothing.

rate of detoxification

Very low. Effects are cumulative. Lethal dosages will typically build up within 15 minutes at most.

decontaminants

Strong alkaline/oxidizer solutions are most effective. Supertropical bleach slurry is the standard. Caustic soda (sodium hydroxide, NaOH) is effective, and should be used with live steam for interior decontamination. Flame may be used as a field expedient.

vapor density

9.2 times as heavy as air.

vapor pressure

0.0007 mm Hg at 25°C(77°F).

liquid density

1.008 g/cc at 25°C(77°F).

persistency

Highly persistent, especially in acidic soils. May last several weeks in temperate climates.

volatility

10.5 mg/m^3 at 25°C(77°F).

latent heat of vaporization

78.2 calories per gram at 25°C(77°F).

freezing point

-51°C(-59.8°F).

boiling point

298°C(568.4°F) with decomposition.

decomposition point

72 hours at 150°C(302°F); 3.2 hours at 200°C(392°F); 8 minutes at 250°C(482°F); 72 seconds at 295°C(563°F).

flash point

159°C(318.2°F).

rate of hydrolysis

Varies with pH. At 25°C(77°F): pH 2-3, 200 days; pH 13, 32 minutes; pH 14, 2.6 minutes.

hydrolysis products

Dimethyl methylphosphonate,
2-diisopropylaminoethyl mercaptan,
ethyl hydrogen methylphosphonate,
bis (ethylmethylphosphonic) anhydride,
bis S- (2-diisopropylaminoethyl) methylphosphonodithioate.

stability in storage

Stable in canisters at normal room temperatures. Unstabilized munitions will begin to decompose at 71°C (159.8°F), at a rate of 5% per month.

action on metals and other materials

None of consequence on common alloys based on iron, copper or aluminum.

molecular weight

267.38

Warning

The above specific data refer to VX is its standard form. Microencapsulation techniques could make this into different forms of poisons presenting profoundly different types of hazards.

Code-designated nerve agents which were not adopted for production

- GF
- VE

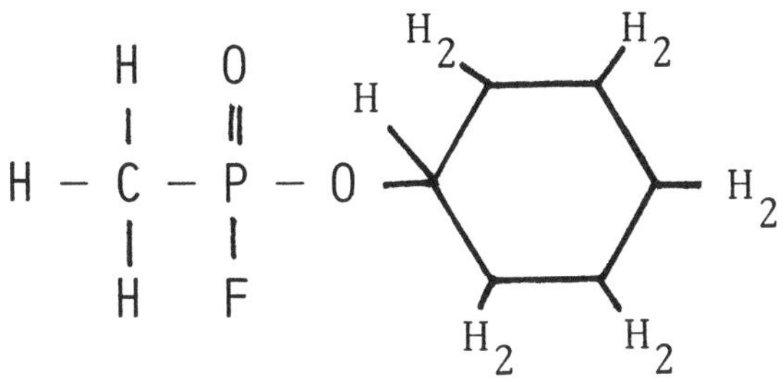

GF

GF was a variation on GB (sarin) in which GB's isopropyl (C_3H_7) group was replaced with an unsaturated benzene ring.

GF offered no advantage in lethality than GB. GF was an attempt to make a naturally thick G agent, allowing persistency without sacrificing volatility. The unsaturated carbon ring tended to revert to a more stable benzene group while in munitions. The result was an agent less effective than GB inside munitions which tended to explode on impact.

During development GF was known as CMPF.

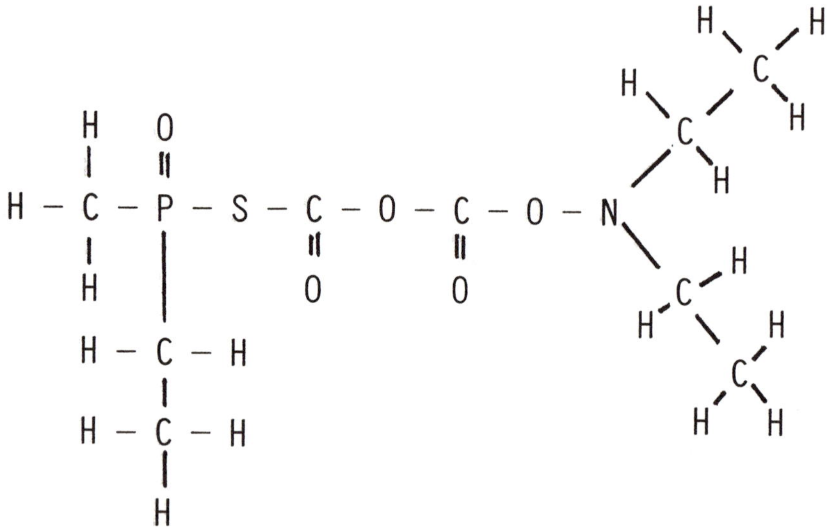

VE

VE was the precursor to VX. It closely resembles Dr Ghosh's origional formula. VE's double ester $(COO)_2$ was replaced by an abbreviated ethyl (C_2H_2) group and the two nitrogen-ethyl bonds were replaced by nitrogen-propyl bonds. The result was a more volatile compound (VX) with better viscosity and better storage characteristics.

New Developments

Binary weapons

Chemical artillery rounds resemble all other munitions, that is they consist of a hollow casing with a filling with fuse on the nose (impact or timed) that sets of the mixture inside. Chemical rounds differ only in that the contents don't explode so there must be a small explosive charge inside to burst open the shell casing.

Most chemical rounds have the actual agent within a glass or some other type of inert liner. Two hazards arise. First, as munitions are inspected and restacked/repacked over the years, the liners *may* break and the rounds *may* begin to leak. Secondly, chemical ammunition dumps are tempting wartime targets (and peacetime targets for terrorists). A third problem is both social and political. Most people realize the hazardous potential of toxic chemical munitions, and in the western nations they urge their elected representatives to keep the things in somebody else's district, presuming they want to tolerate them at all.

A practical proposal to safely store chemical munitions while not really having any is to break down the chemical components into two or more seperate groups. These would be packed into an artillery or rocket casing (or spray unit) immediately prior to use. The concusion of firing would break the containers and the spin of the artillery projectile (a few hundred times per second) would mix the ingredients to produce an agent. For example, sarin (GB) would be produced by combining methyl phosphonyl difluoride and isopropanol (with the proper catalytic compounds) in this manner.

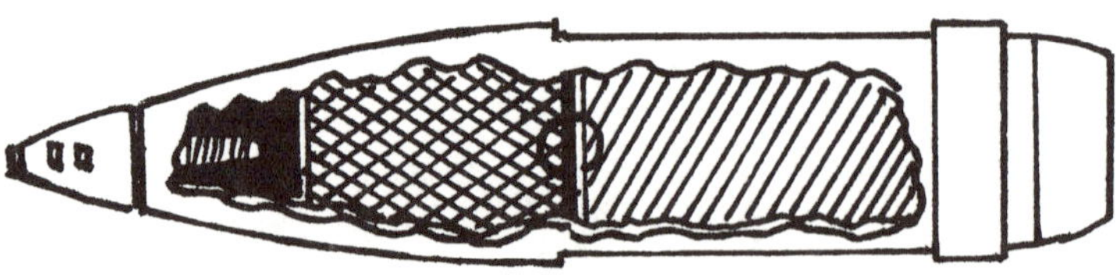

New formulations: bicyclophosphonates

Phosphoric acid is a common, harmless compound used in the manufacture of many things from soft drinks to fertilizers:

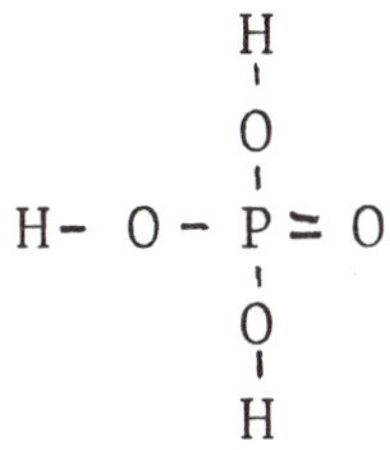

H_3PO_4

produced from phosphonic acid

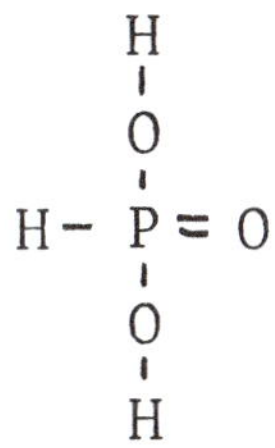

H_3PO_3

Phosphonic acid's esters are the *phosphonates*. A *bycyclic* phosphonate ester could involve replacement of two opposite OH bonds with benzene groups to form biphenyl groups

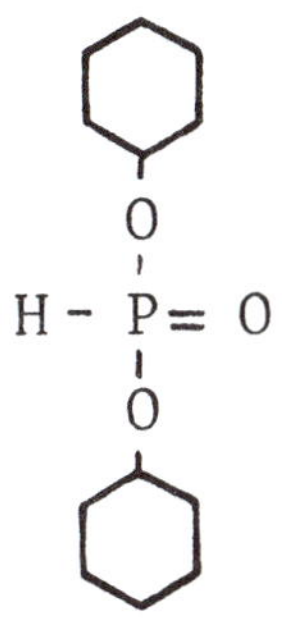

or more properly it would involve two phosphonic radicals back-to-back, joined through double oxygen bonds:

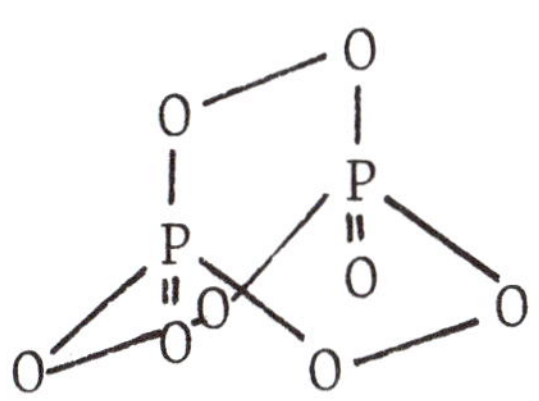

or a pattern of

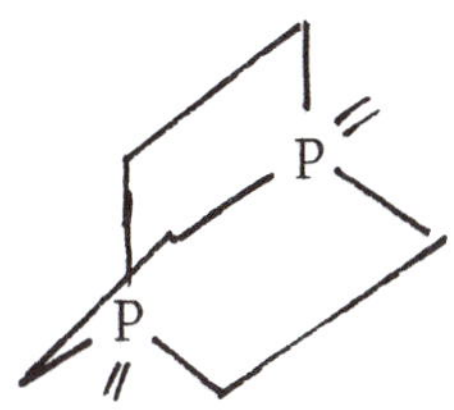

Some O: bonds could be replaced by enzymereactive strings with excellent absorption potential.

The bicyclophosphonates, and the phosphonates in general figure in current pesticide research. They form the basis of compounds which are more reactive than the simple P(:O)O bonds of tabun, sarin, and VX.

Peptides

Peptides, in simplistic terms, are what occur when two or more amino acids collide. They occur naturally in human hormones, forming from the breakdown of proteins in the course of digestion. In short, they are a normal part of human chemistry.

All amino acids contain an acid group (in organic chemistry a carboxylic acid, COOH) and an amino group (NH_2) on the opposing pole. Interaction with another amino acid group causes ~~loss of~~ a loss of the OH group from a COOH and a hydrogen atom from an NH_2 group (precipitating as water, H_2O). The two amino acid groups are joined in a peptide bond (C:OHN). For example:

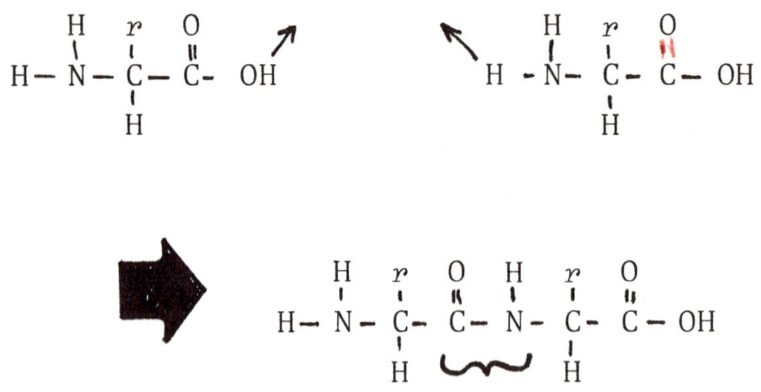

The *r* points represent places where specific reactive groups could be inserted, and would attack whichever body activities that particular peptide is keyed towards. A toxic Trojan horse.

Field treatment for nerve
agent poisoning

atrophine

2-pam chloride

atropine

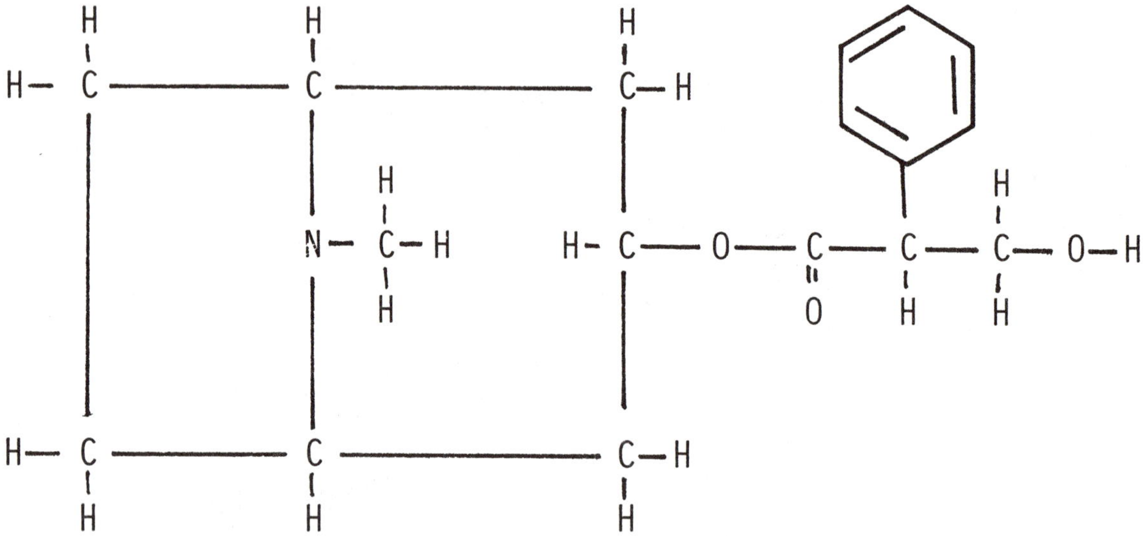

Commerial name: Festalan[R] (20% preparation)
Action: parasympatholytic; anticholinergic; antispasmodic

An alkaloid prepared from various plants of the nightshade family, or by sympathetic preparation. Usually in 30% solution in ethyl alcohol.

As a nerve agent antidote, atropine is used in 2-milligram autoinjectors. Two such dosages are used, one each applied to the large muscles of the legs. Administration should follow first symptoms or immediately after known unprotected exposure.

Substitutes for cholesterase. Acts on parasympathetic nerve endings to inhibit the actions of acetylcholine on smooth muscles, exocrine glands and the heart.

May present its own medical hazard to persons with glaucoma, gastric retention, prostrate hypertrophy, pyloric (stomach to intestine) and bladder obstruction, and congestive heart problems.

Directly injected atropine briefly acts as a central nervous system stimulant. For about ten minutes a moderate feeling of euphoria occurs, known as atropine intoxication. As the body adjusts to this enzyme substitute and attempts some Cholinesterase production the feeling of euphoria is replaced by a pronounced feeling of depression, especially with the 4-milligram (or more) dosages required to counteract nerve agent poisoning. Difficulty in speech, blurred vision, hot dry skin, marked thirst and stupor will occur within 15 minutes of injection.

Atropine is the first part of a two part treatment. Whereas it is used to counteract the effects of nerve agents, medical administration of 2-pam chloride (or a similar cholinesterase reactivator) is required as an antidote to atropine.

Lastly, a final precaution. Atrophine has strong psychoactive side effects. It is a member of the acetylcholine mimicking psychedelics, which includes such compounds as scopolamine and muscarine. More than one auto injecter dosage (which may be neccessary) will probably cause severe confusion or hallucinations (auditory and possibly visual) in victims. This should always be kept in mind when treating nerve gas casualties.

2-pam chloride

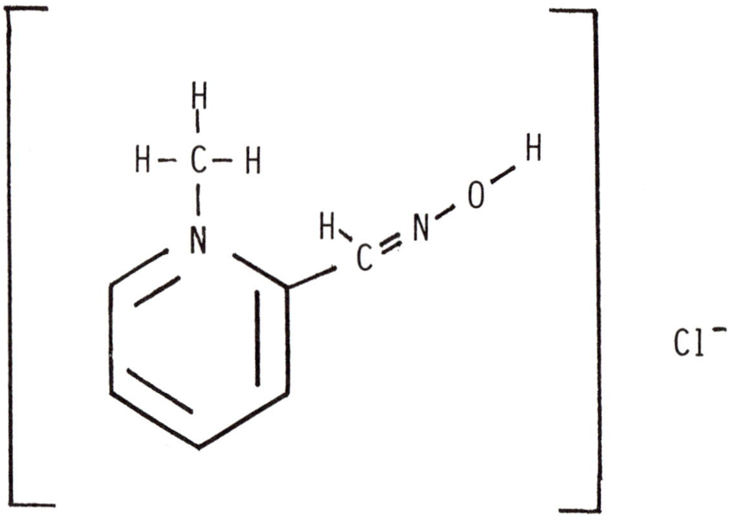

Chemical name: 2-hydroiminomethyl-1-methylpyridinium chloride

Synonyms: 2-pam chloride, protopam chloride, 2-FMPOCl, 2-PAMCl, 2-pyridine aldoxime chloride, pralidoxime chloride

Commercial name: Protopam Chloride

Reactivates cholinesterase which has been deactivated due to phosphorlation from organophosphate compounds. Also detoxifies organophosphate residues which remain in the neural synapses.

Typically the follow-up to atrophine treatment in both military and civillian applications. Atropine acts as an emergency substitute for cholinesterase and 2-pam chloride restores the action of that enzyme and clears away enzyme residues. Marginally effective against the carbamate anticholinesterases. Not effective against phosphorus or the inorganic phosphates. Developed as an antidote for the organophosphate pesticides developed in the late 1930s through the 1950s. By connection it proved to be effective against the military nerve agents which grew out of those compounds.

2-pam chloride is administered by regular medical personnel, which in military terms means combat support hospitals, evac hospitals, or field hospitals. Whereas atropine is auto-injected, 2-pam chloride must be administered intravenously. The usual dosage is 1 to 2 grams in 100 mL of saline over a 15 to 30 minute period. Repeated dosages may be required. In emergency cases, a direct injection may be given consisting of 1 gram of 2-pam chloride dissolved in 20 mL distilled water. The injection should be intravenous, but may be intramuscular or subcutaneous (between skin and muscle tissues). In severe cases additional doses may be needed every three to eight hours. The patient should be administered 2-pam chloride for as long as poisoning symptoms persist.

Recovering patients, once out of the initial atropine stupor, may exhibit irrational behavior. Care should be taken that they be strapped down or otherwise placed under restraint during treatment. This is highly likely in nerve agent victims, where a heavy atropine dosage will have been given and a long delay in secondary treatment would be typical under conditions of war.

Comparative Tables

nerve agents — comparative data

agent	*rate of action*	*state at 68°F*	*odor*	*volatility (mg/m^3)*	*LCT_{50} ($mg\text{-}min/m^3$)*	*ICt_{50} ($mg\text{-}min/m^3$)*	*vapor density (x air)*	*vapor pressure (mm Hg)*
GA	very rapid	colorless liquid	faintly fruity; none when pure	610 at 77°F	400	300	5.63	0.07 at 77°F
GB	very rapid	colorless liquid	almost none when pure	22,000 at 77°F	100	75	4.86	2.9 at 77°F
GD	very rapid	colorless liquid	fruity; camphor odor when pure	3900 at 77°F	100	35	6.33	0.4 at 77°F
VX	rapid	colorless ot pale amber liquid	odorless when pure	10.5 at 77°F	100	50	9.2	0.0007 at 77°F

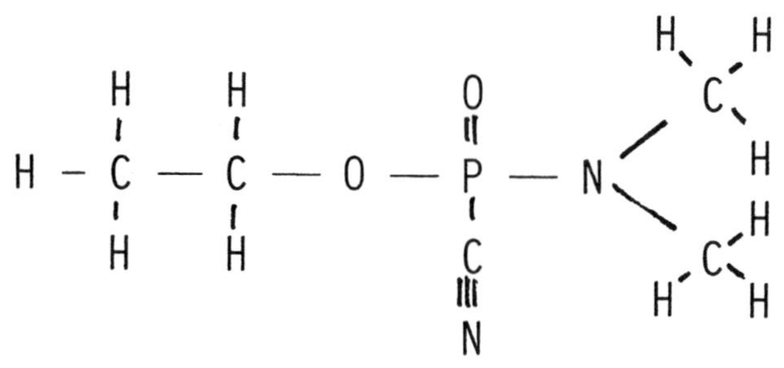

Tabun (GA)

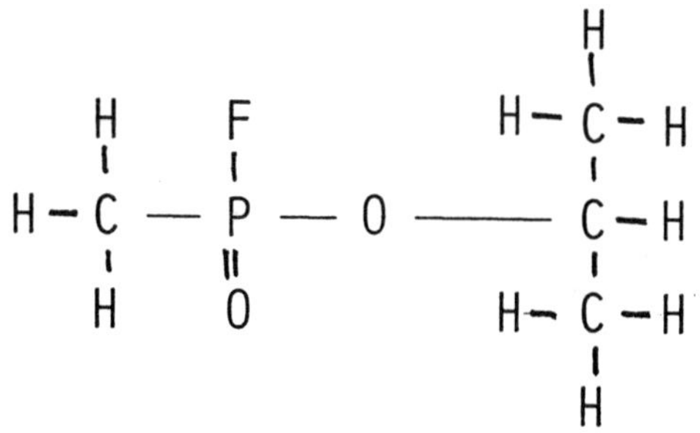

Sarin (GB)

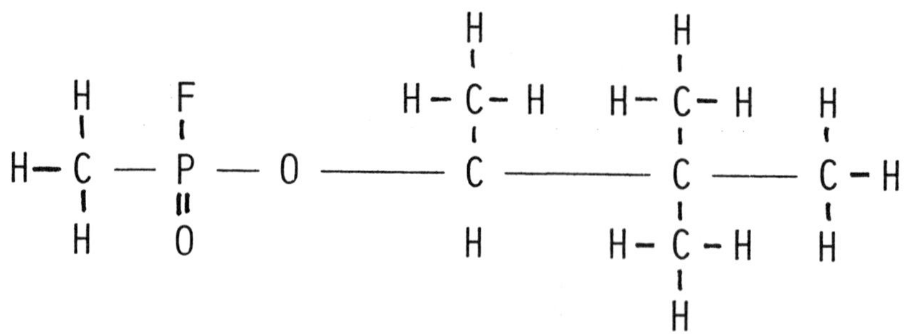

Soman (GD)

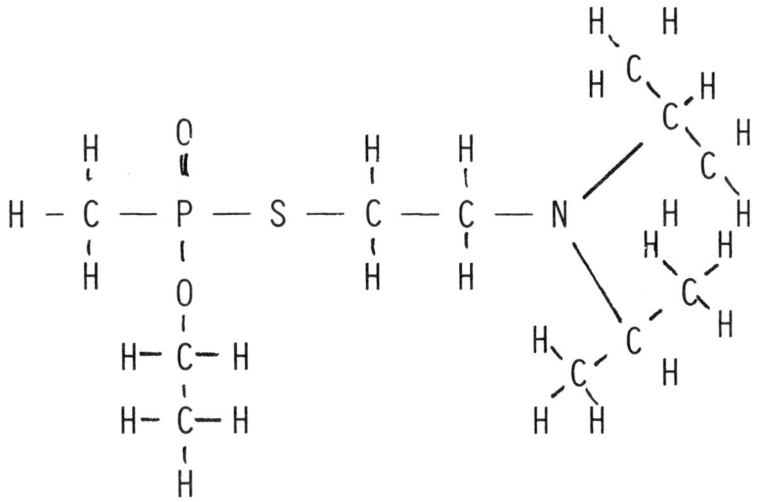

VX

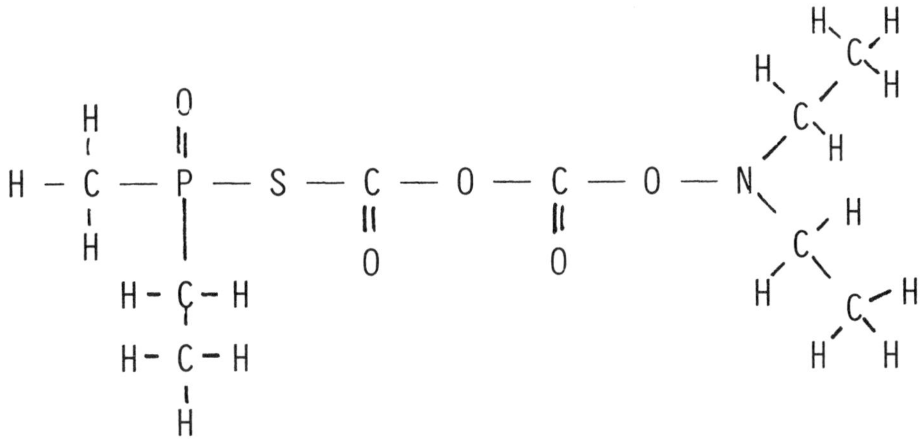

VE *obsolete*

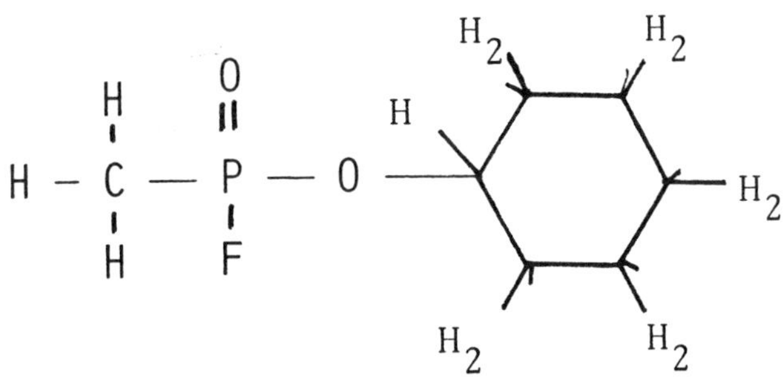

GF *obsolete*

RECOMMENDED READING

Agnew, L.R.C., et al, eds. *Dorland's illustrated medical dictionary 24th edition.* Philadelphia. W.B. Saunders Co. 1965.

American Medical Association, AMA Department of Drugs, with the American Society for Clinical Pharmacology and Therapeudics. *AMA drug evaluations, 3rd edition.* Littleton, MA. PSG Publishing Co. 1977.

Barnaby, Frank. *Future war: armed conflict in the next decade.* New York. Facts on File Publications. 1984.

Clarke, E.C.G., ed. *Isolation and identification of drugs.* London. Pharmaceutical Press. 1978.

Daintith, John, ed. *Dictionary of chemistry, derived from the Oxford University Press concise science dictionary.* New York. Warner Books. 1968.

Douglass, Joseph D. Jr. *Biochem warfare: new dimensions and implications,* in Defense and Foreign Affairs, p.41. April, 1987.

Douglass, Joseph D. Jr and Livingstone, Neil C. *America the vulnerable: the threat of chemical and biological warfare.* Lexington, MA. Lexington Books. 1987.

Gad, Shayne C. *Accute toxicology testing.* Caldwell, NJ. Telford Press. 1987.

Gad, Shayne C. *Behavioral and neurotoxicity testing,* chapter in *Handbook of product safety evaluation, Shayne C. Gad, ed.* New York. Marcel Dekker. 1987

Harris, Robert and Paxman, Jeremy. *A higher form of killing, the secret story of chemical and biological warfare.* New York. Hill and Wang. 1982.

Huff, Barbara, et al, eds. *Physician's Desk Reference, 41st edition.* Oradell, NJ. Medical Economics Co. 1987.

Jaycock, M.A. and Gad, Shayne C. *Hazard and risk assessment,* chapter in *Handbook of product safety evaluation, Shayne C. Gad, ed.* New York. Marcel Dekker. 1987.

Lingeman, Richard R. *Drugs from A to Z, a dictionary.* New York. McGraw-Hill. 1974.

McGeorge, Harvey J. II. *Chemical Warfare: seeking an east-west balance,* in Defense and Foreign Affairs, p.29. April, 1987.

Masterton, William, et al. *Chemical principles.* Philadelphia. Saunders College Publishing. 1981.

Meyer, Eugene. *Chemistry of hazardous materials.* Englewood Cliffs, NJ. Prentice-Hall. 1977.

Research and Education staff. *The organic chemistry problem solver.* New York. Research and Education Association. 1986.

Windholz, Martha, et al, eds. *The Merck index, an encyclopedia of chemicals and drugs, 10th edition.* Rahway, NJ. Merck & Co. 1983.

PERTAINING TO FUTURE DEVELOPMENTS

Gefter, Ye. L., Institute of Element-Organic Compounds, Academy of Sciences of the U.S.S.R. *Organophosphorus monomers and polymers.* Translated from the Russian by J. Burdon, PhD. Oxford. Pergamon Press (distributed by MacMillian Co, NY). 1962.

Gordon, James J., Inns, Robert H., et al. *Delayed neuropathic effects of nerve agents and some other organophosphorus compounds.* Archives of toxicology, vol 52 pp 71-82. 1983

Zervas, L. ed. *Peptides, proceedings of the sixth European symposium, Athens, 1963.* Oxford. Pergamon Press. 1966.

Chapter Five

RIOT CONTROL AGENTS

Vomiting Agents

official definition

The vomiting compounds are normally solids which, when heated, vaporize and condense to form aerosols. Under field conditions vomiting compounds cause great discomfort to victims; when released indoors they can cause serious injury or death.

FM 3-9

Vomiting agents (compounds) are arsenic-based riot control agents devised near the end of the first world war. None of them is authorized for use, by mutual agreement, by any of the NATO signatories for any use whatsoever. This is not to say that they do not have a potential use by someone else.

They share this basic bonding pattern:

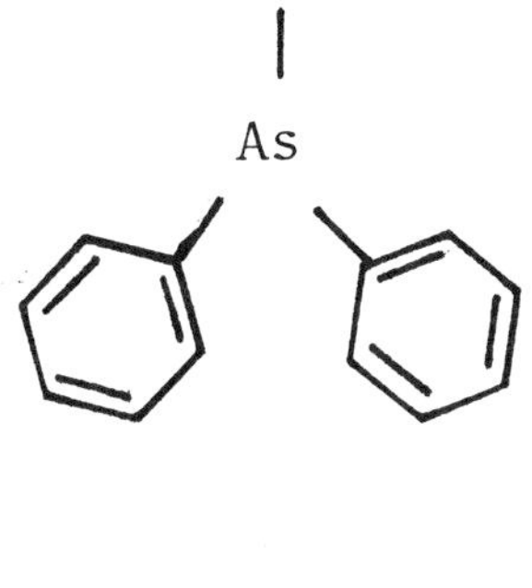

The following are those agents which have seen wide usage, in historical order of appearence:

- DA
- DC
- DM (adamsite)

Diphenylchlorarsine

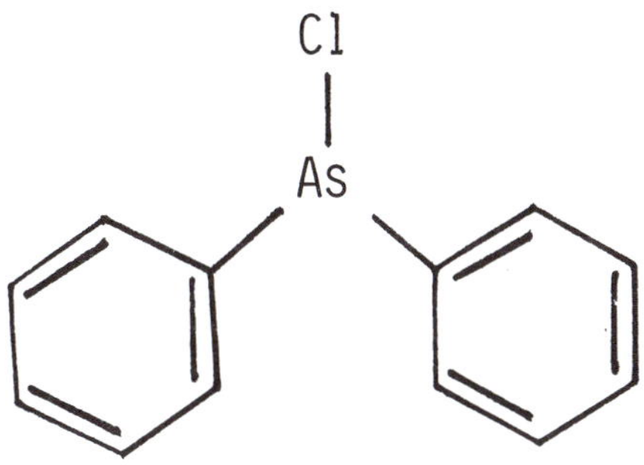

DA

Standard NATO agreement (STANAG) code: DA

Chemical name: diphenylchlorarsine
Common name: diphenylchlorarsine
Formula: $(C_6H_5)_2AsCl$

Family: riot control agent
Type: vomiting agent

In pure form, a colorless and odorless white powder. As dispersed as an aerosol, irritating to the eyes and respiratory system. Causes nausea and vomiting within two minutes. By mutual treaty, it is not to be used by any of the NATO members.

History

Diphenylchloroarsine was developed in 1918 by the British army for use in a smoke generator known as the M-Device. Lethality was not so much a consideration in its development as was this compound's extreme irritating effects and the fact that it readily penetrated the gas mask filters then in use.

The isolation and development of this particular compound came within the same program which developed the ethyl and methyl chloroarsine compounds belonging to the blister subtypes of the casualty agent class. It saw some limited use as a riot-control agent up to the 1930s. Its nausea-creating effects and toxic by-products led to a universal ban against its use against civilians, at least by the western nations.

Structure

Diphenylchloroarsine is prepared from trichloroarsine ($AsCl_3$):

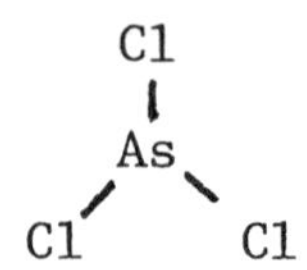

Two chlorine ions are replaced by benzene groups, forming a stable compound which may be safely stored under all field conditions:

Pathology

The immediate effects of diphenylchloroarsine are those associated with tear-gas compounds: severe irritation to the eyes, nose and throat. If this compound is inhaled for about one minute, severe headache and the feeling of tightness of the chest and of the bowels occurs. The headache rapidly develops into a general nausea which results, depending on the tolerance of the individual, in vomiting within three minutes.

In closed or confined spaces diphenylchloroarsine can produce fatalities through first causing unconsciousness and then asphyxiation.

The human body will effectively detoxify this compound within a time frame of exposure. The effects of mild exposure will normally last about 30 minutes after evacuation. Severe exposures may take several hours to detoxify and minor sensory disturbances may persist for up to one day.

Field behavior

In pure form, diphenylchloroarsine is a solid. To form a gaseous mass heat must be applied to it. Therefore it is used either as a filling in thermal-type grenades or used in conjunction with thermal smoke generators.

In open areas it forms no significant vapor mass and dispersion/dilution is effected by air movement, as effects are directly proportional to vapor concentration and not due to any specific toxicity of the compound itself. Will remain in closed or confined spaces for up to a day before aeration of the gaseous solution will cause it to break down into various arsenious oxides.

Specific data

median lethal dosage (LCt_{50})

15,000 mg-min/m^3 (estimated)

median incapacitating dosage (ICt_{50})

12 mg-min/m^3 (over ten minutes)

skin toxicity

Irritating. Non toxic in open areas or in short exposures.

eye toxicity

Irritating. Non toxic in open areas or in short exposures.

rate of action

Immediate irritation to eyes and respiratory tract. Nausea within 2 to 3 minutes of exposure.

protection required

Protective mask/respirator in open areas. In closed or confined spaces additional protective overclothing should be used.

rate of detoxification

The human body will detoxify DA inhaled in brief exposures within 1 to 2 hours. See text.

decontaminants

None needed in open areas. In closed or confined spaces, use bleaches or caustic soda.

vapor density

Forms no significant vapor mass.

vapor pressure

0.0036 mm Hg at 45°C (113°F).

solid density

1.387 g/cc at 45°C (113°F).

persistency

Short duration. Practical dissemination only by aerosol.

volatility

48 mg/m^3 at 45°C (113°F).

latent heat of vaporization

56.6 calories per gram.

melting point

41°C (105.8°F).

boiling point

333°C (631.4°F) with decomposition.

decomposition point

300°C (572°F).

flash point

350°C (662°F)

rate of hydrolysis

Slow in opened container. Rapid when disseminated (in gaseous form).

hydrolysis products

Principally hydrochloric acid and diphenylarsenious acid (both toxic).

stability in storage

Very stable when in pure form.

action on metals and other materials

None, when dry. See Hydrolysis products, above.

molecular weight

264.5

Diphenylcyanoarsine

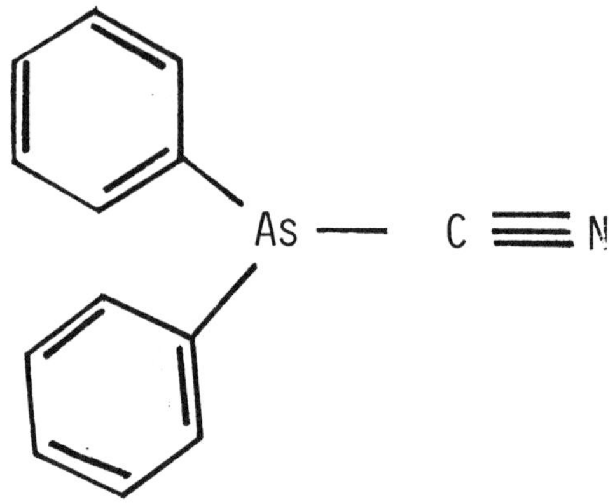

DC

Standard NATO agreement (STANAG) code: DC

Chemical name: diphenylcyanoarsine
Common name: diphenylcyanoarsine
Formula: $(C_6H_5)_2As\ CN$

Family: riot control agent
Type: vomiting agent

In pure form a white powder. Both as a powder and as a burning aerosol it has an odor often described as resembling that of garlic and bitter almonds. Causes nausea and vomiting in under one minute. By mutual agreement, it is not to be used by any of the NATO members.

History

Diphenylcyanoarsine was the last of the series of arsine based agents developed by the British army at the Porton Down laboratories. It reached its final development in 1920. It was intended that the vomit potential of diphenylchloroarsine and adamsite would be combined with the lethality of cyanide in a single compound. However, by 1920 filter elements had improved to the extent that the two earlier compounds no longer had their effectiveness in the field. Furthermore, the cyanide radical as attached to a central arsenic atom did not prove particularly lethal in tests. This marked the end of the development of diphenylarsine-based compounds for military applications.

Its nausea-causing effects and toxic by-products led to a universal ban against its use against civil populations by the 1930s, at least by the Western nations.

Structure

Diphenylcyanoarsine is a close relative of diphenylchloroarsine and is manufactured through the same process from *tri*chloro-arsine ($AsCl_3$). It is more difficult to manufacture than diphenylchloroarsine, but is less so than the manufacture of adamsite, and does not involve the explosive hazard of the latter.

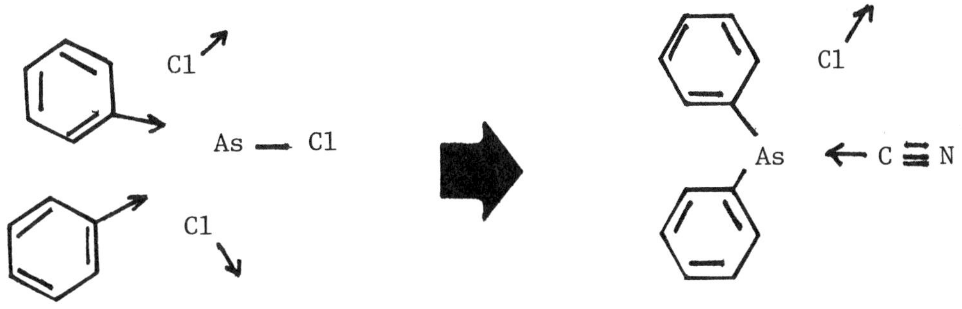

Pathology

The immediate effects of diphenylcyanoarsine are identical to those of diphenylchloroarsine and like those associated with tear-gas compounds: severe irritation to the eyes, nose and throat. Inhaled for 1 to 2 minutes in open areas, severe headache and tightness of the chest and of the bowels occurs. Depending on individual tolerences, vomiting may occur within three minutes.

In closed or confined spaces fatalities may occur through unconsciousness and exphyxiation.

The human body will detoxify the effects of moderate inhalation within an hour. Severe exposures require several hours to detoxify. Minor sensory disturbances may persist for up to one day.

Field behavior

In pure form, diphenylcyanoarsine is a solid. To form a gas, it must be heated. It would be used as a filling for thermal-type grenades or in a thermal smoke generators.

In open areas this compound forms no significant vapor mass. It will disperse/dilute in the wind. Its effects are proportional to vapor concentration rather than any toxic qualities of the compound itself. The vapors will remain in closed or confined spaces for up to a day before hydroylsis begins to break the vapor down into hydrochloric acid and various arsenic oxides.

Its cyanide radical gives diphenylcyanoarsine a very pronounced odor similar to a mixture of garlic and bitter almond extract, decreasing its surprize value. Some test solutions and machinery may register positive for the two main casualty-blood agents, hydrogen cyanide and cyanogen choloride, when exposed to this compound.

Specific data

median lethal dosage (LCt$_{50}$*)*

10,000 mg-min/m^3.

median incapacitating dosage (ICt$_{50}$*)*

(30 seconds) 30 mg-min/m^3 (5 minutes) 20 mg-min/m^3.

skin toxicity

Irritating. Relatively non-toxic in open areas or to short exposure.

eye toxicity

Irritating. Relatively non-toxic in open areas or to short exposure.

rate of action

Immediate irritation to the eyes and respiratory tract. In high concentrations it may cause incapacitation within 30 seconds.

protection required

Protective mask/respirator in open areas. In closed or confined spaces additional protective overclothing should be used.

rate of detoxification

The human body will detoxify DC inhaled in brief exposures within 1 hour.

decontaminants

None needed in open areas. In closed or confined spaces, use bleaches or caustic soda.

vapor density

Does not form an appreciable vapor mass

vapor pressure

0.0002 mm Hg at 20°C (68°F).

solid density

1.334 g/cc at 35°C (95°F).

persistency

Short duration. Practical dissemination only by aerosol.

volatility

2.8 mg/m^3 at 20°C (68°F).

latent heat of vaporization

71.1 calories per gram. DC must have a constant exposure to a heat source to maintain a concentration.

melting point

31.5°C (88.7°F).

boiling point

350°C (662°F) with decomposition.

decomposition point

Begins at 300°C (572°F).

low

Low.

rate of hydrolysis

Very slow in pure form. Moderate rate when in aerosol form.

hydrolysis products

Hydrogen cyanide and diphenylarsenious oxide, both of which present a toxic hazard.

stability in storage

Very stable in storage.

action on metals or other materials

No action when dry. Slightly corrosive to ferrous alloys when hydrolysed.

molecular weight

255.0

Adamsite

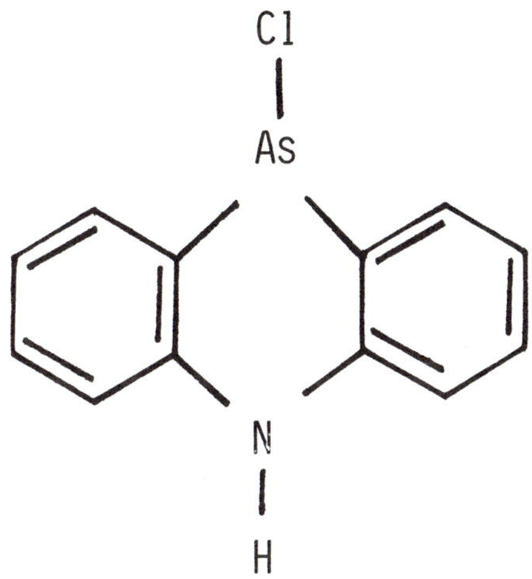

DM

Standard NATO agreement (STANAG) code: DM

Chemical name: diphenylaminochloroarsine, or phenarsazine chloride

Common name: adamsite

Formula: $C_6H_4(AsCl)(NH)C_6H_4$

Family: riot control agent

Type: vomiting agent

In pure form, a yellowish and odorless clear solid. Dispersed as an aerosol, irritating to the eyes and respiratory tract. By mutual agreement, not to be used by any of the NATO members

History

Adamsite was a development of the British army's Porton Down facility in 1919-1920. It was produced worldwide until superseded by the CN series of tear agents. Adamsite was not toxic enough to be an effective battlefield agent while it proved to be too drastic a compound for use against civilian mobs. It was developed as a chemical variation on diphenylchloroarsine (e.v). In its orogional forms it was designed to be disseminated from a thermal smoke generator.

Much of its longevity in production is owed to its effectiveness as a pesticide. As dissolved in benzene, carbon tetrachloride, or xylene it forms the basis of many solutions used to treat wood against marine borers and similar pests.

It was its nausea causing effects and toxic by-products (principally arsine-based compounds, depending on available reactants) which led to a universal ban against its use on civil populations in the 1930s in the Western nations.

Structure

Adamsite is a close relative of diphenylchloroarsine and is manufactured from trichloroarsine ($AsCl_3$). The process involves ammonia bonding, utilizing sharp temperature and pressure gradient increases.

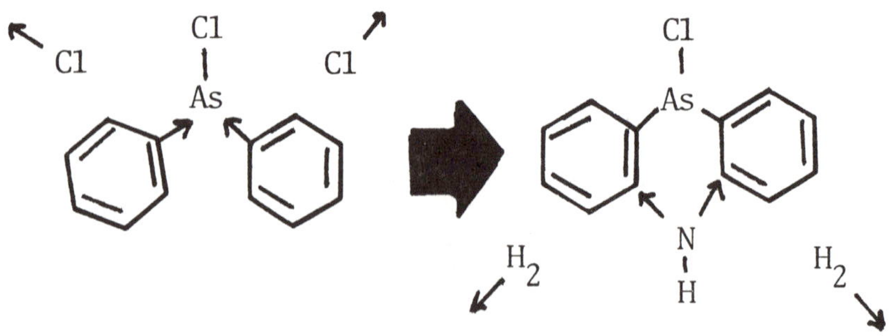

The resulting compound offers no advantage over diphenylchloroarsine as regards its use as war gas or riot control agent either in terms of effects or its stability in storage. The inclusion of nitrogen, however makes Adamsite more useful as an ingredient in pesticide solutions.

Pathology

The immediate effects of adamsite are identical to those of diphenylchloroarsine and like those associated with tear-gas compounds: severe irritation to the eyes, nose and throat. Inhaled for 1 to 2 minutes in open areas severe headache and tightness of the chest and of the bowels occurs. Depending on the tolerance of the individual, vomiting may occur within three minutes.

In closed or confined spaces an incapacitating dosage may occur rapidly. Fatalities may then occur through unconsciousness and asphyxiation.

The human body will detoxify the effects of mild exposures within 30 minutes of evacuation. Severe exposures may take several hours to detoxify and minor sensory disturbances may persist for up to one day.

Field behavior

In pure form, Adamsite is a solid. To form a gas it must be heated. Thus, it must be used as filling for thermal-type grenades or for use in thermal smoke generators.

In open areas adamsite forms no significant vapor masss. The greater the air movement (breezes, wind) the greater its dispersion/dilution. Its effects are proportional to vapor concentration rather than any toxic qualities of the compound itself. The vapors will remain in closed or confined spaces for up to a day before aeration will cause the vapors to break down into various arsenious oxides and acids.

Specific data

median lethal dosage (LCt_{50})

15,000 mg-min/m^3.

median incapacitating dosage (ICt_{50})

(one minute) 22 mg-min/m^3 (one hour) 8 mg-min/m^3.

skin toxicity

Irritating. Relatively non-toxic in open areas or short exposure.

eye toxicity

Irritating. Relatively non-toxic in open areas or short exposure

rate of action

Immediate irritation to the eyes and respiratory tract. In high concentrations it may cause incapacitation within 1 minute.

protection required

Protective mask/respirator in open areas. In closed or confined spaces additional protective overclothing should be used.

rate of detoxification

The human body will detoxify DM inhaled in brief exposures within 1 to 2 hours. See text.

decontaminants

None needed in open areas. In closed or confined spaces, use bleaches or caustic soda.

vapor density

Forms no significant vapor mass.

vapor pressure

Negligible [2×10^{-13} mm Hg at 20°C (68°F)].

solid density

1.65 g/cc at 20°C (68°F).

persistency

Short duration. Practical dissemination only by aerosol.

volatility

Negligible.

latent heat of vaporization

80 calories per gram at 200°C (392°F), with a heat of sublimation at 134 calories per gram.

melting point

195°C (383°F).

boiling point

410°C (770°F) (estimated), with decomposition.

decomposition point

Above 195°C (383°F).

flash point

None. Nonflammable.

rate of hydrolysis

Hydrolyses rapidly when an aerosol. No significant hydrolysis to the solid compound, which quickly forms an oxide coating.

hydrolysis products

Hydrochloric acid and diphenylarsenious acid (both toxic).

stability in storage

Very stable in pure form

action on metals and other materials

Slightly oxidizing when dry. When wet, corrosive to ferrous alloys, bronze, and brass.

molecular weight

277.57

Tear Agents

official definition

The tear compounds cause flow of tears and irritation of the skin. Since tear compounds produce only transient casualties, they are widely used for training, riot control, and for situations where long-term incapacitation is unacceptable. When used against poorly equipped guerrilla or revolutionary armies, they have proved extremely effective. When released indoors they can cause serious illness or death.

FM 3-9

Tear agents (or compounds) came into being at the end of the first world war first to supplement and then to replace the vomiting agents. The following are those agents which have seen large-scale employment, in historical order of appearence:

- CA (obsolete)
- CN (mainly civilian use after 1958)
- CNB (obsolete)
- CNC (semi-obsolete)
- CNS (obsolete)
- CS

α-Bromobenzylcyanide

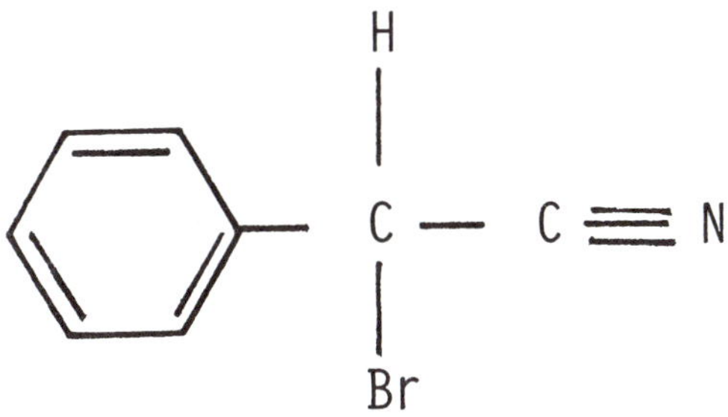

CA

Standard NATO agreement (STANAG) code: CA

Chemical name: α-bromobenzeneacetonitrile
Common name: camite; α-bromobenzenecyanide
Formula: $C_6H_5CHBrCN$

Family: riot control agent
Type: tear compound

In pure form a colorless crystalline solid, a strong eye and respiratory irritant smelling vaguely like rotten fruit. May be in solution in alcohol, chloroform, or acetone. Obsolete.

History

Dating from 1918-1919, CA (bromobenzylcyanide) was the first of the Porton Down supplements/replacements for the D series arsenical vomiting agents. Like the D series, CA was origionally a war agent that didn't prove lethal, or at least as origionally intended. CA did not prove entirely satisfactory in use. It leaves a high proportion of residue in any porous surface and can easily develop lethal concentrations inside buildings, caves, or similarly closed areas.

Outmoded in 1920 with the introduction of the CN series and is currently obsolete in NATO inventories. Too: persistent, toxic, corrosive to metals, and explosive with iron.

Structure

Bromobenzlcyanide is a hydrocarbon based around a ethyl group

$$- C - C -$$

having on its left axis a benzene group

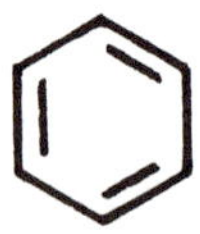

and on its right axis a nitrogen bond $\equiv N$ which forms a cyanide group $- C \equiv N$. The central carbon bond has what should be a hydrogen bond on its p_z orbital replaced with a bromium bond.

CA is commonly manufactured in a three step process: first, toluene is chlorinated to form benzyl chloride; second, by the action of sodium cyanide in an ethyl alcohol solution, benzyl chloride is converted to benzyl cyanide; third, benzyl cyanide is brominated with bromine vapor in the presence of sunlight.

CA is freely soluable in alcohol(s), ether, chloroform, acetone, and other organic solids. Also soluable in phosgene (CG), chloropicrin, and benzyl cyanide.

Pathology

At 30 mg-min/m^3 for physical incapacitation, CA was the most virilent tear-producing compound until the advent of CS in the mid 1950s. It produced a severe burning sensation to the mucous membranes and equally severe lacrimation to the eyes accompanied by headache and nausea. The nausea will quite easily lead to vomiting, although the vomiting is more of a psychological reaction than physiological as is the case with the earlier D series of vomiting agents.

Like the other tear agents, CA will go into solution with human sweat and as such will incur a burning sensation to the face, especially in the areas around the mouth, nose, and eyes. CA is particularly wont to penetrate clothing, making the areas around the neck, armpits, the tender skin areas behind the elbows, knees and around the buttocks and crotch suseceptible to rashes and minor blisters. Care must be taken to bathe after any prolonged exposure.

CA can be lethal to those in the vapors without protection (mask or respirator) who are in enclosed or confined areas for periods of time above a few minutes. Nausea can lead to unconsciousness which may mean suffication. Benzene/cyanide compounds can be toxic in high concentrations, if not from inhalation then by systemic poisoning, although CA lacks the volatility, and hence the ability to create the high vapor mass that the other tear agents (save for CS) typically exhibit.

Field behavior

CA is a solid white, crystalike powder which melts at between 18.5°C and 25.5°C(65.3°F-77.9°F) to create a mildly volatile (271 mg/m^3 at 30°C/86°F). CA was typically used in solution with ether or acetone as an aerosol or as part of a thermal-ignition grenade or gas-projection device.

Almost seven times the weight of air, the vapors may be expected to migrate to the lower points in either the terrain or man-made structures. CA readily penetrates any porus surface including cloth, plaster, dirt, and even some types of paint. Most persistent of all the tear agents. May persist in areas for several days, thus presenting a toxic hazard beyond that normally associated with any other riot-control agent.

Specific data

median lethal dosage (LCt_{50})

8,000 mg-min/m^3.

median incapacitating dosage (ICt_{50})

30 mg-min/m^3.

skin toxicity

Severe irritation from splashed liquid. Non toxic in open areas or short exposures.

eye toxicity

Severe irritation from splashed liquid, which may cause temporary loss of sight. Vapors are non toxic in open areas or temporary exposure.

rate of action

Immediate.

protection required

Protective mask/respirator in open areas. In closed or confined spaces protective overclothing must be worn.

rate of detoxification

Rapid. Irritation from high concentration of vapors may last several hours. Skin rash may last several days.

decontaminants

Little required in open areas. Steam and caustic soda may be required for indoor areas or any areas where human habitation is immanent. See Field Behavior, above.

vapor density

6.7 times as heavy as air.

vapor pressure

0.011 mm Hg at 20°C(68°F).

liquid density

1.47 g/cc at 25°C(77°F).

solid density

1.52 g/cc at 20°C(68°F).

persistency

Most persistent of the tear agents. Heavily splashed liquid will remain for up to two days in open areas. Permeates most porous surfaces.

volatility

17 mg/m^3 at 0°C(32°F); 115 mg/m^3 at 20°C(68°F); 271 mg/m^3 at 30°C(86°F). Fairly low.

latent heat of vaporization

55.7 calories per gram at 20°C(68°F); 79.5 calories per gram at boiling point of 242°C(467.6°F),

melting point

Pure: 25.5°C(77.9°F). With normal impurities: 18.5°C(65.3°F).

boiling point

242°C(467.6°F), with decomposition.

decomposition point

Chloroform solution: begins at 60°C(140°F). Pure CA: 242°C(467.6°F). Hydrobromic acid and dicyanostilbene will be formed.

flash point

None. CA does not burn.

rate of hydrolysis

Very slow.

hydrolysis products

"Complex condensation products," in all sources.

Stability in storage

Special canisters required (another reason for obsolescence). Moderately stable in glass, lead, or enamel-lined canisters. DO NOT STORE IN FERROUS ALLOYS!

action on metals and other materials

The liquid is highly corrosive to all common metals except lead. Reaction with pure iron: EXPLOSIVE!

molecular weight

196.0

Chloroacetophenone

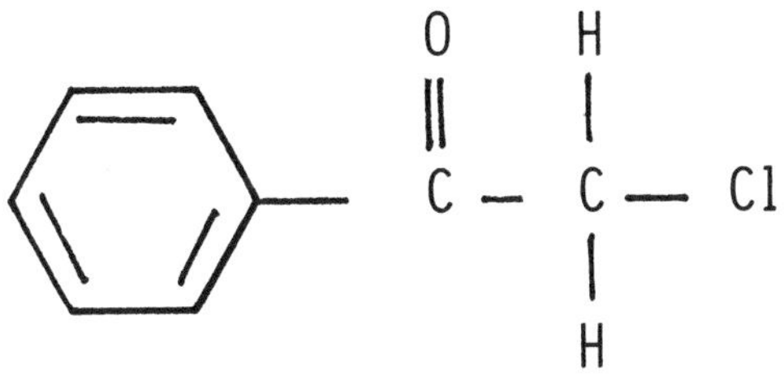

CN

Standard NATO agreement (STANAG) code: CN

Chemical name: 2-chloro-1-phenylethanone
Common name: chloroacetophenone
Formula: $C_6H_5C{:}OCH_2Cl$

Family: riot control agent
Type: tear compound

CN is a colorless crystalline solid with a fragrance similar to pungent apple blossoms. Principal ingredient of the CN series of riot control agents developed after the first world war. Obsolete in US military stores, although common in police agency mixtures.

History

CN was specifically developed to be a non-lethal riot control substance, the earlier compounds such as adamsite having shown themselves to have severe side effects. Riot control agents are designed to be used by police agencies (or military units in support of civil police agencies), or as military training agents. Creating casualties among their citizens does not serve the best interests of any government.

CN was developed at the British Porton Down facility shortly after the first world war. Manufacture in the United States began shortly thereafter. By the 1930s CN, and the CN variants had replaced the D series riot gasses in most countries. The CN series was not surplanted until the 1950s.

CN survives as the principle ingredient in the riot agent under the tradename MACE, derived from *Methylchloroform chloro ACEtophenone*.

Structure

Prepared by chlorination of acetophenone with selenium oxychloride. Commonly found as a solution in which the crystals are suspended in alcohol, ether, or benzene allowing easier dissemination in aerosol form.

In very simple terms a phenyl (benzene) group attached to a propanone (acetone) group, the left CH_3 group replaced by the C_6H_5 and the right CH_3 group chlorinated in a CHClH pattern. The reactivity of the chlorine bond accounts for much of the lacrimatory effect.

Pathology

CN has a pronounced lacrimatory effect, causing a natural reflex to shut the eyes. It is irritating to exposed skin, especially that of the face. Sweat seems to amplify the effect as CN will go into suspension in it and enter into the pores of the skin. Especially vulnerable are the tender skin areas where sweat accumulates, such as under the armpits, knees, elbows, and the area of the crotch and buttocks. High concentrations will cause rashes in these tender skin areas if sufficient exposure with lack of cleansing occurs. In extreme cases minor blistering may occur. Toxic eye and skin effects are highly unlikely to occur in concentrations possible in open or urban terrain, although some individuals may be slightly more susceptible to the efefcts of CN than others. Likewise, some sensitive individuals may experience nausea upon exposure.

CN may form lethal concentrations in closed or confined spaces.

Field behavior

CN must be mixed with alcohol or ether to be used as a liquid aerosol. To be used in normal form as a smoke, it must be heated in the presence of a secondary burning agent either mixed in with the powder or burned in close proximity, such as in a thermal grenade.

At a little over five times as heavy as air, CN vapors could be expected to seek lower levels of terrain or structures. Its volatility is principally a result of the agent used to heat it, so dissipation comes rapidly as the vapor clouds cool. CN presents a severe discomfort to personnel without protective masks. Thermal grenades may cause fires. Vapors may penetrate plaster and ruber-based paints.

Specific data

median lethal dosage (LCt_{50})

Solvent dispersal: 7,000 mg-min/m^3.

Thermal burning: 14,000 mg-min/m^3

median incapacitating dosage (ICt_{50})

80 mg-min/m^3 (both).

skin toxicity

Irritating but non toxic in open areas or in short exposures.

eye toxicity

Irritating but non toxic in open areas or in short exposures.

rate of action

Immediate.

protection required

Protective mask/respirator in open terrain or for short exposure in other areas. For prolonged exposures in closed or confined spaces protective overclothing should be used.

rate of detoxification

Rapid. Respiratory effects disappear within minutes. Skin irritation from high concentrations may last about two hours.

decontaminants

None required in open areas. In closed or confined spaces where powder or residue persist use alkaline solutions and steam.

volatility

0.0026 mm Hg at 0°C(32°F). 0.0041 mm Hg at 20°C(68°F). 0.152 mm Hg at 52°C(125.6°F).

vapor density

5.3 times as heavy as air.

latent heat of vaporization

98 calories per gram. Must have thermal source.

solid density

1.318 g/cc at 20°C(68°F).

liquid density

1.187 g/cc at 58°C(136.4°F).

persistency

Short. Practical dissemination is only by thermal source or aircraft aerosol.

melting point

54°C(129.2°F).

boiling point

248°C(478.4°F), with decomposition.

decomposition point

248°C(478.4°F).

flash point

Very high. Does not interfere with use

rate of hydrolysis

Slow. Not readily hydrolysed.

hydrolysis products

Hydrochloric acid and hydroacetophenone.

stability in storage

Stable in steel and plastic containers.

action on matals and other materials

Slight oxidation to ferrous alloys.

molecular weight

154.59

Chloroacetophenane, carbon tetrachloride, benzene mix

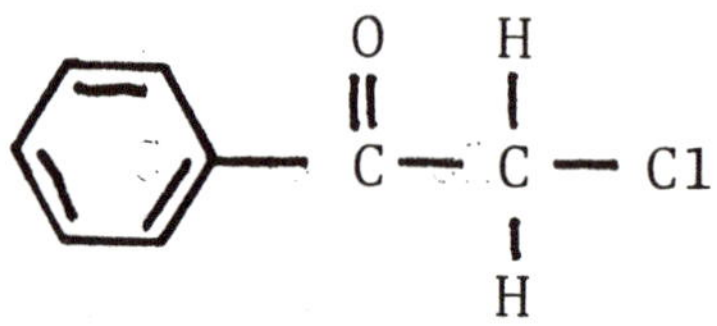

chloroacetophenane (CN)
10 parts

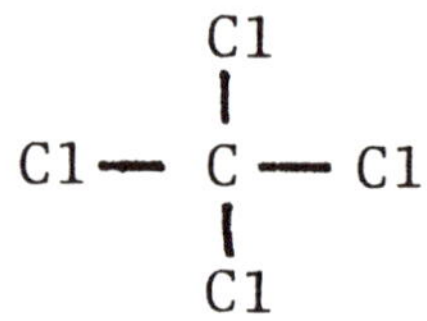

carbon tetrachloride
45 parts

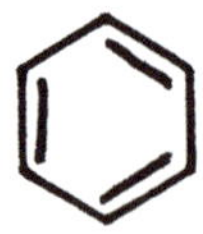

benzene
45 parts

CNB

Standard NATO agreement (STANAG) code: CNB

Chemical name: (none)

Common name: chloroacetophenane, carbon tetrachloride, benzene mix

Formula: $C_6H_5COCH_2Cl + CCl_4 + C_6H_6$

Family: riot control agent

Type: tear compound

A clear, slightly brown liquid smelling heavily of benzene and having an immediate strong irritating effect on the eyes and respiratory tract. Flammable! Obsolete.

History

CNB is a formualtion of CN (chloroacetophenone, qv), CN being the riot control agent formulated at the British Porton Down facility immediately following world war one as a replacement for the D series agents. Whereas those earlier compounds proved too virilent for use against civilized society CN began to recieve complaints from many colonial police agencies alleging lack of effectiveness.

Rather than attempt to develop an entirely new compound, Porton Down developed several formualtions of the origional compound. The main problem with CN was that it had to be in munitions relying on a burning agent to make a vapor of a powder. When the thermal agent refused to burn, due to faulty manufacture or climatic conditions, CN was useless. The obvious response was to make a liquid version of CN which could be dispersed as a spray. CNB was the first of several such formulations, of which agents designated CNB, CNC, and CNS saw actual production. CNB, invented in 1919 and adopted by the United Kingdom and the United States in 1920, is obsolete, being replaced first by CNC, which itself was replaced by CNS and CS, neither of which are flammable.

In the U.S. inventory CNB was used primarily as a training agent, that is something odius to the nose that trained troops in the use of their gas masks without doing bodily harm. A footnote to this is that CNB, being less potent than CNC was the preferred training agent when both were available. The institutional reply to this was to recommend that CNC be used in lesser concentrations, then to drop CNB from the inventory.

Structure

CNB is a suspension of 10 parts (by weight) of CN in a

solution of 45 parts carbon tetrachloride (CCl_4) and 45 parts benzene (C_6H_6). The solution offered two advantages over the origional CN. First, as a liquid solution or suspension, it could be applied directly by any spray apparatus. Secondly, there was no perceptible seperation of components during the formation of the vapor mass, which readily occured under moderate to warm air temperatures.

Pathology

Like CN, CNB has a profound lacrimatory effect, resulting in a natural reflex to shut the eyes. It is similarly irritating to the skin, notably that of the face and such exposed portions of the body where sweat accumulates. CNB will pebetrate clothing or adhere to it under long exposure due to its benzene component. The same rashes caused by CN will be caused by CNB, and due to the carbon tetrachloride and benzene components may be slightly more serious than those caused by CN. CNB has a slightly more powerful gagging or choking effect than CN. Eye toxicity remains about that of CN although, again, some individuals may be somewhat more susceptible to CNB's effects than others. Likewise, some sensitive individuals may experience nausea upon exposure.

CNB can form lethal concentrations in closed or confined spaces, although concentrations in open areas are highly unlikely ever to do so.

Field behavior

Approximately four times as heavy as air, CNB will seek lower terrain elevations and structural levels as it vaporizes. Its volatility dependent upon its components, notably that of carbon tetrachloride. This is responsible for CNB's airborn duration averaging under 15 minutes per concentration. Residual components may remain following dispersal of the vapor mass. CNB may penetrate into porous surfaces such as dirt, plaster, and some paints to leave a typical tear gas keytone-chlorine odor. Vapors may be flammable.

Specific data

median lethal dosage *(LCt_{50})*

11,000 mg-min/m^3.

median incapacitating dosage *(ICt_{50})*

80 mg-min/m^3.

skin toxicity

Irritating but not toxic in open areas or short exposure in other areas. See Pathology.

eye toxicity

Irritating but not toxic in open areas or short exposures in other areas.

rate of action

Immediate.

protection required

Protective mask/respirator in open areas. In closed or confined spaces protective overclothing should be worn.

rate of detoxification

Rapid. Skin irritation from higher concentrations may last several hours.

decontaminants

None required in open areas. In all others CNB components may be broken down by a heated concentration of 5% sodium hydroxide, 20% water, and 75% carbitol.

vapor density

4 times the weight of air

vapor pressure

That of the solvents (above 61mm Hg at 20°C(68°F) for CCl_4/C_6H_6 mix.

liquid density

1.14 g/cc at 20°C(68°F).

persistency

Short. Practical dissemination only be aerosol.

volatility

CNB is a mixture (suspension) so there is no true volatility. CCl_4 has the highest and CN has the lowest.

latent heat of vaporization

Not applicable. See above. Solvents interact.

freezing point

-7°C(19.4°F) to -30°C(-22°F): C_6H_6 and CCl_4, as they interact during cooling. CNB component settle out rather than freeze, per se.

boiling point

Begins 75°C (167°F) for CCl_4 and completes at 247°C (476.6°F) for CN. With decomposition.

decomposition point

Complete above 247°C(476.6°F).

flash point

Below 4.4°C(40°F). One of the main reasons CNB and CNC ceased to be used by police agencies.

rate of hydrolysis

Does not hydrolyse.

hydrolysis products

None. No hydrolyzation.

stability in storage

Fairly stable. Best stored under temperate climatic conditions (60°F to 80°F).

action on metals and other materials

Slightly oxidizing to ferrous alloys.

molecular weight

119.7 (on basis of components).

Chloroacetophenane, chloroform mix

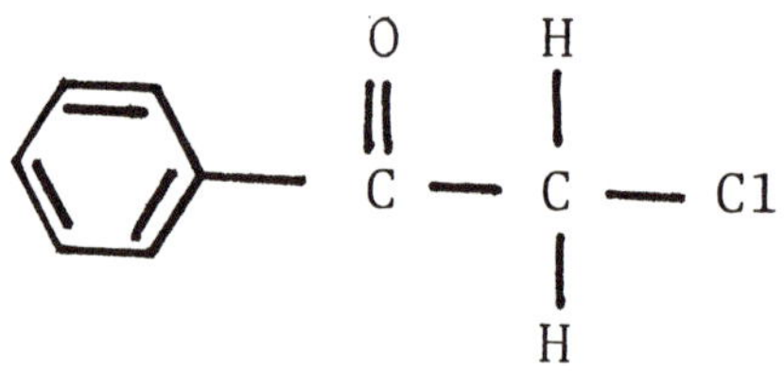

chloroacetophenane
70 parts

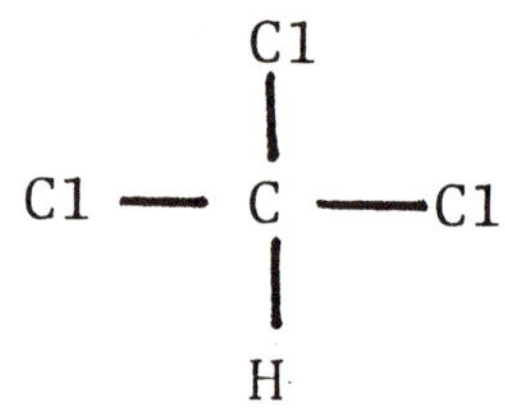

chloroform
30 parts

CNC

Standard NATO agreement (STANAG) code: CNC

Chemical name: (none)
Common name: chloroacetophenane chloroform mix
Formula: $C_6H_5COCH_2Cl + CHCl_4$

Family: riot control agent
Type: tear compound

A clear liquid smelling heavily of chloroform and having an immediate strong irritating effect on the eyes and respiratory tract.

History

The second solvent-based formulation of CN (chloroacetophenone) devised at the British Porton Down facility. Like CNB, it is a suspension of CN in an organic solvent. Pure CN being a crystal-like powder, it cannot be used unless:

- it is heated to form a vapor, using either a burning grenade or some sort of power-driven thermal generator, or,
- it is made into a liquid suspension which may be dispersed as an aersol either by ground or aerial spray.

CNB, although effective in its intended role as a tear gas made use of two seperate organic solvents (benzene and carbon tetrachloride) which were not entirely compatible, tending to seperate after they were released from confinement in the canister.

CNC uses only one solvent, chloroform, which accounts for 70% of its mass. CN accounts for the other 30%. Unlike CNB, CNC proved itself in all climates, giving good performances from the Yukon to India to the South Pacific with even aeration charactoristics.

CNC was not so much superceded by CNS as it was supplemented by it. Lacking the heavy benzene concentration of CNB, CNC is less likely to induce nausea and vomiting than the former. Likewise it does not contaminate its areas of use as does CNB. Of more importance from the user's standpoint, CNB is flammable and was known to explode when initial concentrations were exposed to spark or flame. CNC is *non* flammable, and in fact will extinguish fires. Thus, CNC still survives as a reliable, if old-fashioned, riot control agent and as a training agent for military and police agencies.

Structure

CNC is a mix, or suspension, of CN (chloroactophenone, $C_6H_5COCH_2Cl$) (30%) and chloroform ($CHCl_3$) (70%). CNC, like CNB, shows no perceivable seperation of components during vapor mass formation. Unlike CNB, CNC remains that way until the vapor mass precipitates.

Pathology

CNC has a pronounced lacrimatory effect. It stings the eyes and makes them water. It can be irritating to the more sensitive skin on the body, such as that of the face near the mouth, nose, eyes, and forehead, and the skin of the knee and elbow joints. Minor rashes are possible from high levels of exposure, although the chloroform has somewhat of a cleansing effect so blistering is not common. Chloroform (trichloromethane) can cause liver damage if ingested over a period of weeks, although protected personnel and others coming into temporary contact with CNC do not appear to suffer any pattern of chloroform toxicity.

Field behavior

With vapor density about four and a half times that of air, CNC can be expected to seek the lower levels of terrain and structures as it vaporizes. Effective concentrations last about fifteen minutes (without renewal) with seperation of components occuring on the ground rather than in the air, as might be the case with CNB. CNC is not known for penetrating porous surfaces although CN residual may be deposited in a thin film on such surfaces as it comes to rest upon.

Specific data

median lethal dosage (LCt_{50})

11,000 mg-min/m^3.

median incapacitating dosage (ICt_{50})

80 mg-min/m^3.

skin toxicity

Irritating. Nontoxic in open areas or in short exposures.

eye toxicity

Irritating. Nontoxic in open areas or in short exposures.

rate of action

Immediate.

protection required

Protective mask/respirator in open areas. In enclosed or confined spaces protective overclothing should be worn.

rate of detoxification

Rapid. Skin irritation from high concentrations may last several hours.

decontaminants

None required in open areas. For enclosed or confined spaces, use caustic soda or strong alkaline solutions with steam to remove liquid CNC or CN residue.

vapor density

4.4 times as heavy as air.

vapor pressure

61 mm Hg at 5°C(41°F); 127 mm Hg at 20°C(68°F).

liquid density

1.40 g/cc at 20°C(68°F).

persistency

Short. Practical dissemination only as an aerosol.

volatility

No true volatility, as in the case of a pure compound. Chloroform has a high vapor pressure whereas CN has a low vapor pressure.

latent heat of vaporization

Not applicable. Aerosol application only.

freezing point

0.23°C(32.41°F). Not a freezing point. Chloroform freezes at -63.5°C(-82.3°F) whereas CN begins to come out of solution at 0.23°C(32.41°F).

boiling point

Variable also. Chloroform boils at 60°C(140°F). CN boils at 247°C(476.6°F).

decomposition point

Stable to the boiling points of its components. Ie, begins at 60°C(140°F) and decomposition is complete at 247°C(476.6°F).

flash point

None.

rate of hydrolysis

Very slow. Not readily hydrolysed.

hydrolysis products

Hydrochloric acid and hydroacetophenone.

stability in storage

Fair. Effecting factor is the seperation point of CN from chloroform (0.23°C/32.41°F).

action on metals and other materials

Slightly oxidizing to ferrous alloys.

molecular weight

128.17. Based on proportional weight of components.

Chloroacetophenane, chloroform, chloropictrin mix

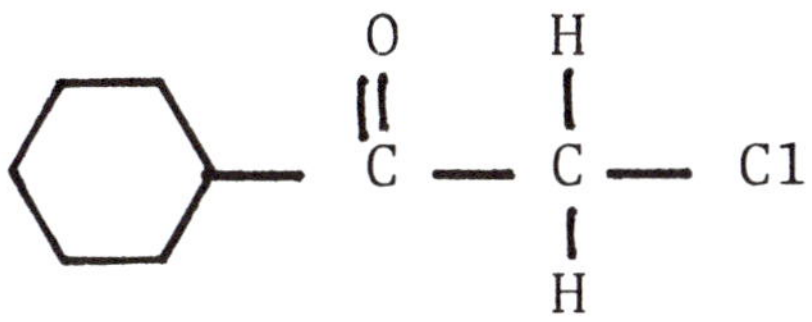

chloroacetophenane
23.0%

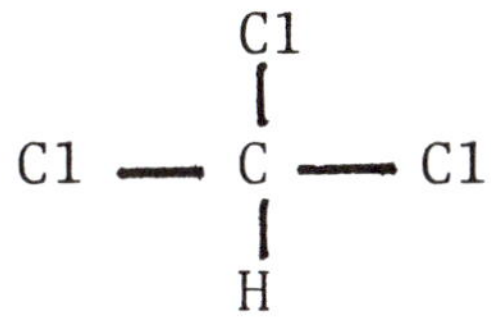

chloroform
38.5%

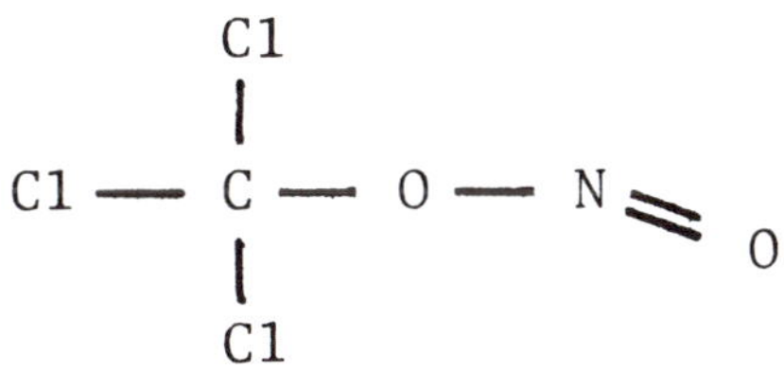

chloropicrin
38.5%

CNS

Standard NATO agreement (STANAG) code: CNS

Chemical name: (none)

Common name: chloroacetophenane, chloroform, chloropicrin mix

Formula: $C_6H_5COCH_2Cl + CHCl_3 + C(NO_2)Cl_3$

Family: riot control agent

Type: tear compound

A clear liquid smelling like flypaper and having an immediate strong irritating effect on the eyes and respiratory tract. May cause severe nausea. Obsolete.

History

The Porton Down CN series went through several variation formulations, out of several hundreds of trial compositions and proportional changes with CN, CNB, CNC, and then finally CNS being those to see major production, storage, and use. The story of the CN series was one to find an agent that was as effective as the older D series, in particular adamsite, without the lethality or contamination of that chloroarsine-based series.

It must be born in mind that the era from 1920 until the mid 1950s was the twilight of the British Empire. This was not only an era of political in-folding but one that saw both nationalistic mobs and communal strife in multi-ethnic areas formerly held together by a political structure that was no longer respected. The earlier CN series no longer seemed effective.

Adamsite's forte was its ability to make the lungs and throat sting (an effect similar to that of phosgene) as well as the eyes and nose. Adamsite also caused immediate nausea, causing vomiting and in many cases, diarrhea. It was found in the 1930s that a *S*pecial formulation of the CN series, using chloropicrin [$C(NO_2)Cl_3$] with the CNC combination of CN and Chloroform ($CHCl_3$), made an agent almost as effective as the old D series vomiting agents but without the chloro-arsenic permanent damage.

CNS, Like its parent formulation, CNC, was not as powerful a lacrimatory as CNB, but like CNC it couldn't ignite under some field conditions. As a general police and military tear agent, CNS replaced all the others in its series (save as a training agent) until it in turn was replaced by CS in the late 1950s.

Structure

CNS is a suspension, or mixture, of CN (chloroacetophenone, $C_6H_5C{:}OCH_2Cl$) in chloroform (trichloromethane, $CHCl_3$) and chloropicrin [$C(NO_2)Cl_2$]. Percentages by weight are:

CN 23%,
chloroform 38.5%,
chloropicrin 38.5%

Chloropicrin is the compound in CNS giving that mixture its pronounced nausea causing effects. Chloropicrin is a chemical relative of picric acid (2,4,6-trinitrophenol, $C_6H_2(NO_2)_3$ an explosive compound. Chloropicrin isn't explosive but its reactivity with hydrocarbons is based on the same $-C-(NO_2)-$ bonding structure.

Pathology

As mentioned above, CNS shares the same lacrimatory effect as CNC, pronounced but noticeably less than the later CS. As also mentioned, CNS was formulated not so much as a tear agent but as a non-arsenical vomiting agent, which function it serves well. It produces nausea within a minute of inhalation by a moderately sensitive person. If inhaled for longer periods, vomiting, colic (severe abdominal pains and cramps), and diarrhea are to be expected in its victims. Persons who are exposed to very large quantities of the vapors or liquid concentrations may suffer these symptoms for weeks, diarrhea being the last of the symptoms to persist.

In addition, CNS is a non-lethal choking agent. It will cause its victims to gasp for air (thus inhaling more CNS) while causing discomfort to the bronchial tubes and lung sacs.

Like CNC, CNS vapors may go into solution with sweat, making it a skin irritant. Especially susceptible is the skin of the face around the forehead, eyes, nose and mouth. CNS will sting shaven areas of skin (mixing with alcohol based after-shaves to heighten the discomfort). If allowed to penetrate the clothing, CNS will cause stinging of the tender skin under the armpits, elbows, knees, and the area around the crotch and buttocks. Skin rashes may result after prolonged exposures, especially in persons with sensitive, or acned skin.

Prolonged eye exposure would not be recommended.

Chloroform is known to cause damage to the liver and other organs, although coming into contact with CNS does not seem to develop any patterns of chloroform toxicity.

Field behavior

Although CNS vapors are about 5 times as heavy as air, CNS has an extremely high volatility (610,000 mg/m^3), thus forming a huge vapor mass above the aerosol. The agent would have an initial tendency to seek lower terrain or levels in structures but this would not be an important factor in areas of mostly open terrain or small structures. Sprayed inside buildings, vessels, or caves the vapors would rapidly infest all unsealed air pockets.

CNS will moderately penetrate such porous surfaces as loose plaster and soil, especially if volatility is a factor in increasing atmospheric pressure. CN and chloropicrin residues may be deposited as a film upon smooth surfaces.

Specific data

median lethal dosage (LCt_{50})

11,400 mg-min/m^3.

median incapacitating dosage *(ICt_{50})*

60 mg-min/m^3. Warning: symptoms include nausea and cholic, at below this level

skin toxicity

Irritating, but non toxic in open areas or short exposures.

eye toxicity

Irritating, but non toxic in open areas or short exposures.

rate of action

Immediate. Pronounced choking effect.

protection required

Protective mask/respirator in open areas. In closed or confined spaces overclothing should be worn.

rate of detoxification

Slow. Trace elements of chloropicrin tend to remain in the body for over a week in most exposures. This accounts for residual gastrointestinal poisoning.

decontaminants

None required in open areas. In closed or confined spaces, gross contamination is possible: use alkaline solutions or a soda ash/solium sulfate solution either heated or in conjunction with steam.

vapor density

Aprox 5.0 times as heavy as air.

vapor pressure

78 mm Hg at 20°C(68°F).

liquid density

1.47 g/cc at 20°C(68°F).

persistency

Short. Practical dissemination is only by aerosol. Vaporizes rapidly. Would remain a hazard within structures or vessels until aerated.

volatility

610,000 mg-min/m^3.

latent heat of vaporization

Aerosol at ambient temperatures. No latent heat.

freezing point

2°C(38.5°F). CNS works best in warm weather. CN seperates.

boiling point

Begins at 60°C(147°F) with chloroform and is complete with boiling of CN at 247°C(476.6°F).

decomposition point

Mixture is stable to the boiling points of its components (begins to decompose at 60°C(147°F).

flash point

CNS does not burn.

rate of hydrolysis

Very slow. Not readily hydrolysed.

hydrolysis products

Hydrochloric acid and hydroacetophenone.

stability in storage

Stable under normal storage procedures.

action on metals and other materials

Very slight oxidation to ferrous alloys.

molecular weight

141.78, based on components.

O-chlorobenzylidene-
malonitrile

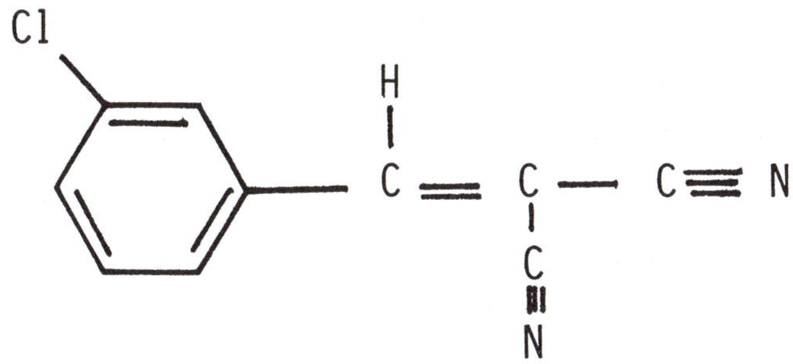

CS

Standard NATO agreement (STANAG) code: CS

Chemical name: O-chlorobenzlidene malontrile
Common name: CS (tear gas); pepper gas (Europe)
Formula: $ClC_6H_4CHC(CN)_2$

Family: riot control agent
Type: tear compound

Clear white solid. Burnt to create a colorless gas with an acrid pepperlike smell, immediately irritating to the eyes and upper respiratory tract. The most common of training and riot-control agents

History

The reasons for the development of CS are the same reasons for the development of CNS. There was an existing need for a riot-control substance that was both more effective than earlier agents, and would be easier to deliver. A third reason, to have an agent which could be used against insurgents or guerrillas, would have been sufficient for the creation of this agent.

The story goes that the British noticed during operations in Korea and later in Cyprus that rioters (and enemy troops without masks) could breathe through alcohol or bleach-soaked cloth, occasionally rinsing their eyes, and continue about their business. CNS, due to its liquidity and high volatility, was also not persistent enough. The Porton Down staff went back to the origional CA formulation and made a more potent version of it which they named CS (see Structure, below). In the Summer of 1958 British forces tested CS on Cyprus (where CNS had failed) and found it very suitable.

The formulation was given to the NATO members, who adopted it as their military standard by Fall of 1958. The U.S. Department of Defense began a crash program resulting in CS's two standard variations, CS1 and CS2. Older stocks of CN variants were completely replaced by CS in the early 1960s. CS became the standard riot control and training agent within the NATO structure.

Structure

CS is a variant of the riot-control agent CA, which dates from about 1920. Similarities can be seen in the comparison of their diagrams. Differences are in *italics*:

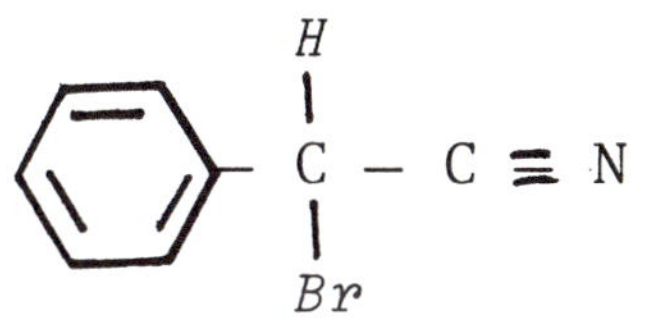

CA

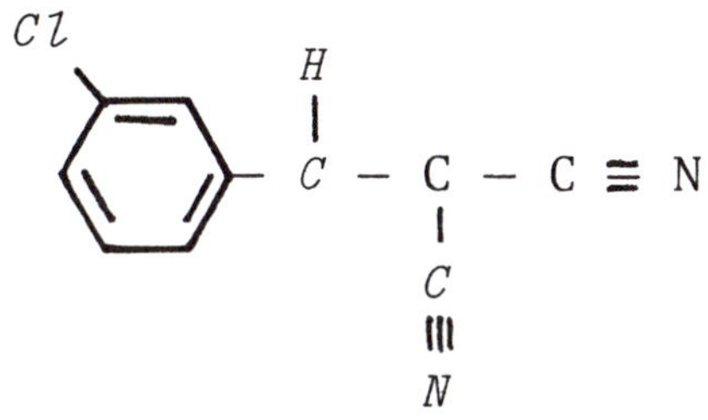

CS

Bond formation is similar to that of CA (qv), CS being formed around a propyl (3-carbon) group to CA's methyl (2-carbon), and having two cyanide (CN) groups, one of which replaces a bromine (Br) bond. Bromine, chemically less active than chlorine, is damaging to throat tissue. Cyanide blocks the uptake of oxygen by the blood through interaction with the iron in hemoglobin, but is not otherwise reactive with tissue. Hence the replacement of the Br bond with a second CN bond. The chlorine attached to the benzene group adds to the gagging effect. The propyl bond seems to add stability to the agent in the environment, and thus makes it more persistent than its predecessors.

Variations on the basic compound

Pure CS is as described above.The two other forms, like those of the CN variations, are mixtures of ingredients with the origional compound, and do not represent changes in CS's chemical structure. CS is not soluble in water or ethanol but is soluble in methylene chloride, CH_2Cl_2 (CHClHCl). CS is used as a filling for burning type grenades. Most commonly used as a training agent in the form of molded capsules containing a burning agent to be ignited in a metal or ceramic pan within a closed room, for the purpose of testing protective ("gas") mask fit. Thermal grenades usually produce large clouds of white smoke (vapor). Vaporization is due to ignitor, not so much to the flammability (above 197°C/386.6°F) of CS, which still represents an advancement over CNS (which CS replaced).

CS1 is a mixture of 95% CS with 5% silica aerogel (similar to common desicants, or moisture-absorbents. The whole is micropulverized to form an extremely fine powder whose particles average from between 3 to 10 microns across. CS1 is dispersed by force-blowing using a vehicle or aircraft mounted generator/blower, or from a hand-held tank in which the propellant is CO_2 or some other non-flammable and non-reactive gas. The micropulversized powder then forms an appreciable vapor mass not dependent on either a thermal agent or the otherwise low volatility [0.71 mg/m^3 at 25°C(77°F) — compare with CNS] of CS itself.

CS2 is a mixture almost identical to CS2. The difference is that CS2 uses a desicant trade-named *Cab-o-sil*. The latter prevents hydrolysis of CS2 in storage or in the despenser as well as preventing the CS2 mix from coagulating, forming hard lumps before usage. CS2 is dispersed the same way as CS1, using the same equipment. Forms the same large vapor mass with the same effects as CS2.

Pathology

CS is extremely irritating to the nose and throat while causing immediate lacrimatory effects. In heavy concentrations CS may create nausea which may result in vomiting. The CN double radical in CS will quickly lead to shortness of breath (thus causing a victim to inhale a lot of the vapor mass). Nausea and the illusion of suffocation typically cause a feeling of dizziness or a "swimming" sensation, so victims unused to tear gas commonly appear highly disorientated.

True CS vapors, caused by the action of a burning agent on the compound, have a pathology differing from the ingestion of unheated micropulverized powder (CS1 & CS2). Warm vapors mix in with human sweat to cause a burning sensation to the skin. Especially effected are the areas of the face around the eyes, nose, and mouth, and the tender areas about the elbows, knees, crotch and buttocks. Attention should be paid to the wrists and ankles as both the vapor and powder like to accumulate. The collar should be closed as CS also likes to filter down to the chest and back. The results are especially annoying to women. The full effects of CS vapors occur within 20 to 60 seconds of exposure. These will endure for up to ten minutes after escape from the vapor, with the possibility of skin rash persisting a day or so after heavy exposures.

CS1 and CS2 have an even more profound respiratory effect. Many sources recommend that dispersal units use a mix of CS1/2 and inert ingredients, at least if the powder is to be blown in the immediate vicinity of anybody. Persons within a few yards of a fixed spray nozzle will feel the full effects of the agent within one to two *seconds*. It is even conceivable that a person hit directly in the face ~~with~~ by a blast of powder could take in an immediate lethal dose (or suffer systemic shock to the same effect), even given the high immediate lethal dose rate of 61,000 mg-min/m^3.

Victims of CS1/2, may be covered with a fine dusting of the stuff. The immediate effects on the eyes are similar to that of CS vapor. Effects on the skin are not as pronounced, at least not until the powder has had a while to go into solution with body sweat and mucous. Great care must be taken to bathe after exposure to powder. All CS solids are persistent. Old training areas, where the agent has been in regular usage, are known to keep their pungency for years after use of the agent has ceased there. Thus, CS may represent a toxic hazard to persons remaining in CS1/2 contaminated areas.

Field behavior

Vapor density for CS is a function of its means of dispersal. Pure vapors are several times as heavy as air and would probably tend to flow down into lower terrain and into the lower levels of structures. In this regard, CS in grenades represents the greater hazard in mixed terrain and in built-up areas. Likewise, thermalized CS would be the most apt to penetrate porous surfaces.

Vapor density to CS1/2 is meaningless. Concentrations are dependent entirely on wind conditions and the presence of rain or snow, which would flush the agent from the air.

As a final general rule, CS would be the agent of choice for both training and tactical military use. CS1/2 would be the best formulation for use against large, unruly mobs in the open.

Specific data

median lethal dosage (LCt_{50})

61,000 mg-min/m^3.

median incapacitating dosage (ICt_{50})

10 to 20 mg-min/m^3.

skin toxicity

Irritating, but not toxic in open areas or short exposures.

eye toxicity

Extremely irritating, but not toxic in open areas or short exposures.

rate of action

Immediate. Vapor: full effects within one minute. Dust: full respiratory/eye effects within seconds.

protection required

Protective mask/respirator for field exposures. In closed or confined spaces, protective overclothing should be used. Personnel in direct contact with agent should wear rubber gloves .

rate of detoxification

Rapid. Incapacitating dosages lose their effects within ten minutes. Accumulates in the landscape, not the body.

decontaminants

None required for vapors in open areas. Persons exposed to powder should bathe using a strong soap. In closed or confined spaces use strong alkaline solutions or caustic soda (sodium hypochlorate) with live steam.

vapor density

See Field Behavior.

vapor pressure

See Field Behavior.

solid density

CS: 1.04/cc for crystalline solid.
CS1/2: 0.24 to 0.26 g/cc for bulk mix (US military policy is to use CS1/2 mixed with inert ingredients, and never in full CS strength).

persistency

Varies with concentration and degree of contamination. Chemically, CS is the most persistent of the tear agents, especially in open areas. It will absorb into most porous surfaces, including soil, plaster, and many organic solids.

volatility

0.71 mg/m^3 at 25°C(77°F). Relies on either a burning agent or pressurization for dissemination.

latent heat of vaporization

53.6 calories per gram.

melting point

93°C(199.4°F).

boiling point

310°C(590°F), with decomposition.

decomposition point

310°C(590°F).

flash point

197°C(386.6°F).

rate of hydrolysis

Very slow. CS2 has no practical hydrolyzation.

hydrolysis products

o-chlorobenzaldehyde and malonitrile.

stability in storage

Stable.

action on metals and other materials

Very slightly corrosive to ferous alloys.

molecular weight

188.5

Riot control agents: new substances

The agents listed in this section work on the basis of producing noxious fumes having irritating, caustic sensations on the respiratory system. They provide their victims with motivation towards either flight or fight. Short of asphyxiation they do little else.

The technology of heated gasses could be used to create a new series of agents based on current analgesics or analogues of those compounds. Such substances, especially those patterned on morphine or the peptides, work as well through inhalation as they do through injection. [see Chapter 3]

Until recently this notion has been strictly science fiction. Such agents could be manufactured but would have neither suitable vapor mass nor would they be guaranteed non lethal. Furthermore, in open societies there would be a public clamor against such things.

But then, not all societies are open. Nor are all governments of highly structured governments all that fastidiously concerned with nonlethality.

Riot control agents: new technologies

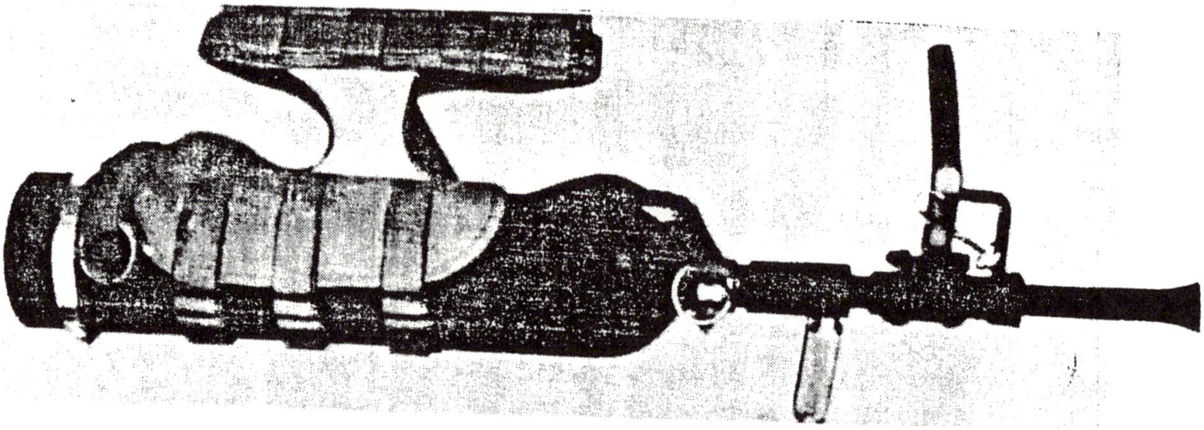

Israeli Military Industries
Model 5 Projectojet

Designed as a man-portable tear-gas disperser to either supplement or replace vehicle-mounted units. A simple but highly effective device consisting of a refillable five liter cannister designed to hold CS2 powder in a CO_2 suspension. Cannister connects through a regulator valve to a nozzle assembly with a throttle trigger. Designed to be suspended under one shoulder by means of a carrying strap. Aimed by use of a grip with one hand as the throttle is operated by the other hand.

Effective range is between twenty and thirty yards, projecting a densly concentrated cloud of CS2.

Can be used to project any type of agent that has been made into a micropulverized powder, with little or no modification. The chemical equivalent of a flame thrower.

SOURCE: Douglass, Joseph D Jr and Livingstone, Neil C. *America the vulnerable, the threat of chemical/biological warfare*. Lexington, MA. Lexington Books. 1987.

Comparative Tables

riot control agents: vomiting   comparative data

agent	*rate of action*	*state at 68°F*	*odor*	*volatility* *(mg/m³)*	LCT_{50} *(mg-min/m³)*	ICT_{50} *(mg-min/m³)*	*vapor density (x air)*	*vapor pressure (mm Hg)*
DA	very rapid	white to brown crystalline solid	none	48 at 113°F	15,000	12	very little of own	0.0036 at 113°F
DC	very rapid	white to brown crystalline solid	none	insignificant	15,000	8-22	very little of own	insignificant
DM	very rapid	white to brown crystalline solid	bitter almond-garlic mixture	2.8 at 68°F	10,000	20-30	very little of own	0.0002 at 68°F

vomiting agents comparative structures

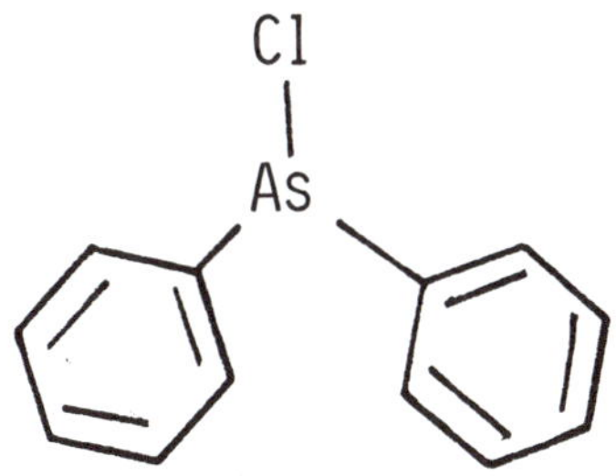

diphenylchloroarsine
(DA)

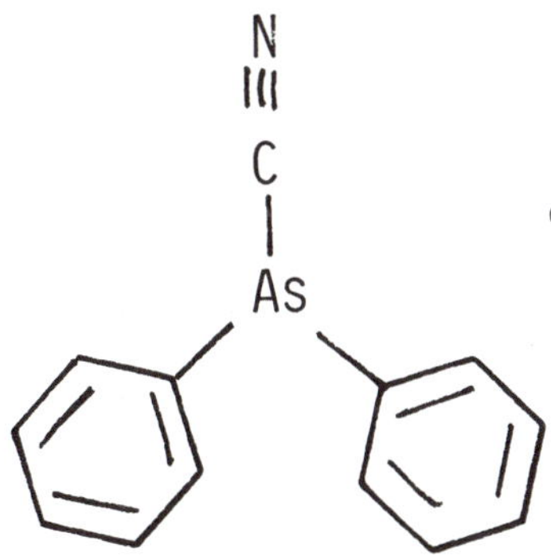

diphenylcyanoarsine
(DC)

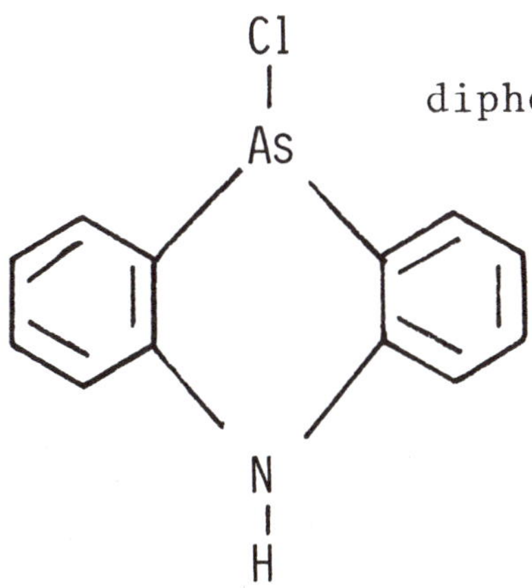

diphenylaminochloroarsine
(DM)

riot control agents: tear agents   comparative data

agent	*rate of action*	*state at 68°F*	*odor*	*volatility* (mg/m^3)	LCt_{50} $(mg\text{-}min/m^3)$	ICt_{50} $(mg\text{-}min/m^3)$	*vapor density (x air)*	*vapor pressure (mm Hg)*
CA	instantaneous	usually in liquid solution	rotten fruit	115 at 68°F	8000	30	6.7	0.011 at 68°F
CN	instantaneous	solid	apple blossoms	343 at 68°F	14,000	80	5.3	0.0041 at 68°F
CNB	instantaneous	liquid	benzene	varies	11,000	80	aprox 4.0	variable. mostly solvent
CNC	instantaneous	liquid	chloroform	varies	11,000	80	4.4	127 at 68°F
CNS	instantaneous	liquid	flypaper	610,000 at 68°F (due to solvent)	11,400	60	aprox 5.0	78 at 68°F
CS	instantaneous	colorless solid	pepperish	0.71 at 77°F	61,000	10-20	varies with burn agent	varies with burn

tear agents — comparative structures

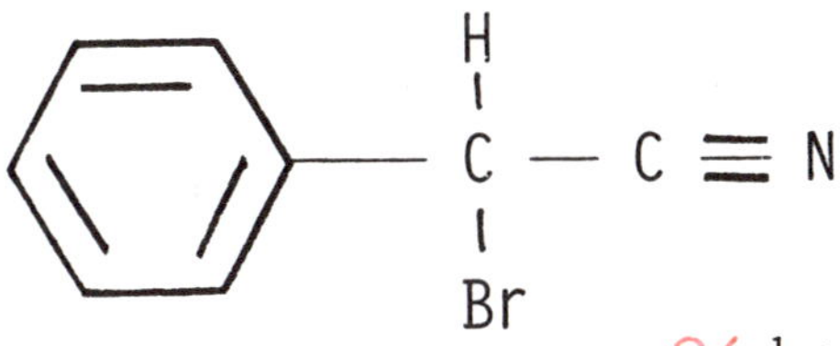

bromobenzylcyanide
(CA)

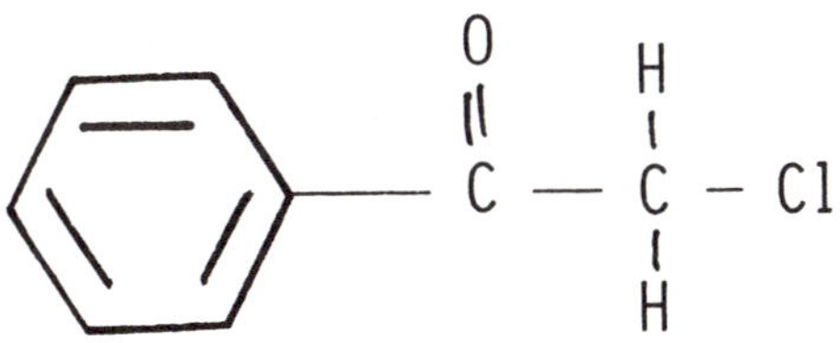

chloroacetophenone
(CN)

forms the basis of CNB, CNC, and CNS

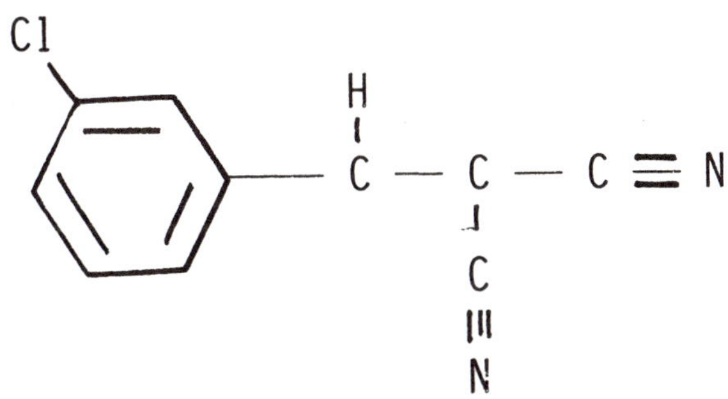

0-chlorobenzylidene-
malonitrile
(CS)

RECOMMENDED READING

Agnew, L.R.C., et al. *Dorland's illustrated medical dictionary. 24th edition.* Phildelphia. W.B. Saunders Co. 1965

Clayton, George D. and Clayton, Florence E, eds. *Patty's industrial hygiene and toxicology. Third revised edition.* New York. John Wiley & Sons. 1978

Daintith, John, ed. *Dictionary of chemistry, derived from the Oxford University Press concise science dictionary.* New York. Warner Books. 1986.

Douglass, Joseph D Jr. *Biochem warfare: new dimensions and implications, in* Defense and Foreign Affairs, p.41. April, 1987.

Douglas, Joseph D Jr and Livingstone, Neil C. *America the vulnerable: the threat of chemical/biological warfare.* Lexington, MA. Lexington Books. 1987.

Gad, Shayne C. *Evaluating irritation and corrosion hazards, chapter in Handbook of product safety evaluation (Shayne C Gad, ed).* New York. Marcel Dekker. 1987

Harris, Robert and Paxman, Jeremy. *A higher form of killing: the secret story of chemical and biological warfare.* New York. Hill and Wang. 1982.

Hayes, A W, ed. *Principles and methods in toxicology.* New York. Raven Press. 1987.

Jaycock, M A and Gad, Shayne C. *Hazard and risk assessment, chapter in Handbook of product safety evaluation (shayne C Gad, ed).* New York. Marcel Dekker. 1987.

Masterson, William and Slowinski, Emil. *Chemical principles.* Philadelphia. Saunders College Publishing. 1981.

Meyer, Eugene. *Chemistry of hazardous materials.* Englewood Cliffs, NJ. Prentice-Hall. 1977.

Research and Education Association staff. *The organic chemistry problem solver.* New York. Research and Education Association. 1986.

Windholz, Martha, et al, eds. *The Merck index: an encyclopedia of chemicals and drugs, ninth edition.* Rahway, NJ. Merck & Co. 1976.

Chapter Six

I N C A P A C I T A T I N G

A G E N T S

Pharmaceutical substances
of potential
military significance

Official definition

An incapacitating agent is an agent producing physiological or mental effects that may persist for hours or days after exposure to the agent has ceased.

FM 3-9

The motivation for such agents came from the desire to create some substance that would make an enemy cease fighting without death or injury. This is an old idea, popularized in science fiction. However, the world is no closer to producing H.G.Well's Sleep Gas or Aldus Huxley's Soma than it was when they wrote. To achieve the desired effect, such an agent must:

- Produce effects that would endure a significant period of time, measurable in hours or days.

- The substances must not endanger life, either in application or residual effect. Nor could any permanent injury result, toxicologic or physical.

- Recovery would not require medical treatment nor aid from any other individual.

- Such agents must be highly potent, easy to store, and deliverable as a practical munition.

These agents would *not* include:

- Sublethal doages of otherwise lethal substances.

- Any substance which would cause long-lasting or permanent injury, or any immediate damage to the human organism.

- Any pharmaceuticals requiring large dosages for effective individual results.

No chemical substance has been created or isolated which meets the above criteria. Studies have been made into the following substances, all of which are psychoactive. None, except agent BZ, has ever been seriously considered for deployment (at least in the west) and even BZ has been removed from stocks as being both unpredictable and potentially lethal.

If anything in the way of psychoactive military agents ever does surface in the world, it would probably be based on the following agents.

This chapter does not purport to be a complete listing of existing or potential incapacitating, but rather as an attempt to acquaint the reader with potentialities. The three main amphetamines are covered only because of their common currency in medical and criminal affairs. which impend upon military matters.

None of the chemical substances listed in this chapter are military agents of any of the NATO nations, nor is any contemplated for use.

Pharmaceuticals have not until recently been considered under the heading of military chemical agents. Whereas there are any number of test solutions for nerve agents, detection of, say, opiates would be left to an overburdened medical service rather than chemical field labs. For this reason this chapter has abstracted *en bloc* individual DETECTION sections from Clarke's *Isolation and identification of drugs* so that some lives might be saved following some future incident. The encyclopedic work edited by E.C.C. Clarke should be considered *the* standard work in this field and a copy belongs in the library of every serious student of chemical affairs.

Central Nervous System Stimulants

official definition

Agents which cause excessive nervous activity, often by boosting or facilitating transmission of impulses that might otherwise be insufficient to cross certain synapses. The effect is to flood the brain with too much information, making concentration difficult and causing indecisiveness and inability to act in a sustained, purposeful manner.

FM 3-9

For purposes of discussion, the catagory is limited herein to cocaine and the amphetamines. These would show the most promise with new technologies and methodologies.

The four substances under discussion origionated under military circumstances. Cocaine was first refined from coca leaves in 1844 but remained a curiosity until a physician issued it experimentally to Bavarian troops in 1883. It was only at that point that the rest of the world took notice, indeed making cocaine a late 19th century fad. Similarly, amphetamine was synthesized (by accident) in 1887 and languished until 1927 when tried as an anti-asthmatic, which by 1935 showed practical use against narcolepsy. The next year the German army began its experimental use much as it had tried cocaine 53 years earlier. By the second world war all sides issued amphetamines as "pep pills," thus introducing these drugs to large populations.

The ability of these substances to disrupt behavior did not go unnoticed.

Until recently, use against opposing forces was viewed strictly in the light of cloak-and-dagger escapades and as a medical and safety hazard when otherwise friendly troops used them "recreationally" or as a pick-me-up.

The amphetamines are related to a natural neurotransmitter *noradrenaline (norepinephrine)*, 4-(2-amino-1-hydroethyl)-1,2-benzediol, $(OH)_2C_6H_5OHCHCH_2NH_2$.

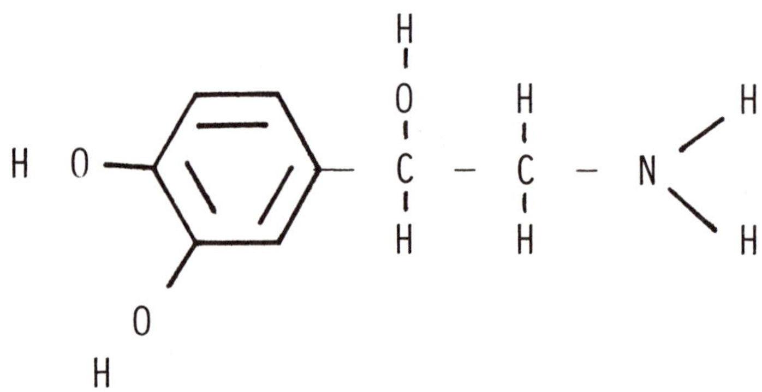

Central nervous system stimulants covered are:

- cocaine
- amphetamine
- dextramphetamine
- methylamphetamine

Noradrenaline stimulates the release of adrenaline (epinephrine), a powerful body vascopressor that increases muscle activity, including the cardiovascular system, and sensitize certain neural synapses. The action of the amphtamines is twofold. First, they mimic the action of noradrenaline. Secondly, they interfere with other enzymes which normally break down noradrenaline or aid its reabsorption. Whereas noradrenaline breaks down and is reabsorbed within minutes, the amphetamines, as a foreign substance, will remain within the body in reactively significant quantities for up to several hours and will not be fully excreted for up to about a week.

Death from cocaine overdose is more common than that resulting from the amphetamines, but in either case appears to be a rarity. Persons suffering from cardiovascular diseases would be those at greatest risk. Persons with low tolerances might be killed by sudden massive dosages, made possible by new biotechnologies but formerly unlikely.

Chronic and excessive dosages of any of these substances may cause permanent changes to both the nervous and endocrine systems.

methyl benzolyecgonine

(cocaine)

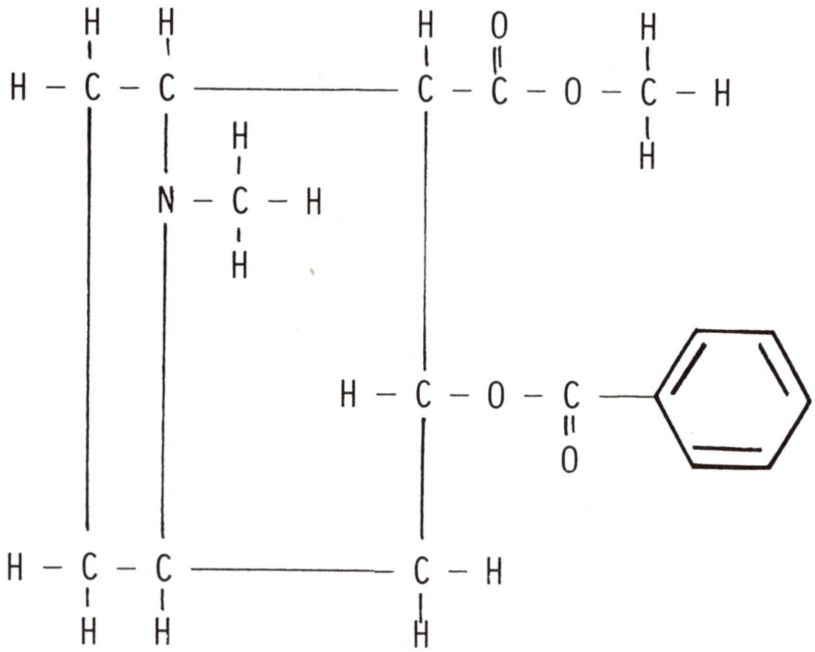

Chemical names: 3-(benzoyloxy)-8-methyl-8-azabicyclo-[3.2.1]octane-2-carboxylic acid methyl ether; 3α-hydroxy-1α-H,5αH-tropane-2α-carboxylic acid methyl ether benzoate.

Type: central nervous system stimulant.

Use: CNS stimulant; topical anesthetic.

Military hazards

Refined cocaine in its pure form of a crystalline white solid or powder offers little real hazard to large bodies of personnel or their equipment. It is not of itself absorbed through the skin (unless aided by $DSMO_2$ or a similar biosolvent). It must be absorbed through ingestion, inhalation, or injection. Excessively large quantities of cocaine would be required to contaminate foodstuffs and the like, although excluding sealed or canned rations.

Likewise, its use against individuals, even in covert application, would require sizable quantities and a disproportionate amount of time.

Cocaine itself is cheap to produce, given a source of coca leaves. To synthesize this drug in areas where no sources of natural materials exist would not be economic. The same production facilities could produce amphetamines even more cheaply and amphetamines are more potent. However, most areas in nothwestern South America might be able to make this into a serious anti-personnel weapon, if even clandestinely. Microencapsulation (reactive enzyme coating of submicron sized particles to create an ultra-fine dust with a liquid suspension at the heart of every mote) of cocaine or cocaine with other reactants would result in an insidious inhalant with lethal potential.

Metabolism and pathology

As mentioned above, cocaine in pure form is administerd orally, by injection, or through inhalation. Injection may involve either alcohol or ethanol solutions, the latter being the most efficient. Cocaine, and its common compounds (cocaine hydrochloride, cocaine nitrate, and cocaine sulfate) are legitimately used as topical or local anesthetics rather than as CNS stimulants in general application. Nerve endings are anesthesized by cocaine and blood vessels are constricted. As the drug detoxifies, effected muscles, blood vessels, and membranes relax. Following detoxification and relaxation of blood vessels membrane bleeding is not uncommon, especially in areas where the drug had come in direct tissue contact.

Cocaine readily crosses the blood-brain barrier, first effecting the cortex. The victim's sense of awareness is increased, and sensations of muscle fatigue are blocked.

Concurrently, the release of adrenaline is facilitated due to cocaine's mimicking of noradrenaline. At this point cocaine's metabolic effects are like those of the amphetamines. There is an increase in muscle activity as the victim undergoes a sort of adrenaline "high."

Military usage would emphasize toxicity associated with overdosage. Desired results would be those which precluded normal activities, behavior, and motor skills. Cocaine overdose can produce auditory and visual hallucinations often accompanied by paranoid delusions. There would be a tendency to excitement and agitation, hypertension and hyperventilation. Constant dialation of the pupils (degrading daytime vision), chills, fever, headache, tremors, exaggeration of the reflexes and failure of muscle coordination should be normal. Persons with weak cardiovascular systems would be more prone towards pulmonary collapse from cocaine than they would be from amphetamines.

Withdrawal symptoms include mental depression, gastrointestinal disturbances and general weakness. Chronic fatigue (with tremors) would eventually give way to extreme drowsiness and and prolonged sleep. If massively inhaled as a dust, cocaine might cause minor capillary bleeding in the lungs.

Cocaine is excreted slowly through the kidneys. Up to

12% of an injected dose is excreted within 24 hours with most rapid elimination within the first 5 to 6 hours. Both unmetabolized cocaine and by-products may remain in the body for extended periods of time and will eventually have adverse effects on the endocrine system.

Cocaine has been known to cause neuropoisoning involving adverse cholinesterase reactions not unlike the phenomenona associated with the casualty nerve agents. Dosages as low as 20 mg have caused death in some victims. Dosages would not exceed 1 gram without severely adverse effects. 2 grams would probably be fatal in any case.

In regards this last cocaine phenomenon, certain South American rodents native to the same areas as the coca plant have long been known to be immune to the neuroactive components of coca. In the 1980s the isolation of a substance these rodents evolved within themselves, cocainesterase, resulted in its chemical resynthesis. This new substance, cheap and easy to manufacture, is currently known as *pseudococainesterase*. It appears to work well in treatment of drug addiction. Furthermore, as part of a bioengineered mixture of enzymes and microspores, entire coca growing areas could be aerial-sprayed to produce future plants incapable of producing cocaine.

Extraction

From the leaves of *Erythroxylan coca* or through synthesis. Main alkaloid compounds include cocaine, cocaicine, cocaamine (isatropylcocaine), truxillococaine. Grown in Bolivia, Peru, and Columbia. Transplanted from that area to Java. Javanese has higher (1.2-2.5% vs 0.5-1.0%) alkaloid composition;negligible cocaine formation, instead producing ecgonine derivatives, and tropococaine (which does not form in South American coca).

Other formulations

Cocaine hydrochloride, also known as cocaine muriate. Used as a topical anesthetic. Soluble: 1 gram in 0.4 ml water; 3.2 ml cold ethanol, 2.0 ml warm ethanol; 12.5 ml chloroform (toxic). Soluble in glycerol and acetone. Insoluble in ether or oils. Saline, bitter taste. Forms a crystaline solid. Numbs the tongue. Along with cocaine sulfate the most common pharmaceutical form. Requires more storage integrity than parent compound as HCl will precipitate out under heat or through vaporization, resulting in nonactive solids.

Cocaine sulfate. Used as a topical anesthetic. Pharmaceutical formulation readily soluble in water or ethanol. A white crystalline solid. Does not require the delicacy of storage required with cocaine hydrochloride. In H_2SO_4.

Cocaine nitrate. Third pharmaceutical preparation of cocaine using nitric acid. Used also as a topical anesthetic.

"Free base" cocaine refers to pure cocaine, unabsorbed into any organic acid. Common street form of cocaine (not counting chalk, talcum powder, flour, and other things used to "cut," or dilute cocaine to increase dealer profits). Pharmaceutical use in in oil-based solutions (•HCl •H_2SO_4 •HNO_3 formulations not being fat-soluble).

Detection

CHROMATOGRAPHY

Paper: use system P1-Rf 0.38 (location under strong UV light)

Location reagent: *iodoplatinate spray*: strong reaction.

Thin-layer: use system T1-Rf 0.60

Location reagent: *acidified iodoplatinate spray:* positive reaction.

Gas: use system G6 retention time 0.57 relative to codeine.

CRYSTAL TESTS

Micro: *gold chloride solution:* serrated needles (sensitivity 1 in 3000); *lead iodide solution:* feathery rosettes (sensitivity 1 in 3000).

ULTRAVIOLET ABSORPTION SPECTRUM

Cocaine in *ethanol*: maxima at 230 mμ; 274 mμ; and 281 mμ; minima at 217 mμ; 260 mμ, and 233 mμ; in 0.1 N *sulphuruc acid:* maxima at 233 mμ (E 1% 1 cm 470); and 275 mμ (E 1% 1 cm 38), with inflection at 281 mμ.

Cocaine hydrochlorate in *water*: maxima at 233 mμ and 274 mμ; minima at 211 mμ and 261 mμ.

INFRARED ABSORPTION SPECTRUM

Cocaine. *Potassium bromide disk:* principal peaks at A 1275; B 1700; C 1106 or 1728.

QUANTITATIVE ESTIMATION (spectrophotometry)

Cocaine in biological materials, following reaction with *bromocresol purple* solution or *methyl orange* solution.

Specific data

lethal dose

0.5 to 2.0 grams.

incapacitating dose

About 20 mg or more

solubility

Cocaine (and see Other Formulations) soluble in organic fats (may be stored in human body fat),One gram cocaine soluble in: 600 ml water (33°F); 270 ml water (80°C); 6.5 ml ethanol; 0.7 ml chloroform; 3.5 ml ether; 12 ml olive oil; 12 ml turpentine; 30-50 ml petroleum. Also in acetone, ethyl acetate, carbon disulfide.

volatility

Visibly above 90°C(194°F). Condensation products are not crystalline.

taste

Slightly bitter. Numbs lips and tongue.

pH

Aqueous solutions are alkaline.

molecular weight

303.35

alpha-methylbenzeethanamine

(amphetamine)

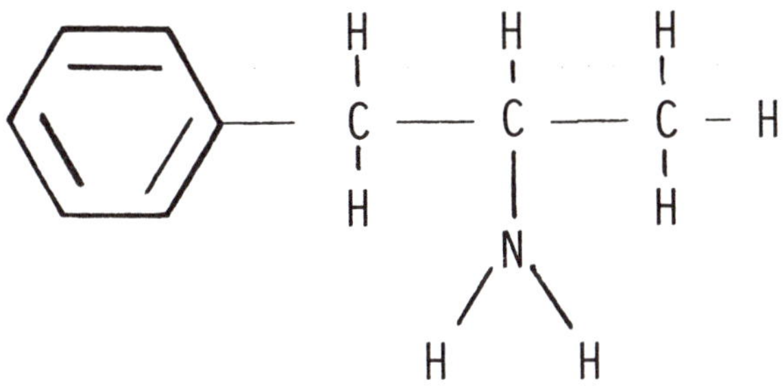

NOREPINEPHRINE-ACTING

Common name: amphetamine, benzedrine

Trade names: Actedron, Allodene, Benzedrine, Adipan, Sympatadrine, Psychedrine, Isomyn, Isoamyne, Mecodrin, Norephedrane, Novydrine, Elasonon, Ortedrine, Phenedrine, Profamina, Sympamine, Simpatedrin.

Formula: $C_6H_5CH_2CH(NH_2)CH_3$

Type: central nervous system stimulant

Use: CNS stimulant; appetite suppressant

Military hazards

Amphetamine in its pure form as a crystalline white solid or powder offers little real hazard to large bodies of personnel and no hazard to most equipment. In and of itself it is not obsorbed through the skin. Large quantities would be required to contaminate foodstuffs, and those would not include sealed or canned rations.

It could be used against targeted individuals in pure form, requiring some sort of covert activity.

Amphetamine fell out of initial consideration due to its unpredictable effects on large groups of persons and the problem of suitable munitions. Initial considerations for use envisioned it being used against rioters or minor insurgents who might be made unfit to fight without their suffering injury or death.

Microencapsulation techniques and the accidental development of skin penetrating solvents, such as $DSMO_2$, may have given amphetamine a new use. In an oil suspension, then made into sub-micron sized protein capsuled dust (a method used since the mid 1970s for certain insecticides), amphetamine could become a profound hazard to rear-area support functions or home civillian populations. Suspended in a $DSMO_2$ solution small but significant dosages could be applied by aerial spray much in the manner of blister or liquified nerve agents. Either method (among others) would overcome the dosages problem inherent with the pure compound. However, in this sort of application amphetamine would cease to be an incapacitating agent and become a casualty agent.

Metabolism and pathology

Pure amphetamine is commonly administered through oral dosage, although solutions (such as amphetamine hydrochloride) may be given intravenously. Ingestion is rapid through the gastrointestinal tract. Amphetamine remains in the human system for a considerable period, and may be detected for about seven days following injestion. Detoxification of sub-lethal dosage is rapid, 30-40% of such dosages being excreted through the kidneys within 48 hours.

In action, amphetamine causes an increase in the spontaneous release of the neurotransmitter noradrenaline (norepinephrine 4-(2-amino-1-hydroethyl)-1,2-benzenediol, and further increases the latter upon each release in proportion to the amount of available amphetamine, and finally, blocks the uptake of noradrenaline. The result is an increase in muscle activity, especially that of the cardiavascular system as the victim undergoes a secondary adrenoline (epinephrine) "high" through neuroreactions in the cerebral cortex. In cases of high dosage (in excess of 200 mg in adult males) a distinctive amphetamine psychosis may occur, characterized by a certain paranoia, compulsive picking at the skin, and possible auditory and visual hallucinations.

Accute overdosages are characterized by these hallucinations accompanied by paranoid delusions, a tendency to excitement and agitation, hypertension, hyperventilation with rapid pulse, constant dialation of the pupils, slurred speach, chills, fever, headache, tremors, exaggeration of the reflexes, and failure of muscle coordination. Death through heart failure is not common, but is possible to those in poor health.

Withdrawal symptoms include chronic fatigue, mental depression, tremors, gastrointestinal disturbances and general weakness. This will be later followed with extreme drowsiness and prolonged sleep.

Extraction

Amphetamine is prepared by the action of the oxime

benzyl methyl ketone, or by the reaction of this keytone with formamide.

Common formulation variations

Amphetamine 4-chlorophenoxyl acetate, $C_{17}H_{20}ClNO_3$, an anorexix or appetite suppressant.

Amphetamine phosphate (1-phenyl-2-aminopropane monophosphate)$C_9H_{13}N{\bullet}H_3PO_4$. This is an acetone solution of amphetamine treated with phosphoric acid. Used as a general central nervous system stimulant.

Amphetamine tannate. Amphetamine in a hydrochloric acid solution. Used as a general central nervous system stimulant, commonly for narcotic poisoning. Most common amphetamine formulation.

Amphetamine sulfide (± alpha-methylbenzene-ethanamine sulfate) $C_6H_5CH_2CHCH_3NH_2{\bullet}H_2SO_4$. Central nervous system stimulant.

Amphetaminil alpha[(1-methyl-2-phenylethyl)amino] benzeneactonitrile $C_6H_6CH_2(CH_3)CHNHC(CN)CHC_6H_5$, a psychotropic.

Detection

CHROMATOGRAPHY

Paper: use system P1-Rf 0.51

Location reagents: *iooplatinate spray:* white. *bromocresol green spray:* strong reaction.

Thin layer: use system T1-Rf 0.48.

Location agent: *potassium permanganate spray:* positive reaction.

Gas: use system G2/120: retention time 0.28 relative to ephedrine.

COLOR TEST

Micro: *sulphuric acid-formaldehyde test:* orange ⟶ brown.

CRYSTAL TEST

Micro: *platinic bromide solution:* masses of irregular plates, weakly birefractive (sensitivity: 1 in 200). *platinic iodide solition:* masses of irregular plates (sensitivity: 1 in 400).

ULTRAVIOLET ABSORPTION SPECTRUM

In 0.1 N *sulphuric acid:* maxima at 251.5 mμ (E1% 1 cm 5.5); 257 mμ (E 1%, 1 cm 15); 263 mμ (E 1% 1 cm 8).

INFRARED ABSORPTION SPECTRUM

In liquid film, principal peaks at A 695, B 737, C 1452.

Specific data

lethal dose

.2-2.0 g (adult, 150 lbs), *immediately* absorbed.

incapacitating dose

In excess of 100 mg (adult, 150 lbs), *immediately* absorbed.

solubility

High in all organic acids, alcohols, and ethers. Low in distilled water.

volatility

Volatizes slowly at 20°C(68°F).

taste

Very acrid. Ammonialike odor.

pH

Aqueous solutions are alkaline.

molecular weight

132.56

d-alpha-methylbenzeethananamine

(dexamphetamine)

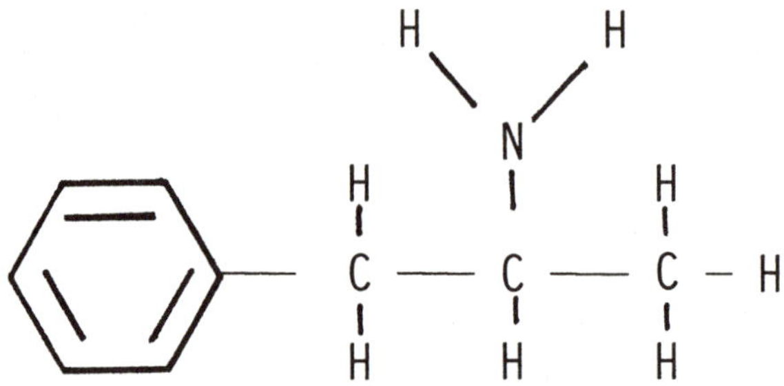

(enantiomer of amphetamine)

NOREPINEPHRINE-
ACTING

Other names: dextroamphetamine, (+)-α-methylphenylamine

Trade names: *principal component in* Alfatin, Dexamphetamine, d-Amfetasul, Obesedrin, Dexten, Maxiton, Sympanin, Simpamina-D, Albemap, Dadex, Ardex, Amsustain, Betafedrina, d-Betaphredine, Diocurb.

Formula: d-[$C_6H_5CH_2CH(NH_2)CH_3$]

Type: central nervous system stimulant

Use: CNS stimulant; appetite suppressant

DEXAMPEX
DEXEDRINE SULFATE
DOMAFATE
DEXALONE

Military hazards

Dexamphetamine, like the other amphetamines, in pure form is a crystalline white solid or powder that presents little hazard to personnel or equipment. In and of itself it is not absorbed through the skin. Large quantities would be required of the pure compound to achieve highly marginal results. Its greatest threat would be its covert use against specific individuals, and then only if some means were found to administer it either orally of intravenously in some appreciable anount.

Its effects on large bodies of personnel would be unpredictable, if used soley as an incapacitating substance. It would cause confusion, disorientation, and possibly some psychotic side effects. The enemy would not come marching in, hands up, singing The Star-Spangled Banner, as one military authority hoped in the 1950s when this agent and amphetamine were considered for military use.

New technologies such as microencapsulation, and such organo-solvents as $DSMO_2$ [see *Amphetamine* for explanations] would make this a fesible casualty agent although its application would require more planning (involving higher eschelons of command) than the normal casualty agent use. However, potential use against support elements and rear-area populations would make this an insidiously effective substance.

Metabolism and pathology

Dexamphetamine is identical in application to amphetamine, although the substance itself is somewhere between two to four times as humanly reactive as amphetamine (depending on which source you read). It is commonly administered orally, although solutions may be administered intravenously. Ingestion through the digestive tract is rapid.

Dexamphetamine remains in the human body about the same length of time as amphetamine. It may be detected in either blood or urine samples for about a week. Detoxification of sub-lethal dosages (the norm) proceeds slightly faster than that for amphetamine, over 50% of absorbed dosage being excreted through the kidneys within 48 hours given (as with amphetamine) somewhat acidic body pH.

Like amphetamine, dexamphetamine causes an increase in the neurotransmitter noradrenaline (norepinephrine), a chemical relative to the man-made amphetamines. Similarly, it blocks the body's natural uptake of the neurotransmitter causing oversimilation of the body's metabolism.

The toxic effects of dexamphetamine are those of amphetamine, only more pronounced, including the CNS overstimulated "high" to the cerebral cortex. Likewise, withdrawl symptoms may be more pronounced than with the former substance.

Dezamphetamine poisoning is characterized by auditory and visual hallucinations with occasional paranoid delusions. There will always be the signs of systemic overstimulation such as excitement and agitation, hyperventilation with rapid pulse, exaggeration of the reflexes with tremors and failure of muscle coordination. The pupils of the eyes will be constantly dialated, speech will be slurred, and cills, fever and headache are to be expected. Death through heart failure can occur in extreme cases.

Withdrawl symptoms include chronic fatigue, mental depression, tremors, gastrointestinal disturbances and general weakness. This will be followed with extreme drowsiness and prolonged sleep.

Extraction

Dexamphetamine is prepared through resolution of amphetamine with d-Tartic acid (d-threo-2,3-dihydroxysuccinci acid).

Common formulation variations

Dexamphetamine sulphate. Most common form of dexamphetamine. Treatment of dexamphetamine with 10% wt of sulphuric acid (H_2SO_4) to make a compouns with improved shelf life.

Dexamphetamine phosphate. Acetone solution of dexamphetamine treated with phosphoric acid (H_3PO_4). Used as a general CNS stimulant and appetite suppressant.

Carboxyphen. Compound formed from dexamphetamine and carboxymethylcellulose. By weight, makes a more effective appetite suppressant.

Detection

CHROMATOGRAPHY

Paper: use system P1-Rf).51

Location reagents: *iodplatinate spray* with *bromocresol green spray:* strong reaction.

Thin layer: use sysytem T1-Rf (0.48)

Location reagent: *potassium permangate spray:* positive reaction.

COLOR TEST

Micro: *sulphuric acid-formaldehyde* test: orange ⟶ brown (sensitivity 1 in 200).

CRYSTAL TEST

Micro: *platinic bromide solution:* long, rhomboidal plates and prisms, strongly birefractive, (sensitivity 1 in 200). *platinic iodide solution:* plates, mostly hexagonal in shape, (sensitivity 1 in 400).

ULTRAVIOLET ABSORPTION SPECTRUM

In 0.1 N *sulphuric acid:* maxima at 252 mμ (E 1% 1 cm 15), 257.5 mμ (E 1% 1 cm 19), 265 mμ (E 1% 1 cm 14).

INFRARED ABSORPTION SPECTRUM

For dextroamphetamine *sulfate: Potassium bromide disk:* Principal peaks at A 118, B 1495, C 1582.

Specific data

lethal dose

.2-2.0g (adult, 150 lb), *immediately* absorbed.

incapacitating dose

In excess of 100.0 mg, *immediately* absorbed.

solubility

High in organic acids. Formulation variations show greater tendency for water absorption than alcohol or ethers.

volatility

Slow.

taste

Slightly bitter taste, followed by a feeling of numbness.

pH

Pure dextroamphetamine pH= 5.0. Aqueous solutions are between 5.0 and 6.0 (slightly acidic).

molecular weight

135.2

N, alpha - dimethylphenethylamine
(methamphetamine)

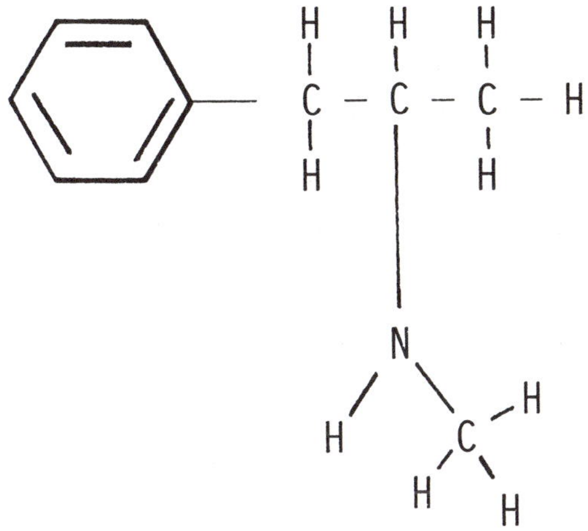

(isomer of phentermine)

NOREPINEPHRINE-
ACTING

Other names: d-deoxyephedrine; desoxyphedrine; methamphetamine; phenylmethylaminpropane; (+)-N,α-dimethylphenethylamine.

Trade names: Norodin.

Formula: $C_6H_5CH_3CH(NH[CH_3])CH_3$

Type: central nervous system stimulant

Use: CNS stimulant; appetite suppressant

Military hazards

Both methylamphetamine and its more common formulation, methylamphetamine hydrochloride (commonly known as "meth" or "speed") present no direct threat to large numbers of personnel or equipment in their pure form.

Microencapsulation techniques would render methylamphetamine into an extremely fine powder. Inhalation of such a powder would have a greater effect than ingestion. In solution with $DSMO_2$ or a similar solvent, a viable aerial spray could be made. Methylamphetamine, due to its greater rate of action, would probably be a better base for such a psychoactive chemical agent. Microencapsulation would probably be the most practical means of dissemination. Key targets would probably be rear-area support activities or selected enemy home populations. Delivery could be by ballistic munitions or through personnel planted in an opponent's home area, there dispersed through newer types of CS delivery systems [see Riot Control Agents]. Probable targets would include defense industries, military activities, police agencies, local and national governmental agencies, airports, harbor facilities, hospitals, etc. Probable deployment would be done either just prior to, or at commencement of hostilities.

Use of this and other types of revamped incapacitating agents might be more cost-effective than the use of lethal casualty agents against civilian populations and in terms of areas of concentration would probably be more efficient as well. Civil defense agencies please note.

Metabolism and pathology

Methylamphetamine, like all the amphetamines, is readily absorbed through the digestive tract. It is more efficiently absorbed through the lungs or direct intravenous injection, either allowing for direct blood absorption. Mindful that methylamphetamine acts more quickly than the other two amphetamines herein discussed, the pathology is the same. Stimulation of adrenaline begins and the action of noraepinephrine is suppressed. Blood flow to body organs decreases as flow to the muscles increases resulting in agitation, increased (involuntary) respiration and heartbeat, possibly leading to tremors, muscle spasms, irritation and exaggeration of the reflexes under increasing dosage or in the effects of strong initial dosages. In toxic dosages (generally those over 200 mg) an initial "whole-body orgasm" usually gives way quickly to both auditory and visual hallucinations, hypertension, hyperventilation, constant dialation of the pupils, slurred speech, chills, fevers, and failure of muscle coordination. Persons with heart disfunctions could suffer cardiovascular collapse. These latter reactions do not occur when regular therapeutic dosages (usually below 30 mg) are administered, but frequently occur in "recreational" drug users. Administered as a military agent, methylamphetamine overdose would be the prime intent. And like the recreational drug user on an overdose, personnel suffering toxic effects would be a danger both to themselves and those around them, especially if they suffer induced/enhanced paranoia.

Aftereffects include chronic fatigue, metal depression, tremors, gastrointestinal disturbances and general weakness. this will be later followed by extreme drowsiness and prolonged sleep.

Body pH has a significant effect on methylamphetamine retention. With neutral to alkaline body pH there is a 16 hour excretion cycle. If body pH is acidic, this cycle may be shortened to about half an hour. The body metabolizes less of methylamphetamine into N-demathylation products than it does amphetamine or deamphetamine, although there may be sufficient by-products and residual for detection up to about a week.

Extraction

Methyamphetamine is made as a condensation product of benzyl methyl keytone and methylamine.

Other formulations

Methylamphetamine hydrochloride. Common commercial preparation of methylamphetamine. Crystalline structure, soluble in water, alcohol, and chloroform. Almost insoluble in water. Found under trade names: Amphedroxyn, Desfedrin, Desoxyn, Destim, Dexoval, D-O-E, Dexephrin, Drinalfa, Efroxine, Gerobit, Hiropon, Isophen, Madrine, Methampex, Methedrine, Methylisomym, Pervitin, Semoxydrine, Soxsympamine, Syndrox, Toneedron. Methamphet in HCl. Used as CNS stimulant and appetite suppressant.

Detection

CHROMATOPOGRAPHY

Paper: location under UV light absorption. Location reagent *idoplatinic spray:* strong reaction; *bromocresol green spray:* strong reaction; *marquid reagent:* orange; *ninhydrin spray:* purple.

Thin layer: use system T1-Rf 0.28. Location reagent: *acidified idoplatinic spray:* positive reaction; *marquis reagent:* positive reaction; *potassium permanganate spray:* positive reaction.

Gas: use system G2/120. Retention time 0.40 reletive to ephedrine.

COLOR TEST

Micro: *sulphuric acid-formaldehyde test:* orange (sensitivity 0.50 μ).

CRYSTAL

Micro: *platinic iodide solution:* blades, some serrated (sensitivity 1 in 400); *potassium bismuth iodide solution:* elongating plates, forming in 8-12 hrs (sensitivity 1 in 200).

ULTRAVIOLET ABSORPTION SPECTRUM

Methylamphetamine in H_2SO_4: maxima at: 251.5 mμ (E 1% 1 cm 8); 257 mμ (E 1% 1 cm 10); 263 mμ (E 1% 1 cm 8), with inflection at 266 mμ.

Methylamphetamine hydrochloride: maxima at: 251 mu (E 1% 1 cm 8); 257 mμ (E 1% 1 cm 10); 263 mμ (E 1% 1 cm 8). Minima at 226.5 mμ; 254 mμ; 261 mμ.

INFRARED ABSORPTION SPECTRUM

For methylamphetamine hydrochloride: *potassium bromide disk:* principal peaks at A747; B698; C1475.

Specific data

lethal dose

Between 0.2 and 2.0 grams *immediately* absorbed. Very rare.

incapacitating dose

Over 200 mg *immediately absorbed.*

solubility

Pure methylamphetamine only slightly soluble in water, soluble readily in ethanol, chloroform, and ether (unlike methylampht·HCl)

volatility

Very slow. Crystalline solid.

taste

Bitter.

pH

Neutral to slightly acidic, depending on plant purity.

molecular weight

149.24

Central Nervous System Depressants

official definition

Compounds that have the predominant effect of depressing or blocking the activity of the central nervous system, often by interfering with the transmission across [neural] synapses. High doses produce toxic delerium which completely destroys the ability to perform any military task.

FM 3-9

A single incapacitating agent has been chosen as representitive of its class. This is morphine, the first major opiate derivative. Morphine has served as the basis of a series of opiate-based substances, including heroin, methadone, and a few others. Narcotic is too general and inaccurate a term for many substances which include both stimulants, depressants, and hallucinogens.

(5α,6α)-7,8-didehydro-4,5-epoxy-17-methylmorphinan-3,6,-diol

(morphine)

NOREPINEPHRINE, SEROTONIN, AND DOPAMINE - ACTING

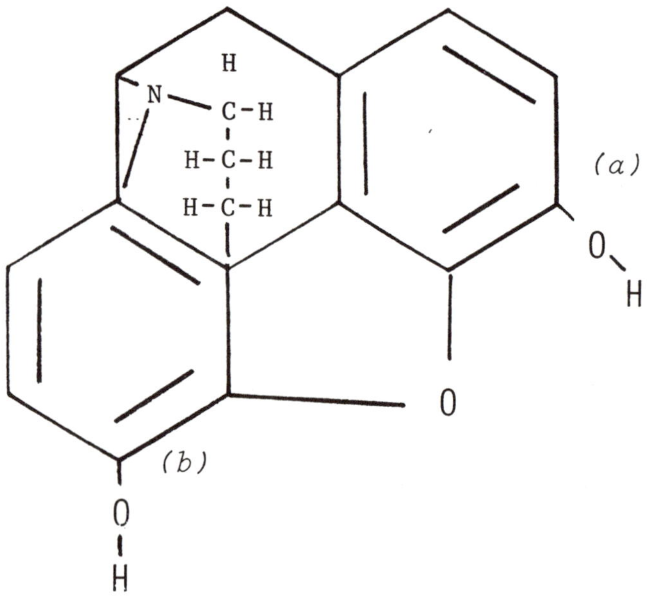

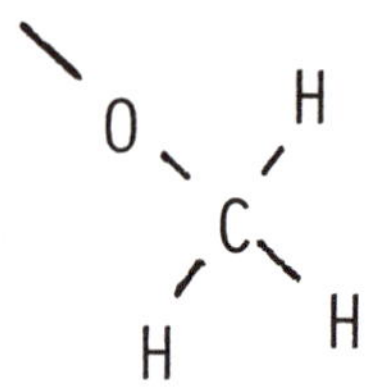

replacement bond at point (a) forms *codeine*

replacement bond at point (*a*) (oxygen replacing carbon in C_2H_5 ring and unsaturating same) with:

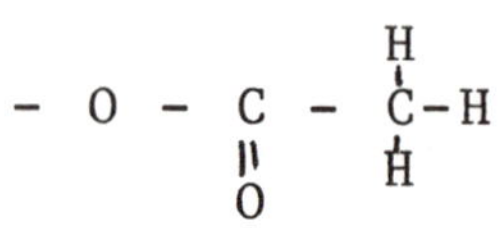

forms *heroin*

while replacing bond at (*b*) (not touching C_2H_5 group) with

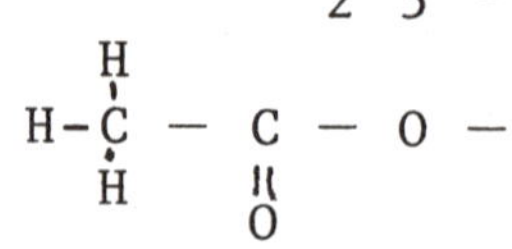

Chemical names: (5α,6α)-7,8-didehydro-4,5-epoxy-~~3,6-dihydroxy-N-~~ 17-methylmorphinan-3,6-diol

Common names: morphine, morphia

Type: central nervous system depressant

Use: analgesic (pain killer)

Morphine is the principal alkaloid of opium, a derivative of the Asian opium poppy *papaver somniferum*. In pure form it is a white crystalline solid having a slightly bitter taste which may be slightly numbing to the tongue.

Military hazards

Morphine in pure form offers little if any tactical military hazards. Morphine is most effectively absorbed into the body as an intravenus hydrochloride, sulfate, mucic or tartrate solution. Effects through oral ingestion are minimal due to low, erratic, and unpredictable absorption through the intestinal tract.

Morphine is thought to act on the peripheral nervous system before it breaks through the brain-blood barrier [see Metabolism and Pathology, below].

However, inhallation appears to be equally as effective as injection. In the past this would have meant morphine could be a burning agent, as raw opium extract has been used for millenia.

However, the most important thing about morphine has proved to be its chemistry. When morphine was first synthesized in the early part of this century, the possibility of synthetic analogues came into being. Morphine from opium is expensive. Similar analgesics from scratch would not be, given time and effort towards production facilities.

The final consequence of narcotics chemistry may not be in the form of new incapacitating agents. Narcotic opiates do not produce the violent physical and psychological changes possible with the amphetamines, cocaine, or the hallucinogenic substances. On the other hand, their chemistry could be incorporated into an entire new generation of riot control agents and so expand the applications of that seperate catagory of chemical substances.

Metabolism and pathology

Oral dosages are inefficient where analgesic effects are required. Morphine is not readily intestinally absorbable. Formulations which are (such as morphine sulfate), are designed principally for injection. Morphine and its derivatives are not the substances in opium tinctures which are used for gastrointestinal disorders (with the slight exception of the $\bullet H_2SO_4$ formulation).

Morphine and its compounds appear to be equally effective injected or inhaled.

Morphine appears to have its most profound effects through the peripheral nervous and cardiovascular systems through direct action with neural functions found there. Morphine may take 30 to 60 minutes before sizable amounts (and then less than 20% of total) penetrate the brain-blood barrier. The morphine derivatives heroin and codeine act much more efficiently in this regard, as to the synthetics meperidine and propoxyphrene. The nine formulations listed below [Other Formulations] were likewise devised for this ability.

The opiates are readily fat-soluble and commonly enter the bloodstream through this route. Trace elements will be found in, and precipitated from, fatty body tissues for a prolonged period. The opiates, and their analogues, are metabolized through the liver before being excreted through the kidneys.

At the lower dosages, morphine and its relative compounds produce a weakening or deadening of acute physical pains and stimulations, while being mildly sedative.

Higher levels of dosage produce a more pronounced sedation, possibly causing severe drowsiness and sleep. At this stage respiratory and cardiovascular depression become obvious.

Acute dosages produce a severe depression of respiratory

and cardiovascular activity as sedation may slip into coma. Chronic constipation should be evident. The pupils of the eyes will be pinpointed, making night vision impossible in those still conscious.

As morphine and the other opiates penetrate the brain and the central nervous system, psychological phenomena come into play. This is usually concurrent with the onset of stupor. There will be induced mood changes and the clouding of mental images (concepts, emotions, observation and analysis of facts and events). Visual and auditory hallucinations occur and the victim will slip in and out of the dream state before becoming unconscious.

In anything above moderate dosages many individuals develop a profound feeling of euphoria. However, this is far from universal and may be dependent on many other psychological and environmental factors.

Extraction and derivation

Morphine is the principal extract from the gum of the flowering body of the Asian poppy *papaver somniferum*. It may also be synthesized although legitimate demand is not such that this is economic. Codeine and heroin are derived directly from morphine (see structural diagram). Morphine is commonly used in any of several formulations (see Other Formulations, below) designed for specific applications and absorption characteristics.

Morphine has been supplemented, although not supplanted, by a number of synthesized analgesics (pain killers) which pose less of an addictive hazard.

Other formulations

Morphine acetate. (morphine •CH_3COOH). Soluble in water and ethanol; insoluble in ether. Narcotic analgesic.

Morphine hydrobromide (morphine $\bullet BrNO_3$). Soluble in water and ethanol. Molecular weight 366.27. Narcotic analgesic. Photosensitive: store away from strong light.

Morphine hydrochloride (morphine •HCl). Soluble in water, ethanol. Slowly soluble in glycerol. Insoluble in chloroform or ether. Molecular weight 321.81. Narcotic analgesic, more common in Europe than in North America. Photosensitive: store away from strong light.

Morphine methylbromide (morphine $\bullet CH_3Br$). Soluble in water. Only slightly soluble in ethanol or chloroform. Insoluble in ether. Molecular weight 380.28. Narcotic analgesic. Photosensitive: store away from strong light.

Morphine mucate (morphine $\bullet HOOC(CHOH)_4COOH$): salt of morphine and mucic acid (compare with morphine tartrate, below). Narcotic analgesic having prolonged action upon injection. Photosensitive: store away from strong light.

Morphine N-oxide (morphine $\bullet NO_4$). Soluble in ammonia/water. Slightly soluble in water, ethanol. Almost insoluble in acetone, benzene, and chloroform. Narcotic analgesic.

Morphine oleate (morphine 20% insolution of oleic acid, $C_{17}H_{33}COOH$). A brown, oily solution soluble in ethanol and insoluble in water. Highly effective narcotic analgesic but deteriorates rapidly.

Morphine sulfate (morphine $\bullet SO_4$). Soluble in water, ethanol. Insoluble in chloroform, ether. Molecular weight 6668.76. Incompatable with: alkalies, tannic acid, iodic acid, potassium permanganate, borax, chlorates, ferric chloride, iodides, lead acetate, magnesia, spirit nitrous ether, mercury bichloride, gold salts. Common North American formulation. Turns brown color in storage - no effect on structure or potency. Narcotic analgesic, sedative, preanesthetic, and gastric sedative. Photosensitive: store away from strong light.

The following are the principal hydrate forms of morphine:

Morphine monohydrate. Refers to refined (free base) morphine.

Morphine acetate trihydrate. Morphine $\bullet 3H_2O$. Forms a yellowish-white powder. Slit acetic odor. Soluble in water ethanol, glycerol, chloroform. Little or no solubility in ether. Volatile and photosensitive: store away from strong light and keep tightly sealed. (2 extra oxygen bonds)

Morphine dihydrate. Morphine $\bullet HI\,2H_2O$. Forms pale yellow crystals (aligned rhomboids) needles. Prone to oxydize in the manner of morphine sulfate. Soluble in water.

Morphine lactate. Morphine $\bullet C_3H_6O_3$. Forms opaque fine crystalline powder. Soluble in water and slightly soluble in ethanol.

Morphine meconate pentahydride. This is the form that unrefined morphine takes in raw opium gum. Morphine, double bonded $\bullet C_7H_4O_7 \cdot 5H_2O$. Soluble in water, ethanol. Yellow crystals.

Morphine nitrate. Morphine $\bullet HNO_3$. White needle-shaped crystals. Soluble in water. Photosensitive: store away from strong light.

Morphine monobase phosphate hemihydrate. Morphine $\bullet$ $H_3PO_4 \cdot \frac{1}{2}H_2O$. From equal parts of morphine (monohydrate) and phosphoric acid. White stick-like crystals. Soluble in water.

Morphine polybase phosphate heptahydrate. Morphine $\bullet$ $2H_3PO_4 \cdot 7H_2O$. Needle-like crystals. Slightly soluble in water, dilute acids, and fixed alkalai hydroxide solutions.. Photosensitive: protect from light (darkening indicates breakdown).

Morphine phthalate pentahydride. Morphine, double bonded $\bullet C_6H_4(COOH)_2 \cdot 5H_2O$. Yellowish powder.

Morphine valerate. Morphine $\bullet C_5H_{10}O_2$. White crystals with acidic odor that darken with exposure to light. Soluble in ethanol. Volatile and photosensitive: keep tightly closed and away from strong light.

MORPHINE TARTRATE TRIHYDRATE

Structurally related opiates:

codeine
heroin

Synthetic narcotic analgesics (unstructurally related but serving same functions):

meperidine (Demerol)
methadone
pentazocine
propoxyphene (Darvon)

Structurally related opiate antagonists (narcotic action suppressants):

cyperenorphine
nalorphine
naloxone

Detection

CHROMATOPOGRAPHY

Paper: use system P1-Rf 0.14. Location under UV light, strong absorption). Location reagennts: *iodplatinate spray*, strong reaction; *bromocresol green spray*, weak reaction; *marquid reagent*, purple; or use system RP1a-Rf 0.88. Location reagents: *iodoplatinate spray*, positive reaction; or use system RP1b-Rf 0.81, location as for system RP1a.

Thin-layer: use ststem T7-Rf 0.11. Location reagent *iodoplatinate spray*, positive reaction; or use system T8-Rf 0.27, location as for system T7.

Gas: use system G1/250 - retention time 1.28 relative to cocaine; or using system G2/225 - retention time relative to codeine; or use system G6 - retention time 1.21 relative to codeine.

COLOR TESTS

Micro: *sulphuric acid - formaldehyde test-* purple (sensitivity 0.05 µg); *ammonium molybdate test:* purple — blue — light green (sensitivity 0.05 µg); *Vitali's test:* yellow/yellow/orange (sensitivity: 0.05 µg).

CRYSTAL TESTS

Micro: *potassium cadmium iodide solution:* sheaves of fine needles (sensitivity 1 in 3000); *potassium tri-iodide solution (I):* plates (sensitivity 1 in 1000).

ULTRAVIOLET ABSORPTION SPECTRUM

Morphine in *ethanol*: maximum at 287 mµ (E 1% 1 cm 55); minimum at 263 mµ (E 1% 1 cm 22); morphine in 0.1 N *sodium hydroxide:* maxima at 250.5 mµ (E 1% 1 cm 255) and 296 mµ (E 1% 1 cm 116); morphine in 0.1 N *sulphuric acid:* maximum at 284 mµ (E 1% 1 cm 43.4) and an inflexion at 279 mµ. *Morphine hydrochloride & morphine sulfate in water:* maximum at 285 mµ (E 1% 1 cm 41), minimum at 261 mµ.

INFRARED ABSORPTION SPECTRUM

Morphine (base): *potassium bromide disk:* principal peaks at A 805, B 1243, C 945 or 118 or 1475.

Specific data

lethal dose

Between 200 mg and 2 grams (adult, 150 lb).

incapacitating dose

About 20 mg.

solubility

Soluble 1 to 500 of water and 1 to 500 of boiling water. 1 to 250 of ethanol; 1 in 1500 of chloroform. Insoluble for all intents in ether. Slight in ammonia or benzene.

For morphine formulations, see Other Formulations, above.

volatility

Pure morphine a crystalline solid to about 254°C(489°F).

taste

Slightly bitter taste. May be numbing to the tongue.

pH

Slightly alkaline in pure form.

molecular weight

285.3

Opium derived substances structurally similar to morphine

acetorphine	narcotic analgesic
acetyldihydrocholine	narcotic analgesic
benzylmorphine	narcotic
desmorphine	narcotic analgesic
diamorphine	narcotic analgesic
dihydrocodeine	narcotic analgesic
dihydromorphine	narcotic analgesic
ethylmorphine	narcotic analgesic
etorphine	narcotic analgesic
hydrocodone	narcotic analgesic, antitussive
hydromorphinol	narcotic analgesic
hydromorphone	narcotic analgesic
methyldesmorphine	narcotic
methyldihydromorphine	narcotic
metopon	narcotic analgesic
myrophine	narcotic

neopine	opium alkaloid
nicodine	narcotic, antitussive
nicomorphine	narcotic analgesic
norcodeine	narcotic (codeine metabolate)
normorphine	narcotic
oxycodone	narcotic analgesic
oxymorphone	narcotic analgesic
phohcodine	antitussive
thebacon	narcotic analgesic
thebaine	narcotic

Psychedelic Drugs

Psychedelic drugs are a group of heterogeneous compounds, all with the ability to induce visual, auditory, or other hallucinations and to seperate the individual from reality. These agents may induce disturbances in cognition and perception and, in some instances, may produce behavioral patterns that have been described as being similar to components of psychotic behavior. Because of this wide range of psychological effects, it is difficult to assign a single term that will adequately classify these agents.

Robert M. Julian. *A primer of drug action.*

To present a general cross-section of available types, the following substances are presented, along with related drugs:

- Agent BZ
- mescaline
- psilocybin
- lysergic acid dimethylamide
- phenylcyclidine (PCP)

3-quinuclidinyl benzilate

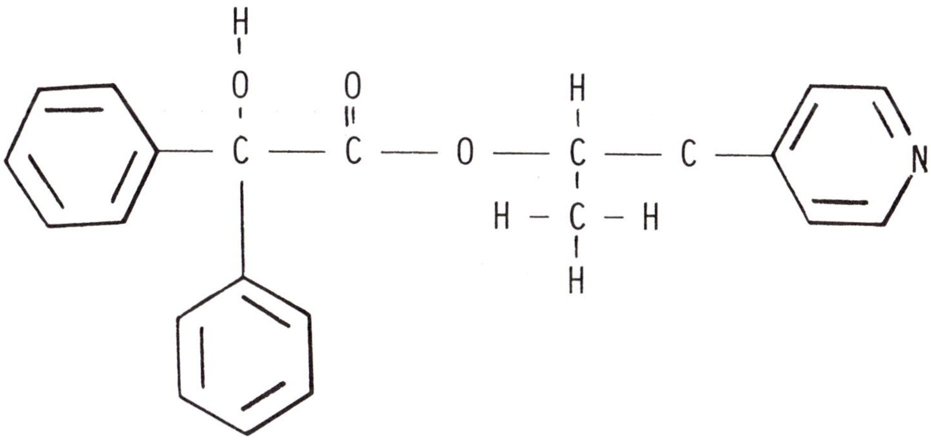

BZ

NOREPINEPHRINE-
ACTING

Standard NATO agreement (STANAG) code: BZ
Chemical name: 3-quinuclidinyl benzilate
Common name: BZ, or "buzz"
Older names/production codes: Ro 2-3308 (La Roche); QNB

Type: central nervous system depressant (hallucinogen)

Status: removed from NATO, and NATO member, inventories

BZ is a crystalline solid produced through actions through acetone or ether from 3-quinuclidinol. In its former applications it was used primarily through thermal disperson, although *never* made in the form of grenades. Production in bulk was for aerial fog dissemination. Vapors colorless with slight benzene smell.

Background

On May 5th, 1952 *The Journal of the American Chemical Society* (74: 2215) published a two part treatise on antispasmotic basic bicyclic alcohols[1] by Drs L.H. Sternbach and S. Kaiser, based on researches done the previous year at Hoffman-La Roche. In the second part, covering the esters of such compounds, they explored several which the editors commented as showing "an antiacetycholine activity equalling or surpassing that of atropine."

Speculation has it that the word *atropine* rang a few bells at Aberdeen and Porton Down. It was at this time that a new generation of nerve agents (the V-series) was under consideration. A super-atropine antidote would be appropriate for super nerve-agents.

However, bicyclic alcohols, and esters thereof formed the basis of a whole new generation of synthesized non-barbituate tranquilizers as well as of antispasmodics. Many of these formulations proved to have the same intoxifying effects as atropine and the 3-quinuclidynl benzenes had pronounced hallucinogenic side effects through, among other reactions, effects on the neural transmitter *norepinephrine* similar to many other CNS active substances.

Tests showed that 3-quinuclidinol benzenes were not acceptable atropine substitues, but that unlike the rest of their bicyclic alcohol ester relatives, stabilized forms could be vaporized through thermal grenades in a manner similar to that of riot control agents.

Between 1953 and 1957 U.S./British studies were made into nonlethal battlefield agents. A dl-benzilate ester form of 3-quinuclidinol (3-quinuclidynl benzilate, first known by the manufacturer's code Ro 2-3308) and a form of mescaline (known by its Edgewood Arsenal lab code EA 1298) were the two main contenders for formal adoption.

1. It is somehow appropriate that the Sternbach and Kaiser article was followed with one by James D. Dutcher on curare alkaloids.

Bear in mind that the whole notion of psychedelic drugs was something new. It was not until the late 1960s and early 1970s that detailed studies of these substances over significant periods were completed. All that was known in the 1950s is that certain natural and synthesized compounds produced extremely disoriented and mostly benign (if silly) behavior. EA 1298 proved lethal. LSD could cause severe psychosis. So Ro-3308, alias QNB, became agent BZ or "agent buzz."

BZ was produced at Pine Bluff Arsenal between 1962 and 1964. It was dropped from the chemical arsenal firstly because its effects on enemy front-line troops would be varied and unpredictable (based on observation of the civillian psychedelic community) and usage of chemical substances against an opponent's civillian sector has *always* been contrary to NATO philosophy.

Military hazards

BZ is a military field agent that has been dropped from the NATO inventory. Such stocks as exist may be counted in grams rather than in tons. This is not to say that it might not be manufactured elsewhere. The formulation and process have been known since 1952 and the bicyclic alcholo esters/ 3-quinuclidnols have been in use as hypotensives and cholinergics since the mid 1950s.

BZ is a crystalline solid in pure form, and as a military agent was mixed with inert solids, so formulated to be used with thermal type munitions or dispersal units. Its use against front line troops would be marginal. How, ever with new techniques and formulations (again, making use of such methodoligies as microencapsulation and sub syances such as $DSMO_2$ and the like) this agent could be used against military support and logistical elements, and it might be employed against home populations through either strategic or covert actions. The more open the society the greater its threat from such actions.

Metabolism and pathology

BZ blocks the action of acetylcholine in both the peripheral and central nervous systems. As such it lessens the degree and extent of the transmission of impulses from one nerve fiber to another through their connecting synaptic junctions. It stimulates the action of noradrenaline (norepinephrine) in the brain, much as do the amphetamines and cocaine, although concurrently depressing hypertensity or hyperactivity associated with the latter substances. BZ thus may induce vivid hallucinations as it sedates its victims. Toxic delirium is very common.

This is an effect associated with atrophine overdose, although BZ will not suppress the cardiovascular system in the manner of atropine. In an area where both nerve agents and psychochemicals are suspected, medical personnel should avoid hasty diagnosis to avoid mixing nerve agent casualties treated with atropine with victims of CNS depressants. BZ will not have the same types of reactions to 2-pam chloride as will atropine and victims' lives may be endangered.

Extraction or formulation

BZ is the bezililate ester of 3-quinuclidnol, formed through acetone-ether actions on the parent compound, the process described in the origional Sternbach, Kaiser report [see Background, above]. This formulation hydrolyzes, lasting up to a month an neutral (7.0) pH and about 2 minutes under extreme alkalai (pH 13.0) conditions.

Other formulations

Seventeen 3-quinuclidinol esters were investigated by Sternbach and Kaiser. Reference here is made to the 5-5-52 issue of the *Journal of the American Chemical Society* (vol 74, table p.220). BZ (3-quinuclidinyl benzilate) carries the Hoffman-La Roche research number Ro 2-3308. Seventeen compounds are listed covering compounds prepared from 9 bases and eight acids and recrystallized using acetone, benzene, ether, methyl and isopropyl alcohols, pet. ethers and water. Ten crystalline solids were made with hydrochloride structures, one with sulphuric acid. One compound is oil soluble. Melting points for crystalline solids range from between 64°C(147.2°F) and 241°C(465.8°F).

Specific data

lethal dosage

Unknown.

incapacitating dosage

Unknown.

vapor density

11.6 times as heavy as air.

solid density

Bulk: 0.51 g/cc. Lab: 1.33 g/cc.

volatility

About 0.5 mg/m^3 at 70°C (158°F). Insignificant.

latent heat of vaporization

Between 170-194°C (338-381.2°F) 62.9 calories per gram.

melting point

167.5°C(333.5°F) bulk mix. Pure chemical 164°C(327.2°F).

boiling point

412°C(773.6°F) bulk mix.

decomposition point

Begins at 170°C(338°F). Complete at 2 hrs at 200°C(392°F).

rate of hydrolysis

25°C(77°F) at pH 7.0: about 4 weeks; at pH 9.8: 16 days, 16 hours; at pH 13: 1.8 minutes.

hydrolysis products

Reduces to 3-quinuclidinol (base) and hydrochloric acid.

molecular weight

337.4

3,4,5-TRIMETHOXYBENZENEETHANAMINE

3,4,5 - triethylphenylethylamine

(mescaline)

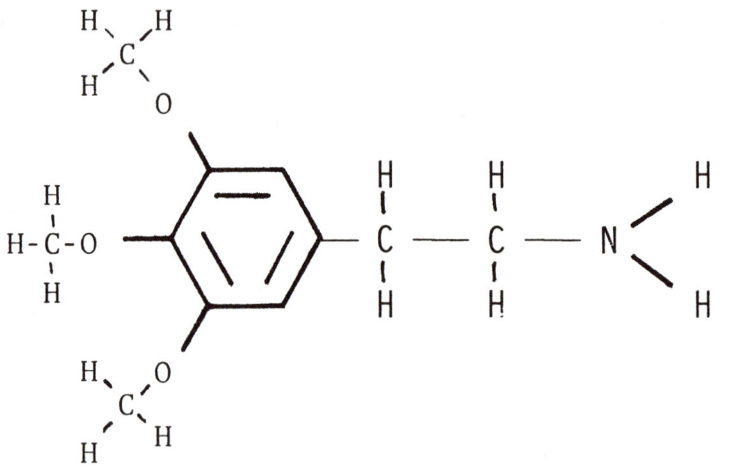

NOREPINEPHRINE-
ACTING

Common name: peyote, mescaline

Formula: 3,4,5$(OCH_3)_3(C_6H_2)C_2H_4NH_3$

Type: central nervous system stimulant (hallucinogen)

Use: naturally occuring hallucinogen

Mescaline is the psychoactive component occuring in, and derived from the peyote cactus *lophophora williamsii* found in northern Mexico and the southwestern United States. Synthetic derivatives of mescaline include DOM (STP, or "speed"), TMA, and MMDA.

Military hazards

Mescaline presents much the same hazard as the amphetamines as regards central nervous system over stimulation. However, whereas the amphetamines are most likely to cause casualties through hypertension and stress, mescaline (and moreso its derivatives) is more likely to present an immediate threat to health and safety. Mescaline is a strong halucinogen which would cause extreme distraction through very vivid audiotory and visual manifestations. Mixed with combat or industrial conditions this would be quite dehabilitating, especially when large numbers of people are involved. The ability to operate machinery, complete tasks involving eye-body coordination, or even to concentrate on a fixed task would be extremely diminished. Injuries and fatalities, unlike those of the amphetamines, from mescaline would be those resulting from physical causes other than from the drug itself. However, the mescaline derivatives such as DOM (STP), TMA, and MMDA would present a direct toxic threat on the order of Methamphetamine and like substances.

In its pure form, mescaline would present a small hazard. However as the principal ingredient in encapsulated dusts or in aerial sprays, a la BZ, it would present a significant hazard to front-line troops, logistical and support elements and to selcted home populations where, as with all pharmaceuticals, disruptions would be tactically more important than fatalities.

Metabolism and pathology

Mescaline is, properly speaking, a central nervous system stimulant. It is a naturally occuring substance similar to, and mimicking the action of, the human neurotransmitter norepinephrine (nor adrenaline) whose purpose is to cause the flow of epinephrine (adrenaline), and more specifically to enable neurotransmissions within the brainstem and the cortexes themselves. It is mescaline's efficiency in substitution for the natural enzyme (having OH and CH_3 bonds on its phenyl group - which all the amphetamines lack) that perhaps accounts for its more unusal properties.

Like too much norepinephrine —— epinephrine (adrenaline) and the amphetamines, mescaline and its derivatives operate to the extent of producing a fright/flight/fight syndrome. This includes a series of strong (unquantifiable) euphoric emotions, increased blood rate and pressure, muscle tremors, rise in body temperature and general EEG rates and behavioral arousal.

Mescaline and its derivatives produce at minimal dosage the hallucinatory effects associated with toxic amphetamine dosages. Moreover, mescaline and its derivatives produce a similarity in type as regards these hallucinations from victim to victim. Brightly colored lights, geometric designs, recall of familiar animals and people occur with color and space perception otherwise unimpaired save for occasional space/time relationships. Otherwise the senses are normal and normal insight and rationality is retained. Unlike such depressants as the opiates, BZ, or even atropine, mescaline and its derivative produce no delirium, amnesia, or clouding of consciousness. Mescaline, unlike its derivatives and toxic dosages of the amphetamines, produces hallucinations which are clear and vivid.

Mescaline is not considered toxic chemically. Over 80% of the total dose is excreted through the kidneys within the first 12 hours. The body metabolizes about 26% of the total dosage into an inactive substance, 3,4,5-trimethoxyphenylacetic acid. Mescaline is readily absorbed from ingestion, injection, or inhalation (mescaline hydrocloride crystals). Absorbed from the gastrointestinal tract, mescaline may remain for short periods in the fatty tissues in the kidneys, spleen and liver. In the liver mescaline can bond to certain plasma and tissue proteins. Dosages of between 400 and 700 mg, via injection, are sufficient to cause hallucinations.

Hallucinations *can* cause serious psychologic disturbances, depending on the mental and emotional status of the victim.

The mescaline derivatives may produce extreme epinephrine (adrenaline) production. They typically produce hallucinations far in advance of mescaline's 30 to 60 minute waiting period. Violent reactions are not uncommon in victims, nor are deaths from neurological or cardiovascular trauma. Hallucination during moments of physical stress could cause deep psychological trauma.

Extraction

Crystalline mescaline is extracted by various organic solvents from the fruiting body of the peyote cactus. Mescaline is soluble in water, ethanol, chloroform. It is almost insoluble in any of the ethers.

Other formulations

Mescaline hydrochloride (mescaline •HCl). Soluble in water and alcohol. Needle-shaped crystals.

Mescaline sulfate dihydrate (mescaline $\bullet H_2SO_4 \cdot 2H_2O$. Soluble in hot water or methanol; slightly soluble in cold water or methanol. Prism-shaped crystals.

Mescaline acid sulfate (mescaline $\bullet H_2SO_4$). Crystalline.

Mescaline aurichloride monohydrate mescaline $\bullet HClAuCl_3 \cdot H_2O$. Soluble in hot water and alcohols. Orange needle-shaped crystals.

Mescaline platinchloride (mescaline $\bullet 2HCl_4PtCl$. Yellow neddle-shaped crystals.

Mescaline n-benzoylmescaline. Clear crystals. Very soluble in water and alcohols.

mescaline n-methylmescaline
mescaline n-acetylmescaline occur naturally

Synthetic derivatives of mescaline. Structurally similar. See diagrams at front of this chapter. *Substituted amphetamines.*

DOM (STP, "speed") α-methyl-2,5-dimethoxy-4-methylphenethylamine. Molecular weight 209.3. 3mg/kg (body wt) produces mild euphoria. Larger dosages may produce hallucinogenic effects lasting to about 8 hours. Soluble in water and chloroform; STP hydrochloride (white powder) soluble in water.

TMA α-methyl-3,4,5-trimethoxyphenethylamine. Molecular weight 225.3. Dosages between 0.8 to 2mg/kg (body wt) produces vivid hallucinations. Above 2.8mg/kg produces, after about 5 hours, hostile behavior embroidered with meglomaniac delusions. Homocidal behavior possible. Chloform sol.

MMDA ?

Detection

CHROMOTOPOGRAPHY

Paper: use system P1-Rf 0.25, location under UV light, absorption.

Location reagents: *idoplatinate spray,* strong reaction; *bromocresol green spray:* weak reaction.

Using system RP1a-Rf 0.90. Same location reagents, location under UV light absorption. Same criteria.

Using system RP1b-Rf 0.94. Same reaction agent, location under UV light, absorption. Same criteria.

Thin-layer: use system T1-Rf 0.22.

Location reagent: *acidified iodoplatinate spray,* positive reaction.

Gas: use system G2/225. Retention time 0.58 relative to *diphenhydramine*.
Using system G6. Retention time 0.21 relative to *codeine*.

COLOR TESTS
Micro: *sulphuric acid-formaldehyde test* — orange (sensitivity (0.1 µg); *ammonium molybdate test* — green → blue (sensitivity 0.025 µg); *Vitali's test* — (dull red) purple/dull red/brown (sensitivity 0.1 µg).

CRYSTAL TESTS
Micro: *potassium bismuth iodide solution*, dense rosettes (sensitivity 1 in 3000); *styphnic acid*, small needles (sensitivity 1 in 3000).

ULTRAVIOLET ABSORPTION SPECTRUM
Mescaline in *ethanol*, maximum at 269 mµ (E 1% 1 cm 75), and an inflection near 225 mµ; in 0.2 N *sulphuric acid*, maximum at 268 mµ (E 1% 1 cm 39).

Specific data

incapacitating dose
400 to 700 mg, in adult male (injection).

solubility
Soluble in water, ethanol, chloroform, benzene. Not soluble in ether or petroleum ethers.

taste
Ammonia-like.

pH
Slightly alkaline.

molecular weight
211.25

3-[2-(Dimethylamino)ethyl]-1H-indol-4-ol dihydrogen phosphate es-

4-phosphoryloxy-NN-dimethyltriptamine

(Psilocybin)

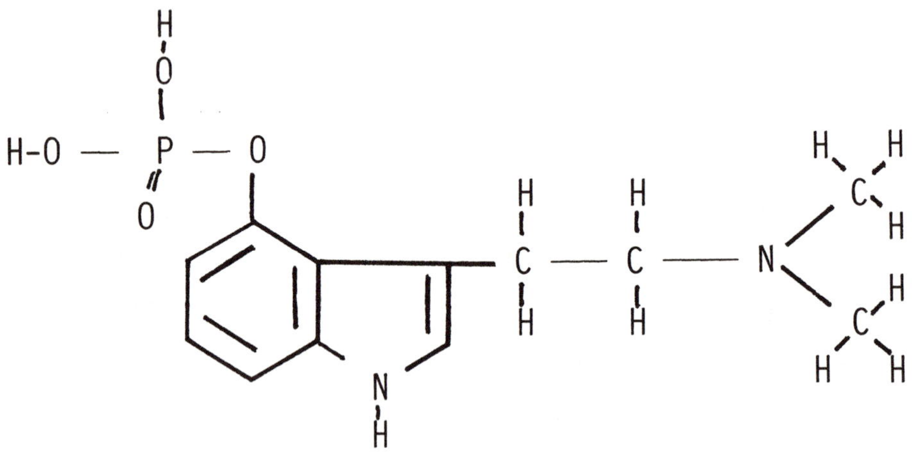

SEROTONIN-
ACTING

Common name: psilocybin, magic mushroom

Type: central nervous system stimulant (hallucinogen)
Use: naturally occuring hallucinogen

Trade name: Indocybin

Psilocybin is the principal active alkaloid in the mushroom *psilocyba mexicana* (known traditionally as *Teonanacatl's flesh* or, in the United States and Europe as *the magic mushroom*). Common lab form is as a refined white crystalline solid. Strong behavior modificant.

Military hazard

Psilocybin is the second most powerful hallucinogen to lysergic acid. Its only drawback is the neccesity for about 15 mg per adult male for adequate dosage insuring hallucinogenic dehabilitation. Unlike lysergic acid (and lysergide, LSD-25), psilocybin's effects only last about four hours maximum and little in the literature indicates this compound produces LSD-like "flashbacks" days, weeks, or years afterwards as a result of dosages absorbed initially into fatty tissues suddenly being metabolized.

Psilocybin would present a safety hazard more than a medical one. Its physiological effects are milder than an amphetamine, or even mescaline syndrome. Yet those under the influence of this substance would not be able to perform complex tasks, especially those requiring concentration and eye-body coordination.

Prior to the late 1970s, this sort of substance would have been limited to the cloak-and-dagger genre. Again, microencapsulation and the (accidental) development of skin-penetrating solvents may have changed the picture. This substance could be delivered by any number of munitions for either inhalation or absorption. Principal targets would be logistical and support elements rather than front line elements. It could be dropped into industrial areas to slow production without directly causing civillian fatalities. It could present a profound hazard if deftly used but haphazard deployment would completely waste it.

Metabolism and pathology

Psilocybin closely resembles the neurotransmitter *serotonin*. The actions of that enzyme are not those of norpinephrine (noradrenaline) and this compound acts in a different manner than the norepinephrine-acting drugs. Psilocybin produces a slight anxiety and the beginnings of the fright/flight/fight syndrome. It does not produce the acute central nervous system reactions associated with the amphetamines or the mescaline derivatives, such as violent behavioral excitation, hyperactivity, and residual psychosises associated with those substances.

What the serotonin-acting substances produce are very powerful emotional-sensory experiences. Psychosis is possible, especially following repeated dosages and depending on other emotional and environmental factors relating to individual victims. However, the damage will be to the psyche and not to the body.

Psilocybin has no special physiological or pharmaceutical advantage over a similar derivative, psilocin. Psilocybin is the main alkaloid component in *psilocybe mexicana* and the one easiestly extracted (simply by treating the stem and cap with methyl alcohol to produce a white crystalline condensation product). Its phosphoric acid group [$OP(OH)_2O$] group is dropped from the molecule during metabolism, creating psilocin, which is the true psychoactive compound.

Psilocybin is usually orally ingested in the form of the raw mushroom. The pure chemical is effectively inhaled or injected as well.

Excretion occurs through the liver and kidneys. A high concentration of psilocybin/psilocin remains in the tissues of those organs for an indefinate period, although generally not psychoactively recycled. About 11% of a total dosage is excreted unchanged; 20% or so is converted to glucuronic acid derivatives; and 4% as indole acid and its derivatives. A further 15-20% of total dosage accumulates in the bile before metabolism is complete.

As mentioned, psilocybin, although very potent, is nowheres as potent as the lysergic acid group. In dosage, up to about 5 mg will produce a mild euphoric state in a male adult (av 150-160 lbs). 5 to 15 mg typically produces (in the same subject) a pronounced increasing intoxication, although without stupor or muscle tone degradation. Above a dose of about 15 mg, there begins the onset of profound perceptual alterations and hallucinations. These may be similar to those which LSD would produce in the same victim, although these produced by psilocybin only last an average of between 2 to 4 hours. During this period the victim may become a danger to himself, his surroundings, and to those around him through his actions.

Extraction

From *psilocybe mexicana* through absorption and filtration with boiling water or boiling methanol. Psilocin minus the phosphoric acid group is insoluble in water.

Related formulations

(see chart at beginning of chapter)

From *psilocybe mexicana:*

Psilocin. Secondary form of the same basic compound, to which psilocybin converts in vitro.

From either *amanita muscaria*, the Fly-agaric mushroom, or *piptadenia peregrina*, a tree native to the Caribbean.

Bufotenine 3-(dimethylaminoethyl)-5-hydroxyindole. Almost identical structure as psilocin, except for placement of hydroxide group on phenyl group. In many ways similar to amphetamine actions: produces increased pulse and blood pressure, dialated eyes and augmented muscle activity at about the 5 mg dosage. Anywhere between 1 and 16 mg it may induce a feeling of light-headedness with stupor in increasing dosage. Not a true hallucinogen. Dosages not exceeding 16 mg may cause staggering, minor paralysis and muscle rigidity. Popular in Haiti where it is known as yopo, cohoba, parica, or epena.

Molecular weight 204.6. Freely soluble in alcohol, less so in ether. Soluble in dilute acids and alkalies.

Dimethyltriptamine 3-(2-dimethylaminoethyl] indole. This compound is not ingested through the gastro-intestinal tract. It is extracted from aqueous alkaline solutions of thr parent mushroom or tree fruiting bodies. It is traditionally inhaled as a powder or smoke, although it could be injected in solution. Unlike Bufotenine, this is a true hallucinogen, although one of limited duration (one to two hours maximum). It further causes alterations in visual perceptions, euphoris, and behavioral excitability. Very popular in the Caribbean where it is known by the same popular names as Bufotenine.

Molecular weight 188.26. Freely soluble in dilute acetic and mineral acids. Also occurs in South American tree *prestonia amazonica*.

Detection

CHROMOTOPOGRAPHY

Paper: use system P1-Rf 0.06. Location under UV light, absorption.

Location reagents: *iodine vapor*, wesk reaction; *marquis reagent*, faint orange.

Thin-layer: use system T1-Rf 0.05

Location reagent: *p-dimethylaminobenzaldehyde spray*, grey ⟶ purple.

COLOR TESTS

Micro: *sulphuric acid-formaldehyde test,* dull orange (sensitivity 0.5 mu); *ammonium molybdate test* — grey-blue → green → yellow (sensitivity 0.5 mu).

ULTRAVIOLET ABSORPTION SPECTRUM

Psilocybin in *methanol:* maxima at 267 mu and 290 mu; minima at 242 mu and 287 mu.

Specific data

incapacitating dose

6 to 16 mg will produce hallucinations.

solubility

Soluble in acetic acid, boiling water, boiling methanol.

taste

Slightly ammonia-like.

pH

Slightly alkaline.

molecular weight

284.27

9,10-didehydro-N,N-diethyl-6-methylergoline-8β-carboxamide

(lysergic acid - 25)

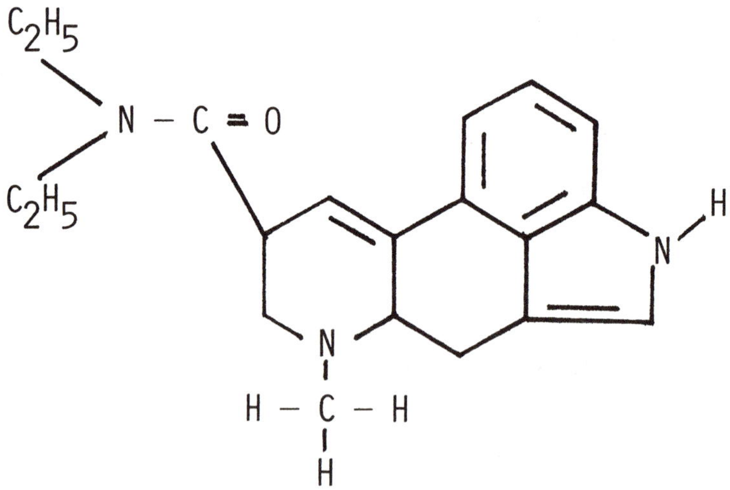

SEROTONIN-
ACTING

Other names: lysergide; lysergic acid diethyamide; LSD; acid

Type: central nervous stimulant (hallucinogen)

Use: psychomimetic, hallucinogen

Trade name: Delysid

Lysergic acid - 25 is a white crystalline solid derived from certain strains of grain ergot. Its hallucinogenic properties were first observed in 1943. In the 1950s and 1960s it achieved notoriety as a social psychedelic. Extremely strong hallucinogen and behavior modificant.

Military hazard

The derivatives of lysergic acid are among the most powerful hallucinatory substances to date, in terms of dosage to effects. Its potency is its main drawback from the military standpoint.

5 µg of LSD had the same effect as 15 mg of mescaline. High concentrations of a chemical substance are required to contaminate large areas of terrain in order to insure adequate contamination of personnel, equipment and stores. Such a concentration would constitute a gross over-contamination and would certainly cause fatalities among the dosed. Furthermore, to insure the survival of the drug against natural deterioration, microencapsulation of the substance would have to be employed. Large quantities of micron-sized dust particles would contribute to a significant downwind hazard for an indefinate period of time.

Thus eliminated as a battlefield agent, an LSD-based agent would have to be used far to an opponent's rear, against theater-area command elements, port facilities, and support elements. There, contamination of personnel, food, medical, and logistical supplies would prove effective. Use against an opponent's home territory would have dire consequences.

Small dosages have profound psychological effects while posing little or no physical threat to their victims. Large dosages (above 1.0-1.5 grams per individual) could concievably cause death through respiratory failure. Any dosage should be considered bio-reactive. LSD-25 causes a profound intoxication-hallucination syndrome within 30 to 60 minutes of oral ingestion. Persons suffering this effect cannot safely operate equipment, perform tasks requiring eye-body coordination, or be capable of rendering rational decisions under conditions of stress. Such individuals would constitute a direct threat to the safety and well-being of those around them.

Metabolism and pathology

LSD-25 is readily absorbed through the gastrointestinal tract and oral ingestion is its traditional route. Inhalation or injection would probably be a more efficient means of absorption. LSD-25, and all the lysergic acids, are central nervous system stimulants which specifically act on the neurotransmitter *serotonin*. The route of transmission is through the bloodstream.

Serotonin-sensitive neurosynapses appear to function differently than those sensitive to norepinephrine. Whereas norepinephrine-mimicking substances (cocaine, amphetamine, mescaline, etc.) stimulate the part of the brain associated with sensory arousal (a reticular formation, the ARAS), LSD and the other serotonin-sensitive substances seem to augment, expand, and otherwise alter the sensory imput itself, especially visual and auditory types. From studies dating back as far as 1943, in reference to this latter regard, it appears that visual and auditory imput are often mixed up. This type of sensory short-circuiting may occur to a lesser extend with the senses of taste, touch, and smell. Hence, subjects have been known to see sounds, hear odors, and the like (or so they seem). Such sensations and the hallucinations caused by them are different than equally vivid hallucinations caused by mescaline and psilocybin. LSD hallucinations do not seem to involve the regular visual patterns and colors common to the latter substances, but rather seem more "personal," involving free-association imagery. This involves an almost random combination of images, memories, and emotions. Psychological and environmental factors play an important part in image formation. Hence no two individuals will have the same reactions to this substance, nor will the same individual have the same "trip" twice.

An interesting effect of the intoxication-hallucination cycle which *does* often occur in diverse individuals is that termed loosely in the popular press as an "out-of-body" experience (OBE) in which the victim may suddenly find him or herself "looking" at themselves from some other vantage point, and having an impression of being able to wander off elsewhere for a brief period. This particular syndome may cause the greatest hazard, especially of the victim is operating a vehicle or machine at that moment.

In LSD caused hallucinations, perceptions of time, space, and events are commonly disassociated to the point of total abstraction. Not all individuals are equally effected; some may "trip off" easily while others may suffer only minor manifestations (such as the abstraction of linear time) and may be otherwise not outwardly effected by the drug.

LSD has a syndrome known as a "flashback," in which a victim may have a toxic reoccurance hours, days, weeks, or in some cases, months following their initial reaction. In virtually all instances this reoccurance will come during a period of normal consciousness. One probable theory is that: a) only a small dosage is required for an episode, b) the manifestation only occurs through serotonin synapses in the brain, and c) LSD may be stored in the body fat where it is not immediately metabolized/detoxified. Therefore a minute residual left in the body could, within some given period of time, find itself re-released into the bloodstream and find its way back to the brain. Flashbacks seem to occur mainly in the primates and not among white rats, which are the traditional toxicologist's study fare. There may be a lesson in this as regards the testing of neurosubstances.

LSD-25 is excreted through the liver and kidneys. After about 8 hours only a small amount remains in the blood. However, only about 8% of the dosage is excreted within 12 hours, fueling speculation as to how much remains in the body and for how long a period.

An initial dose of 1 µg per kilogram of body weight (between 200 and 400 µg in most adults) is sufficient to trigger an intoxication-hallucination syndrome.

LSD-25 is not without adverse effects. Doses as low as 30 µg have been known to cause dizziness, vomiting, intestinal paralysis, along with paralysis of arms and legs. But then, the toxic cycle of this substance has not been fully explored to differentiate the psychological from the psysiological traumas. Deaths have been noted due to respiratory failure although no specific neurological explanations have been uncovered in those cases. Again, severe psychological trauma is possible through LSD-25 and a neurological basis for psychosis has been upheld through experimental models.

Tolerance to LSD-25 can develop but usually exists for two days or less. Dosages up to 1.5 mg have been noted.

Extraction

Extracted by various organic solvents from aqueous alkaline solutions of ergot alkaloids.

Other formulations

Lysergide -25 d-Tartrate. $(LSD)_2 \bullet C_4H_6O_6 \cdot 2CH_3O_6$. Elongated crystals formed in methanol solution. Soluble in water.

Related substances:

Lysergic acid. Structure identical to LSD-25 except that the $NOC(C_2H_5)_2$ group of the latter is replaced by a simple COOH (carboxyl) group. Similar but less intense to LSD-25. Behaves as either an acid or a base. Soluble in pyridine. Slightly soluble in water and pH neutral organic solvents and in dilute sulphuric acid. Completely soluble in sodium hydroxide (NaOH), ammonium hydroxide (NH_4OH), sodium carbonate (Na_2CO_3) and hydrochloric acid (HCl). Molecular weight 268.32.

Detection

CHROMOTOPOGRAPHY

Paper: use system P1-Rf 0.47. Location under UV light, blue fluorescence.

Location reagents: *idoplatinate spray,* weak reaction; *p-dimethylaminobenzaldehyde spray,* deep purple.

Thin-layer: use system T1-Rf 0.66.

Location reagent: *p-diethylaminobenzaldehyde spray,* blue.

System T9-Rf 0.60. Location under UV light, blue fluorescence.

Location reagent: *p-diethylaminobenzaldehyde spray,* blue.

COLOR TESTS

Micro: *sulphuric acid-formaldehyde test:* grey (sensitivity 1.0 µg); *ammonium molybdate test:* grey-green —— grey-blue (sensitivity 1.0 µg); *ammonium vanadate test:* grey (sensitivity 1.0 µg); *Vitali's test:* brown/brown/purple-brown.

Specific data

lethal dose

An single dose of about 2 gr would probably cause respiratory collapse.

incapacitating dose

Between 1 and 4 micrograms (ug).

solubility

Soluble in NaOH, NH_4OH, Na_2CO_3, HCl. Slightly soluble in dilute H_2SO_4, neutral pH organic solvents and water.

taste

Would have an oily, slightly acidic taste. However, a quantity large enough to actually taste would constitute an overdose.

molecular weight

323.4

1-(1-phenylcyclohexyl) piperdine
P C P
(phenylcyclidine)

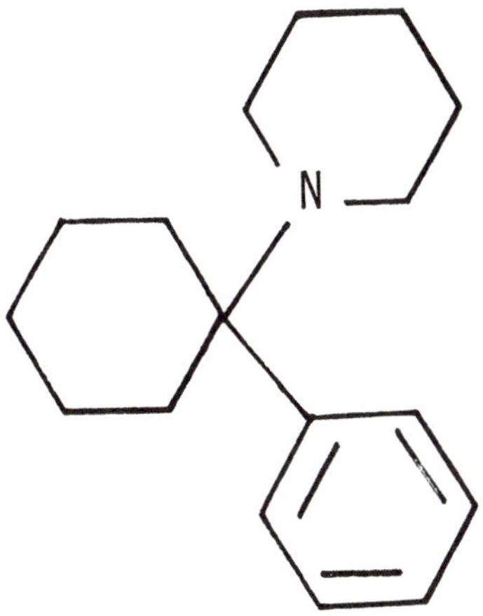

NOT this !

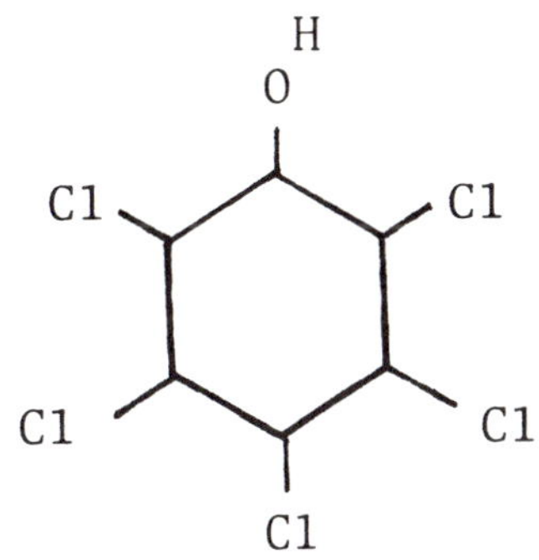

pentachloralphenol
P C P

insecticide - herbicide - wood preservative

Common names: PCP, HOG, angel dust *(note: often illicitly sold under the names "cannabinol" or "THC" which it is* NOT. *See following section for actual cannabis structures.)*

Type: analgesic and anesthetic

Use: analgesic and anesthetic (not FDA approved for human use except under experimental conditions); hallucinogen

Trade names: Sernyl, Sernylan

A crystalline white powder, most commonly found as a hydrochloride. Produces anesthesia through dissociation rather than by neural suppression. Hallucinogen. Bad side effects.

Military hazard

Phenylcyclidine, like LSD, is too potent a substance to be used directly as a military agent. Quantities that would be required for area contamination could produce lethal toxic reactions among victims. Furthermore, although producing auditory and visual hallucinations not unlike those of the amphetamines, phenylcyclidine is an extremely effective anesthetic. It will obliviate its victims to all pain without neccessarily rendering them unconscious. An enemy suffering less than incapacitating dosages would not be near as effective a fighter as when sober, but he or she might have to be killed outright to be stopped.

Effects against the rear of an opponent, to command, logistical, and support functions would be effective much in the way LSD-25 might be, and under the same criteria.

To be made environmentally stable, phenylcyclidine would have to be microencapsulated or the like. This would result in a super fine powder which might present an enormous downwind hazard.

Metabolism and pathology

Phenylcyclidine was first synthesized in 1956 as a potential anesthetic. It became the first in a series of anesthetics which do not induce anesthesia through the neural synapses as with the traditional sedative-hypnotic class of anesthetics. Nor dies it seem to work any effect through norepinephrine, serotonin, or dopamine synapses in the brain..

The actions of this "dissociative anesthetic" occur in the brain rather than in the peripheral nervous system. In ways not completely understood, it seperates its victims from their physical selves, or at least their objective awareness of its functioning or responses. The patient, or victim, usually remains conscious and no significant depression of cardiovascular or respiratory functions occurs at the noraml anesthetic dosage of about 0.2 mg per 1 kg of total body weight.

Above that level toxic overdose effects occur, begining at around a total dose of 10 mg in a 150-160 lb adult. At this stage a mild state of excitement occurs concurrent with all the symptoms of gross intoxication. Amphetamine-like auditory and visual hallucinatations may occur, their impact heightened by the anesthesia. The victim typically recovers from this level of toxicity within 1 to 4 hours, with a general state of mental confusion disappearing between the 4th and 72nd hour.

Although sensitive individuals may incur extreme toxic effects at lower dosages, those effects occur in the 150-160 lb adult with dosages near or exceeding 1 gram. Severe agitation is not uncommon at this point, with the victim becoming belicose and violent. He or she may suffer great physical injury, aided and abeted by an inability to feel pain. As the toxicity takes further effect, muscle rigidity or spasms occur. Cardiovascular and respiratory spasms may occur as anesthesia gives way to stupor which in turn may degenerate into coma. Death is not unknown at this point, especially if further drug interactions are involved. If the victim survives, his or her general state of delusion may last for up to two weeks. Confusion or dissociation may in turn continue for a month or two.

Hospital records of chronic phenylcyclidine users are the principal source of long-term effects of this substance. Their diagnosises commonly contain reference to psychaitric disorders such as severe depression, anxiety, or paranoid psychosis. Conflicting theories exist, as with the case of

LSD, as to whether such phenomena are due to neurological changes, severe psychological trauma, or a mixture of such effects in personality types as are drawn to voluntary drug use.

The metabolism of phenylcyclidine is simple. Ingestion, inhalation, or injection all provide efficient entry for this water soluble substance. It efficiently enters into the bloodstream and quickly passes the blood-brain barrier. It is slowly metabolized and excreted through the liver and kidneys. Detoxification of the substance appears to proceed at a somewhat slow pace, as evidenced by the withdrawal periods associated with overdosage.

Extraction

Phenylcyclidine is synthesized, extracted from alkaline solution by various organic solvents.

Other formulations

Phenylcyclidine hydrochloride. Phenylcyclidine • HCl. Forms crystalline solid soluble in water or ethanol.

Phenylcyclodine hydrobromide. Phenylcyclidine • HBr. Forms crystalline solid soluble in water or ethanol.

Anesthetic similar in structure and action:

Ketamine (trade name *Ketalar*). Does not produce the promounced behavioral changes or hallucinations that are common the phenylcyclidine. Approved as a limited use anesthetic for human. Unsaturated nitro-benzene ring replaced by $NHCH_3$ group; unsaturated C_6H_5 group has oxygen bond; saturated C_2H_5 group has a chlorine bond replacing a hydrogen bond.

Detection

CHROMOTOPOGRAPHY

Paper: use system P1-Rf 0.80

Location reagents: *iodoplatinate spray;* strong reaction.
bromocresol green spray, weak reaction.

Using system RP1a-Rf 0.53. Location under UV light-absorption.

Using system RP1b-Rf 0.00. Location same as RP1a.

Thin layer: use system T1-Rf 0.59.

Location reagent: *acidified iodoplatinate spray,* positive reaction.

Gas: use system G2/225 with retention time 1.3 relative to *diphenhydramine.*

Using system G4 — retention time 0.84 relative to *diphenhydramine.*

CRYSTAL TESTS

Micro: *gold bromide solution.* — small oily crystals — view under polarized light (sensitivity 1 in 1000); *potassium permanganate solution* — small irregular plates (sensitivity 1 in 1000).

ULTRAVIOLET ABSORPTION SPECTRUM

Phenylcyclidine in solution at pH 2, maxima at 253 mμ, 258 mμ, 263 mμ, and 269 mμ (E 1% 1 cm 15); in 0.1 N *sulphuric acid,* maxima at 252.5 mμ (E 1% 1 cm 8), 257.5 mμ (E 1% 1 cm 10.9), 262.5 mμ (E 1% 1 cm 12.3), 269 mμ (E 1% 1 cm 9.2).

INFRARED ABSORPTION SPECTRUM

Phenylcyclidine hydrochloride, *potassium bromide disk:* Principal peaks at A 1466, B 700, C 760.

Specific data

lethal dose

Possible in dosages exceeding 1 gram.

incapacitating dose

Typically, when dosage exceeds the 0.2 mg per kg of total body weight. Common at about 10 mg total dosage (150 -160 lb adult).

solubility

Soluble in water and ethanol.

taste

Oily , slightly ammoniac. Tasting not recommended.

molecular weight

243.38

Substances sometimes considered for deployment or restructure as military incapacitating agents but lacking sufficient potency

Diagrams and descriptions of the following substances:

- cannabis
- methaqualone
- nitrazepam

Cannabis

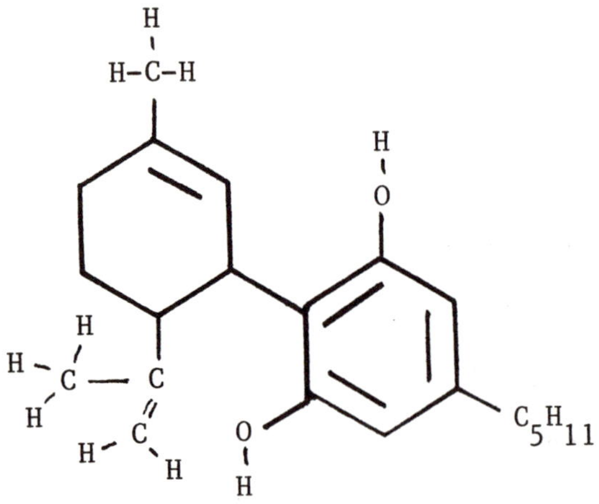

CANNABIDOIL (CBD)

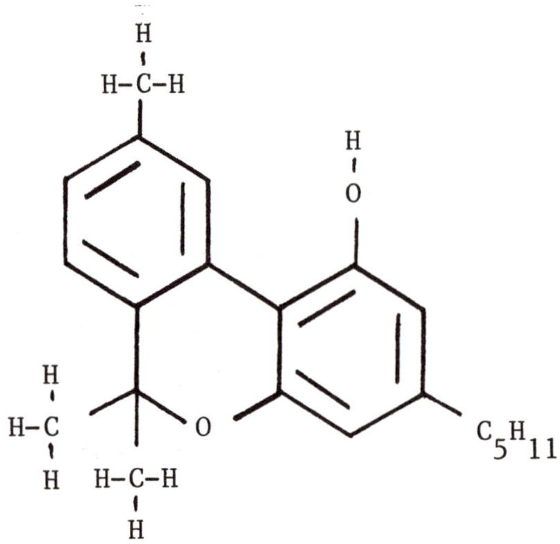

CANNABINOL (CBN)

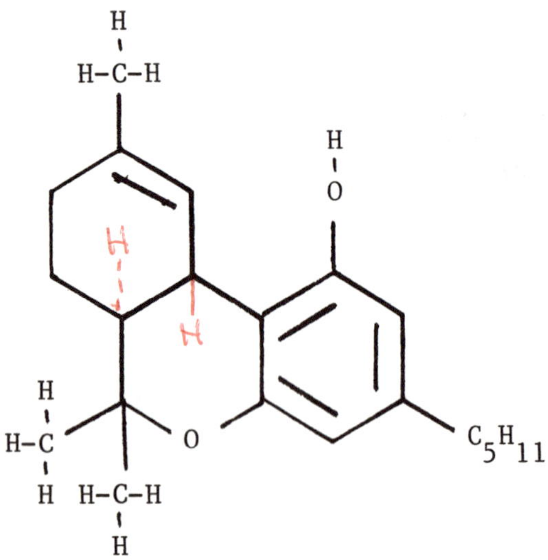

Δ^9-THC (Δ^1-THC)

← ISOMERIC →
TETRAHYDROCANNABINOLS

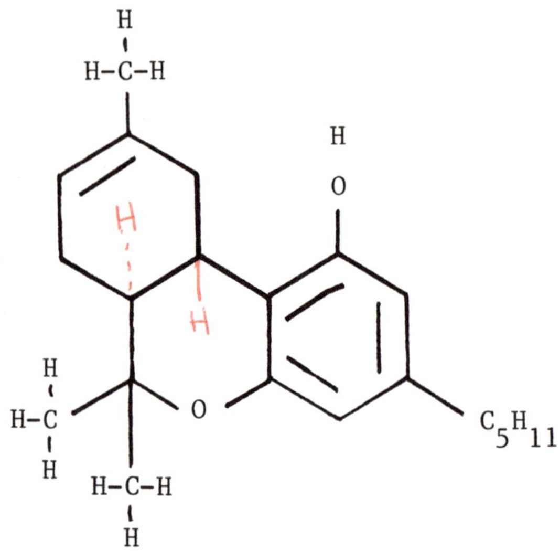

Δ^8-THC ($\Delta^{1(6)}$-THC)

Chemical names: cannabidoil; cannabinol; Δ^9-THC (Δ^1-THC); and Δ^8-THC ($\Delta^{1(6)}$-THC). Principal components.

Found in: dried flowering tips of pistillate plants of *cannabis sativa*, known variously as Indian hemp, India cannabis, marihuana, marijuana, bhang, ganja, charas, kif, hasach, hasish, pot.

Type: central nervous system depressant

Actions: intoxicant; mildly hallucinogenic

2-methyl-3-(2-methylphenyl)-4(3H)-quinazolinone (methaqualone)

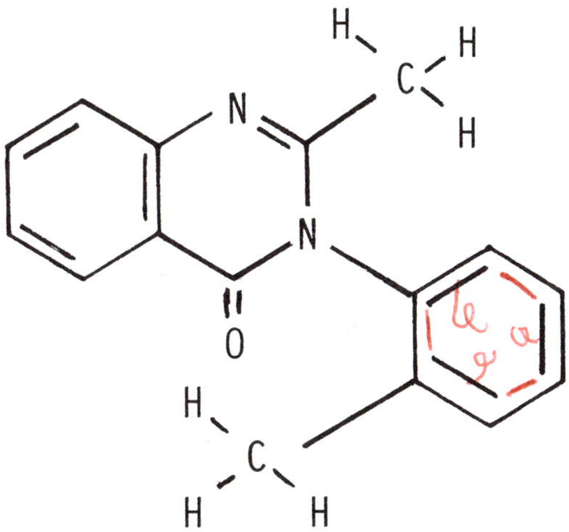

molecular weight
250.3

Other names: metoquizolone; MAOA; MTQ; ortonal; QZ-2; RIC 272; Rorer 148; TR 495; Tuazolon.

Proprietary names: Cateudyl; Citexal; Dormigoa; Dormogen; Dormutil; Dorsedin; Fadormir; Holodorm; Hymnial; Hypocol; Hyptor; Inofil; Melsomin; Mollinox; Motolon; Nobedorm; Noctilene; Normi-Nox; Omnyl; Optinoxan; Parminal; Parest; Quaalude *(the origion of the nickname "ludes")*; Roulone; Rouqualone; Sindesvel; Somnafac; Sonal; Somberol; Somnomed; Sopor; Soverin; Torinal; Tuazolone.

Type: central nervous system depressant.

Actions: similar action to morphine.

1,2-dihydro-7-nitro-2-oxo-5-phenyl-3H-1,4,benzo-diazepine

(nitrazepam)

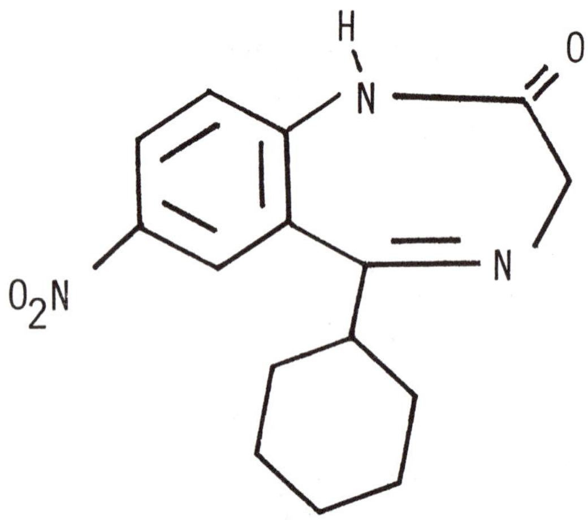

molecular weight
281.3

Proprietary names: Megadon; Mogadon
Type: hypnotic (sleep-inducing substance)

Requires dosages of about 5 mg. Controlled dosages of up to 300 mg show no toxic side-effects. A yellow crystalline powder insoluble in water and thus uneffected by most adverse weather conditions. Also insoluble in ether. Soluble in ethanol and chloroform. Its effects are not as pronounced as the mind-altering substances although it would profoundly amplify the effects of stress and fatigue.

Organic solvent capable
of skin penetration
with
drug assimilation

DMSO

dimethyl sulfoxide
(DMSO)

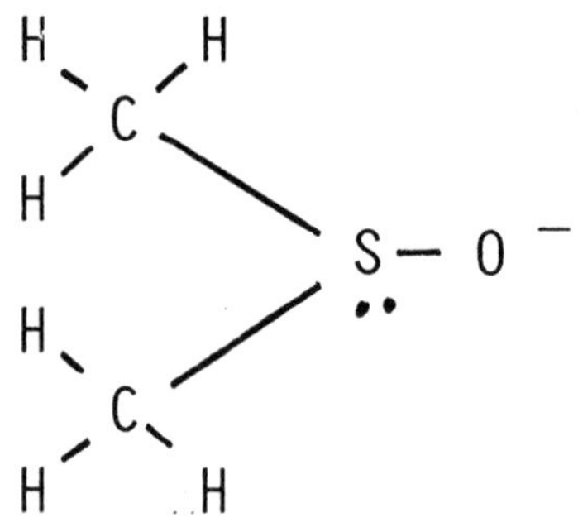

Pharmaceutical quality DMSO is used alone as an anti-inflammatory , or as a penetrant carrier for other drugs.

DMSO was first obtained as a byproduct of paper manufacture from wood pulp when dimethyl sulfide, used to reduce wood fibers oxidized in the presence of certain concurrent nitrogen oxide reduction reactions. The two main patents for DMSO production are held by Aktiebolaget Centrallaboratorium (1952) and Crown Zellerbach (1962), both paper producers.

The origional isolated solvent contained toxic nitrogen compound impurities. Pharmaceutical quality DMSO does not cause the redness, itching, and scaling associated with industrial quality DMSO (used as an industrial solvent).

DMSO is an extremely effective penetrating solvent. Its :S-O$^-$ bond readily combines with, then drops, other hydrocarbon, and many nonorganic bonds. DMSO penetrates the skin of the average person as water might penetrate a sponge, as its unique bonding qualities allow it to carry any number of substances along with it. These could include both casualty and incapacitating agents otherwise incapable of skin penetration. Carried through the skin by DMSO, the effect of such agents would be immediate, if not catastrophic.

Comparative Tables

Structural similarities between certain neurologically active substances having military potential

Neurotransmitter, *noradrenaline* *(norepinephrine)*

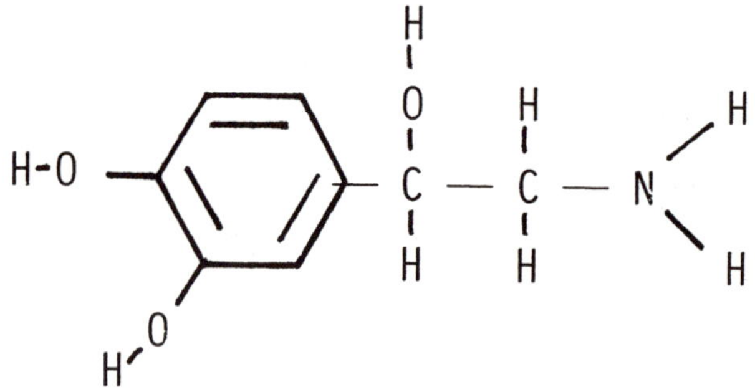

The amphetamines (central nervous system stimulants)

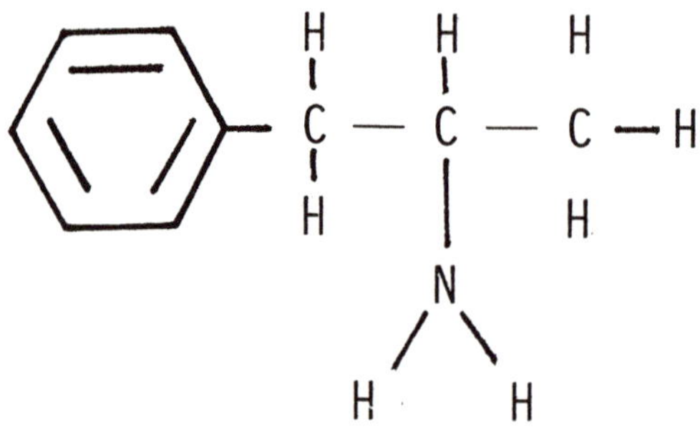

amphetamine

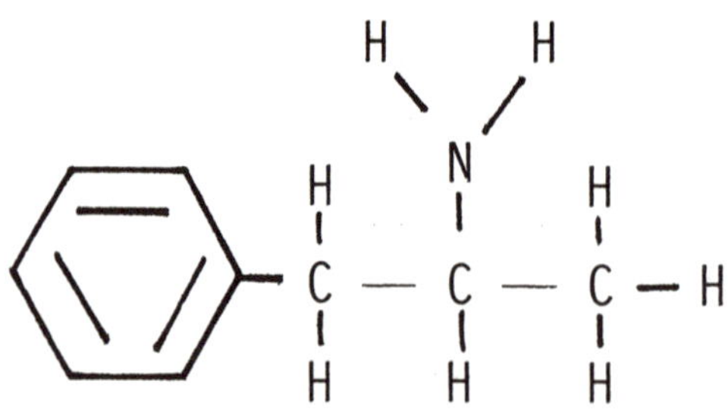

dextramphetamine

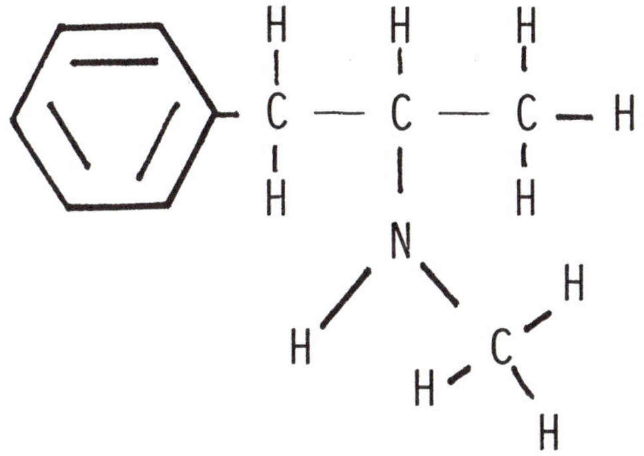

methylamphetamine

Mescaline (psychedelic) and its derivatives

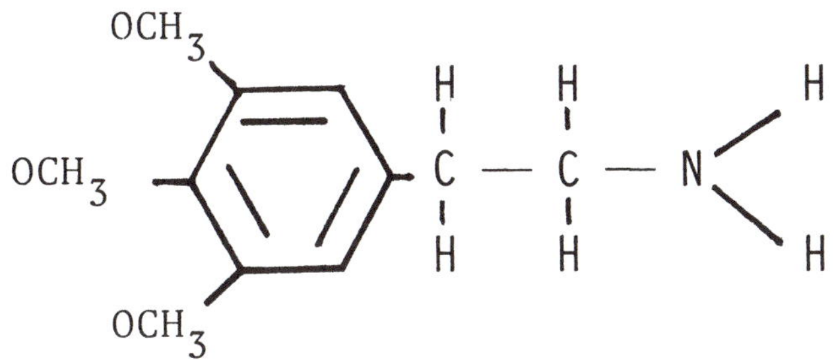

mescaline

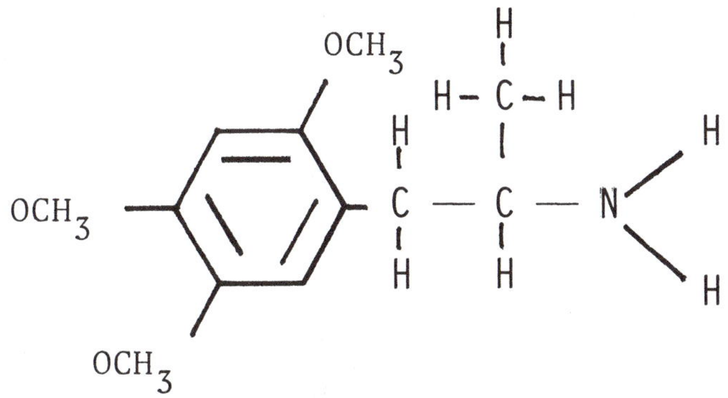

DOM (STP, "speed")

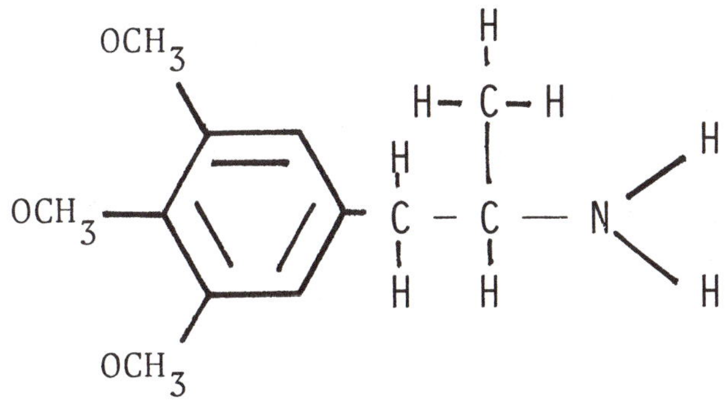

TMA

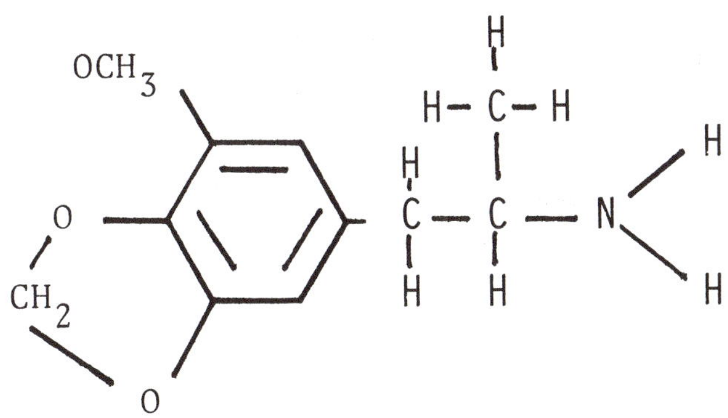

MMDA

Neurotransmitter, *serotonin*

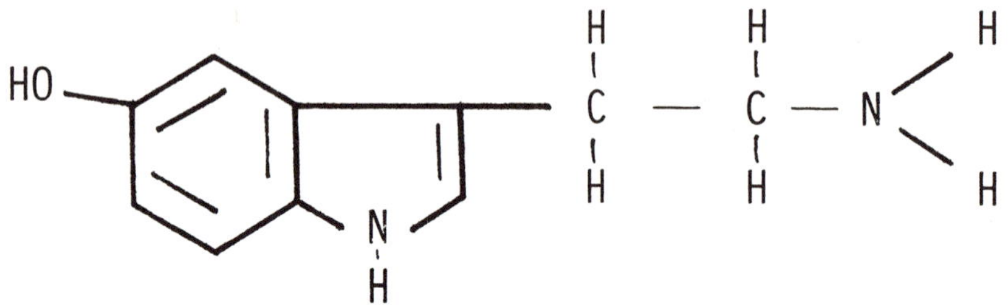

Psychodelic substances resembling serotonin

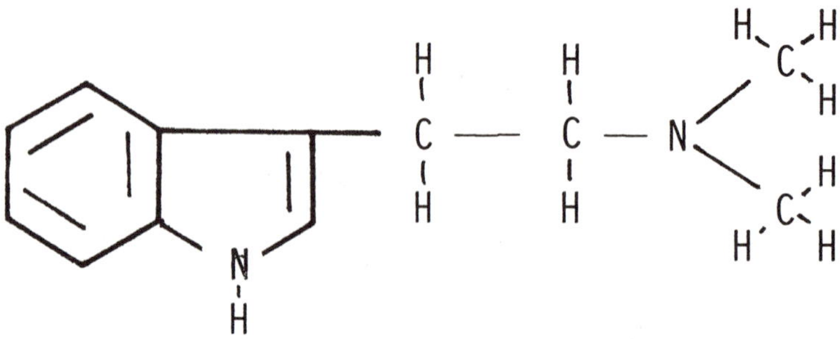

Dimethyltriptamine
(DMT)

from *amanita muscaria*

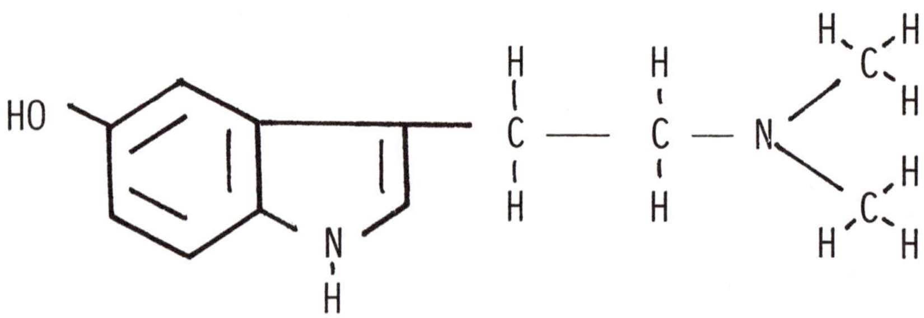

Bufotenine

from *amanita muscaria*

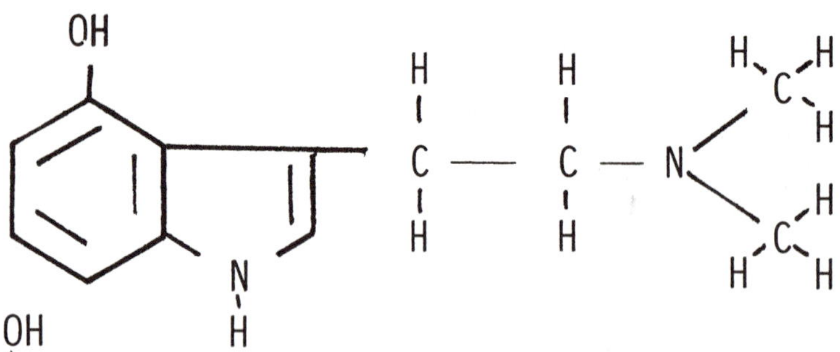

Psilocin

from *psilocybe mexicana*

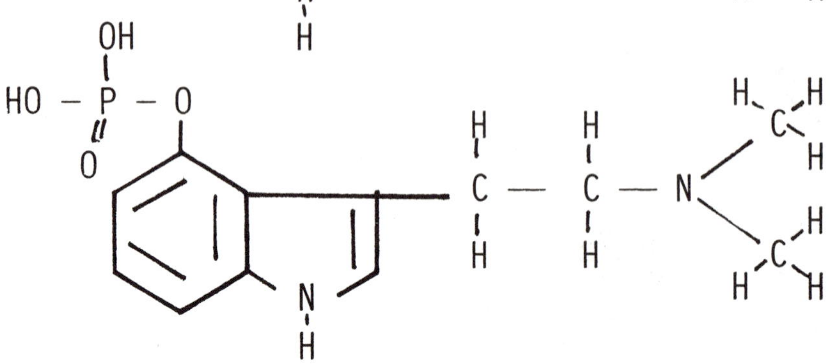

Psilocybin

from *psilocybe mexicana*

REFERENCES

American Medical Association. AMA Department of drugs, with the American Society for Clinical Pharmacology and Therapeutics. *AMA drug evaluations, third edition.* Littleton, MA. PSG Publishing Co. 1977.

Brecher, Edward M. and the editors of Consumer Reports. *Licit and illicit drugs.* Boston. Little, Brown. 1972.

Clarke, E.C.C., ed. *Isolation and identification of drugs.* London. The Pharmaceutical Press. 1978

Clayton, George D. and Clayton, Florence E., eds. *Patty's industrial hygiene and toxicology, third revised edition.* New York. John Wiley & Sons. 1978.

Crone, Hugh. *Chemicals & Society, a guide to the new chemical age.* New York. Cambridge University Press. 1986.

Giese, Friedo. *Beilstein's index, trivial names in systemic nomenclature of organic chemistry.* Berlin. Springer-Verlag. 1986.

Julien, Robert M. *Principles of drug action, second edition.* San Francisco. W.H. Freeman & Co. 1978.

Lingeman, Richard R. *Drugs from A to Z, a dictionary.* New York. McGraw-Hill. 1974.

McCloud, Don, et al, eds. *Drug information primer, an introduction to selected psychactive drugs.* University of Oregon Drug Information Center. 1977

NIOSH. Lewis, Richard and Sweet, Doris, eds. *Registry of toxic effects of chemical substances.* Cincinnati. U.S. Department of Health and Social Services, Centers for Disease Control, National Institute for Occupational Safety and Health. 1985.

Perry, Paul S., et al, eds. *Psychotrophic drug handbook, third edition.* Cincinatti. Harvey Whitting Books.

Sax, Irving and Lewis, Richard J. *Rapid quide to industrial chemicals in the workplace.* New York. Van Nostrand & Co. 1986

Smith, David E., ed. *Amphetamine use, misuse, and abuse.* Boston. G.K. Hall. 1979.

Windholz, Martha, et al, eds. *The Merck index, an encyclopedia of chemicals and drugs, tenth edition.* Rahway NJ. Merck & Co. 1983

SPECIAL REFERENCE

Douglass, Joseph L. and Livingstone, Neil C. *America the vulnerable, the threat of chemical/biological warfare, the new shape of terrorism and conflict.* Lexington, MA. Lexington Books. 1987.

Harris, Robert and Paxman, Jeremy. *A higher form of killing, the secret story of chemical and biological warfare.* New York. Wang and Hill. 1982.

Chapter Seven

B I O T O X I N S

ORDER

The United States renounces offensive preparations for and the use of toxins as a method of warfare.

The United States will confine its military programs for toxins, whether produced by bacteriological or any other biological method or by chemical synthesis, to research for defensive purposes only, such as to improve techniques of immunization and medical therapy. I have directed the destruction of all existing toxin stocks and weapons which are not required for a research program for defensive purposes only.

The United States will have no need to operate any facilities capable of producing toxins either bacteriologically or biologically in large quantities and therefore also capable of producing biological agents.

Richard Milhouse Nixon

President of the United States
14 Febuary 1970

Definition

Toxins, in between the biological and chemical agents, are the poisonous by-products of microorganisms, plants and animals. Toxins tend to be more stable than microorganisms because they are not living. Some toxins have the advantage, such as ricin and botulinus toxin, of being relatively easy to manufacture, and of being extremely toxic — even more toxic than nerve agents on an equal-weight basis.

Douglass, Joseph D. and Livingstone, Neil C.
America the vulnerable, p.13

Soviet military literature views the biotoxins as comprizing a "third generation" of chemical weapons. As they have assigned these such importance, it would not be unreasonable to expect further developments of the biotoxins from the Soviets, who are painstaking in weapons research.

Terrorists in the Western nations have already been known to have at least cultured some of these substances, notably botulinus toxin.

This chapter will discuss three well-researched toxins. The author does not wish to speculate about rumors of even more effective biotoxins, such as those derived from cobra venom or shellfish, until more research data is available. The following three are potent enough:

- botulinus
- ricin
- tricothecene

Botulinus Toxin

once known as Agent BTX

Description

Botulinus toxin is a neuropoison produced by a bacterium, *clostridium botulium*, which effects the release of acetylcholine in a manner similar to the nerve agents.

Unlike the nerve agents, botulinus works slowly in the body, effecting the peripheral system within 12 to 36 hours of ingestion. The toxic syndrome is known as *botulism.* In normal circumstances botulism is a result of eating improperly canned foodstuffs. As a military toxin it would be cultured directly from the bacterium.

Botulinus toxin actually refers to any of eight distinct but related toxins, long amino acid complexes, created by the metabolism of the bacterium as it breaks down organic matter. The eight toxins have been designated A, B, C_1, C_2, D, E, F, and G. Types C_1, C_2, and D are not commonly absorbed through the gastrointestinal tract. Types A, B, and E are responsible for most human poisonings. Type E is produced by the actions of the bacterium with seafoods.

Type E botulinus should not be confused with certain natural toxins produced by some shellfish.

Botulinus toxin(s) will be destroyed by heat. Temperatures at or near the boiling point of water (100°C or 212°F) would be sufficient. The spores of the actual bacterium are heat-resistant short of flame, although it is the toxin and not the bacterium or bacterium spores that cause botulism.

Botulinus toxin is produced by multiplying bacilli at normal room temperatures (20°-30°C or 68°-86°F) in contaminated food having a pH of 6.0 or above (barely acidic to alkaline) in the absense of air. Growing cultures produce gas (mostly carbon dioxide) as a waste product and contaminated canned goods typically bulge, often to the bursting point. The same conditions which produce botulinus by accident may be used to deliberately culture the toxin, which may be seperated from a protein "soup" by centrifuge and filtration. The toxins are easy to produce.

Pathological course

Natural botulinus toxin poisoning involves small dosages and symptoms occur between 12 and 36 hours, with some cases being within as little as 6 hours or as late as 8 days.

Deliberate botulinus toxin poisoning might produce acute symptoms well within an hour. Doses of the toxin(s) as small as one-tenth to one microgram (0.1-1.0 μg) have been known to kill. Significant dosages in grams might prove quickly fatal. Ingestion is a more efficient means of infection than injection or entry through wounds.

Botulinus toxin first effects the gastrointestinal tract causing cramps, constipation, vomiting and finally nausea. Blurred vision and the impression of eyestrain follow next by double vision and a feeling of vertigo. The eyelids will involuntarily droop as the toxin begins to effect muscle coordination and strength.[1] At this point the small muscles of the hands and feet, and then the arms and legs will feel increasingly weak. Throughout these symptoms the victim will maintain normal consciousness and judgement.

Minor poisoning may not progress beyond this point, with a lessening of symptoms over a period of days. The victim may require long periods of inactivity (rest) or light duties.

Severe poisoning progresses to effect the major skeletal muscles and then in involuntary muscles of first the respiratory tract. Breathing must be a deliberate affair. Next to be effected is the cardiovascular system. Most of those who

1. Reported cases of partial facial paralysis are common to acute poisonings.

die from accute botulinus toxin poisoning succumb to heart failure. Those who survive accute poisoning may take several months to recover.

Use as a casualty-producing substance

The effects of botulinus toxin have been known for millennia, ever since man began to store processed foodstuffs, especially meats and gravies. The toxin has been seperated for a number of centuries and has long been used by the professional poisoner and his or her political clients.

Serious study of botulinus toxin as a military agent did not occur until the 1930s, when the father of the Japanese chemical and biological program, major (later general) Shiro Ishii began a study program in occupied China during 1935. Major Ishii had been impressed by a naturally occuring epidemic of cholera among Japanese troops a few months prior (and equine anthrax a few months later). He established a research center at the village of Pinfang in Manchuria for the study of militarily-significant diseases and toxins. The first experiments were on draft animals, then on prisoners. Naturally, the word got out.

A crash program began at the British chemical laboratories at Porton Down to isolate and develop strains of *clostridium botulium* with antidotes and treatments for each. A toxins mix was developed, which recieved the formal code of BTX. This represented the maximum potential which might be encountered from the Axis powers. As of 1987 the research files are still sealed.

Botulinus toxin is thought to have been used by British MI6 (Military Intelligence 6, foreign counter-intelligence operations) to do away with Reinhard Heydrich, Hitler's governor of Czechoslavakia and presumed heir. A group of Czech partisans operating out of MI6 ambushed Heydrich in the countryside. Heydrich was slightly wounded and even chased a few of his ambushers down the road with pistol in hand. Heyrich's Mercedes had been hit with an antitank projectile filled with some sort of semi-liquid mix. Four days later Heydrick, who felt weak in the late AM dropped dead in the early PM of classic botulin poisoning. German lab reports were either lost or destroyed in the war as to both the canister and its contents.

If botulin toxin *did* kill Heydrich, it would be a good example of how the toxin operates through wounds rather than through injestion. The toxin would not slowly penetrate the body from the intestines but would accumulate in the main neural centers until significant dosage(s) existed to take fatal effect, with normal medical treatment mostly ineffective. WITH Most of the Japanese records being destroyed, contemporary collaborative studies are not possible. Other Allied intelligence projects were of small scale. BTX was not used as a military weapon for the same reasons that the chemical casualty agents were not used.

Postwar stuides in the United States, Great Britain, France, and elsewhere determined that botulinus toxin would present a significant contaminant hazard to public water and food supplies. Studies were made up through the early 1960s in which imitation or (normally) non-toxic but easily traceable organisms and their by-products were released on a large scale. The inferences drawn concerning botulin toxin were that although degraded in the environment, it would present a significant hazard for a number of hours. However, microencapsulation techniques developed in the 1970s and 1980s could expand that time frame to weeks or months.

In 1980 French police and intelligence personnel raided a "safe house" used by the German "Red Army Faction" group of terrorists at 41A Chaillot Street in Paris. The apartment contained a very simple but effective "bathtub" operation that was producing botulinus toxin.

Finally, on an equal-weight basis, botulinus toxin is more deadly than the nerve agents.[1] It lacks the rapid action of the nerve agents and is probably less effective than ricin or tricothecene by the same time criteria.

1. It doesn't kill any faster (in fact, toxins work much slower); it just takes a lot less to do the job.

Ricin (glycoprotein toxin)

Description

Ricin toxin is refined from a natural series of glycoproteins occuring in the castor bean plant *ricinus communis* of the family *euphorbiaceae*. The active component of this toxin is *ricinine:*

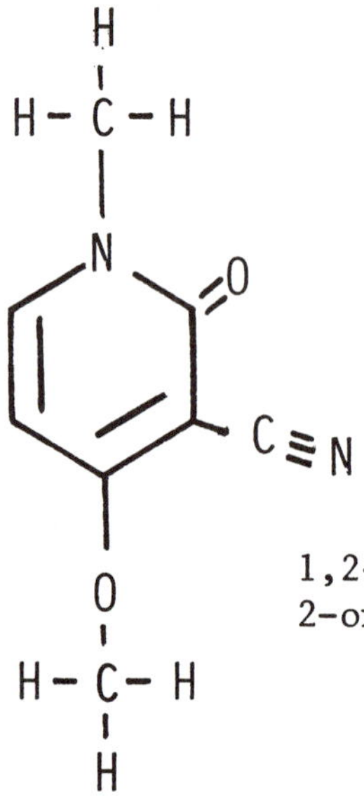

RICININE (ricidine)

1,2-dihydro-4-methoxy-1-methyl-2-oxo-pyridinecarbonitrile

mol. wt. 164.16

Ricin is refined from the seeds and leaves of the plant. The pure chemical would probably BE more effective than the whole glycoprotein, but as some sources claim it may be 1000 times as deadly as VX[1], the point is moot. The substance is more easily derived from the natural source than it is synthesized. Ricin is slightly soluble in water, alcohol, chloroform, and ether. It will not form salts with acids.

Ricin is a phenylcyanide compound with a passing resemblance to certain of the barbituates and other neuroreactive compounds.

1. see ff, p.342

Pathology

The toxicology of ricin depends to some extend on the manner in which it enters the body. If swallowed, some portion of it will be diluted or altered in the intestines, but not before causing bloody diarrhea and (depending on dosage) damage to the liver and kidneys. Its neuroenzyme interruptive effects would be more pronounced if ricin were directly injected into the body. It appears to have a rapid effect on the central nervous system, suppressing heart function to the point of hypotension. Rapidly penetrating the brain-blood barrier, and immediately blocking synapse actions there, ricin typically produces convulsions (which should not be confused with tremors elsewhere due to cholinesterase interference) and death.

Ricin(ine) does not occur naturally in significant quantities to produce more than nausea or vomiting from accidental ingestion. Abnormally large quantities of castor seeds and leaves would have to be eaten, so small is the natural occurence, highly potent though the substance may be. Death from ricin would be a deliberate act.

Use as a casulty-producing substance

Castor-seed poisoning predates the Borgias. Examination of *ricinus communis* and the seperation of ricinine did not occur until early this century and the first major medical analysis is probably that of Böttcher in 1918.

Ricin poisoning does not now constitute a threat to large bodies of personnel or their supplies. This is not to say that facilities for toxin synthesis in bulk do not already exist somewheres or that they might not be built in the future. Microencapsulation to protect it from the elements and make it victim-selective by which enzymes could dissolve the microscopic-sized protein jackets. Rather than use as a general agent, ricin would probably be used against military and civillian command/leadership elements.

Selective deployment fits ricin's role in this century with the cloak-and-dagger set. It makes a better assassin's weapon than hydrocyanic acid (AC)-in-the-eyes and other older methods. Both the British and the Soviets examined ricin for its covert potentials from the late 1930s to the 1960s, and the major published works concerning ricin have origionated in Czechoslovakia and Hungary since the 1940s. Ricin is a current assassin's weapon [see below] which has come to pose a threat in more than military affairs. Counterintelligence agencies of the more militant nations have been familiar with ricin since the 1960s. Terrorists (under the aegis and abilities of their various sponsers) are familiar with ricin. And so are the entrepreneurs. In one publicized event, occuring in the Spring of 1984, two brothers in Springfield, Massachusetts were apprehended by the FBI. Taken in evidence was a 35mm film cannister holding about 1 oz of ricin. The brothers had apparently planned their own retail sales operation, and had founded a company (Specialty Chemicals Inc) that advertised the stuff for public sale.

The ricin umbrella

As we all know, nobody *really* believes in ideology, power politics, and that sort of thing. Given half a chance the world would be one great love fest, and beyond a lot of rhetoric the people of the world are really all brothers and sisters with everything in common. If we would all just hold hands and with faith in heart, sing the songs of peace all the boogey men would go away. Right?

A misunderstanding occured in September of 1978 to the person of Georgi Markov. Georgi was a former Bulgarian journalist and writer who had gone to live in England where he worked for the BBC in London as a commentator. On the 7th of September he walked up the Waterloo Bridge steps to the BBC studios when a stranger bumped into him. Markov was poked in the thigh with the stranger's umbrella. After mutual apologies the two men parted. That evening Markov developed a fever and his blood pressure began to drop. Two days later his heart stopped. His wife had Scotland Yard perform a detailed autopsy in their forensic lab. Removed was a small metal ball, about the size of the "ball" in a ballpoint pen. It was made of a platinum-iridium alloy and had four holes in it.

About this time, a friend of Markov's, and a former Bulgarian writer turned journalist himself, read about his colleague's death. This man, Vladimir Kostov, recalled how he, too, had been jabbed with an umbrella, only on the Paris Metro. He, too, had developed a fever, but it had subsided after about four days. Kostov went to the police, who had a platinum-iridium pellet removed from his back. French police pathologists took the pellet to Scotland Yard who in turn called in a toxicological team from Porton Down.

Kostov's pellet was like Markov's. Apparently it had lodged in fatty tissue and the wax sealing up its pinpoint holes had not immediately melted nor had all the agent, which spectral analysis showed to be ricin, entered Kostov.

In 1980, a Soviet citizen was seeing the sights of Tyson's Corner, Virginia. After being jabbed with an umbrella he quickly called some American friends up the road in Washington, DC. He died en route to the hospital at Fairfax, Virginia. The local police claimed that the death was under suspicious circumstances and that under the laws of the State of Virginia an autopsy had to be performed. The

Soviet embassy protested against one of its citizens being dissected and filed a sharp series of protests with the US State Department. As a coroner's jury looked on, the autopsy was finally performed. A platinum-iridium alloy ball was removed. The ball was kept by the American friends while the victim, Boris Korczak, was sent to his final resting place aboard an otherwise empty Aeroflot plane.

A number of people have died from these mysterious ricin filled metal balls. A number of people, from the British Labor leader Hugh Gaitskell to the Algerian statesman Houari Boumédienne have died from ricin-like symptoms.

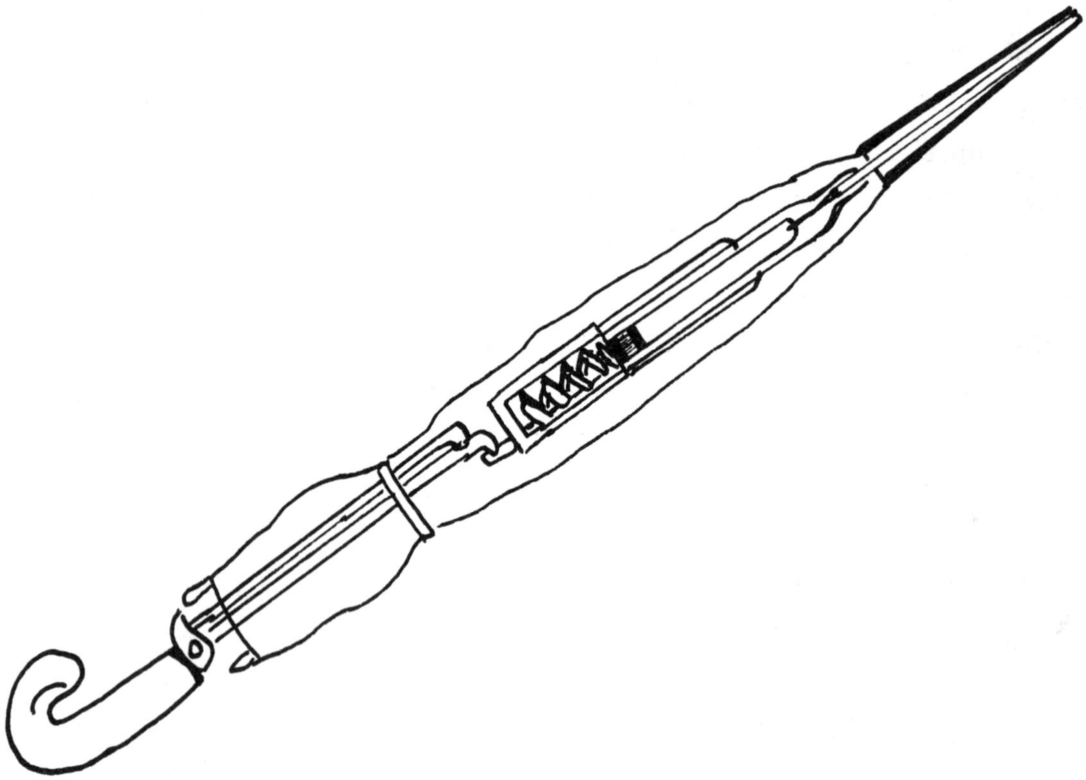

Tricothecene mycotoxins

T-2

Nivalenol

Dedication

This section is dedictaed to Dr R.V. Chalam, head of the Mission Valley [California] Toxicology Center for his assistance. Dr Chalam devised the standard chromotopography test for the detection of T-2 (tricothecene) mycotoxin appearing at the end of this section.

Description

Tricothecene mycotoxins are derived from the toxic contamination of such grains as wheat or corn and are a by-product of rot caused by *fusarium nivale*, *fusarium tricinctum*. These subtances were the cause of Soviet crop blight of the 1930s which killed thousands of persons and tens of thousands of cattle and horses. Tricothecene reamins a hazard to Soviet agriculture in spite of their biological expertise.

Tricothecene need not be laboratory purity to be of military importance. The opposite is true. A mix of a number of naturally occuring toxins is probably more effective.

Crude tricothecene is extracted from fungal contaminated corn or wheat meal slurry. The residue contains a number of related toxins. The final mix may be boosted with aflatoxins [see below].

The two key tricothecene mycotoxins are *Nivalenol* and *T-2*. Each is summarized below:

NIVALENOL 12,13-epoxy-3,4,7,15-tetrahydroxytrichotec-9-en-8-one

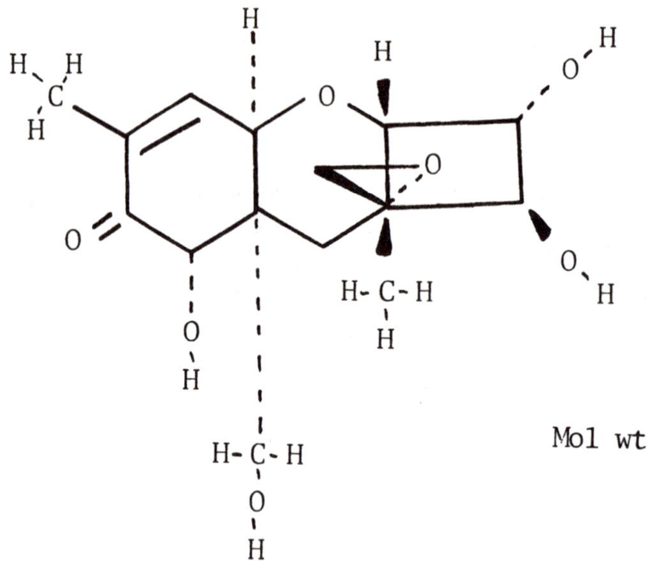

Mol wt 312.33

description

Tricothecene mycotoxin isolated from *fusarium nivale*. Soluble in methanol, ethanol, and other polar organic liquids. Slightly soluble in water.

effects

An extremely strong hemorrhagic substance. Causes immediate tissue necrosis. Also causes blisters, nausea and dizziness, vomiting and diarrhea. Untreated, it may lead to death. Its systemic toxicity is proportional to dosage.

T-2 12,13-epoxytricothec-9-ene-3,4,8,15-tetrol 4,15-diacetate 8-(3-methylbutanoate)

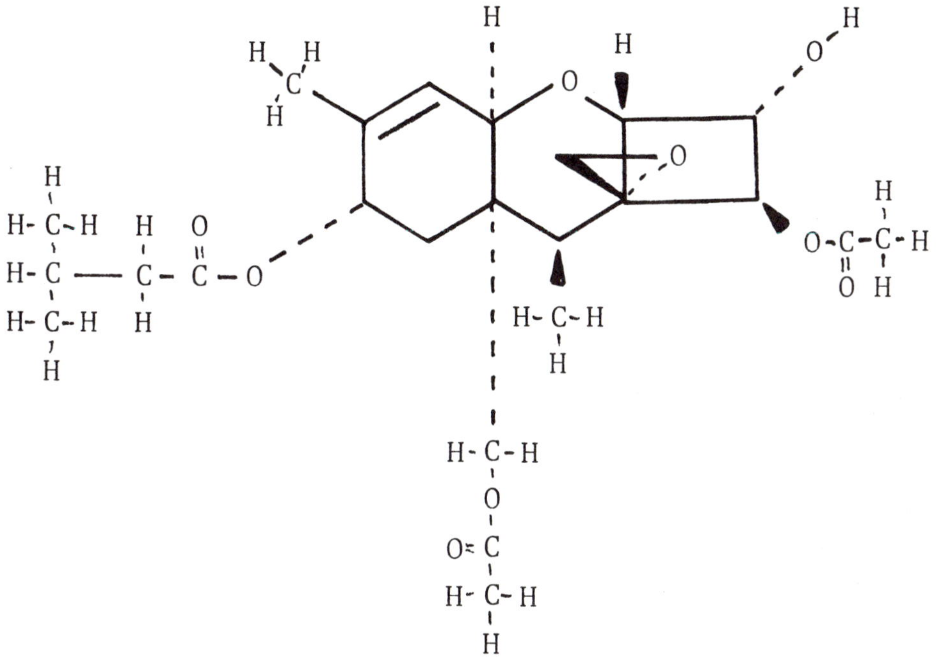

description

Tricothecene mycotoxin isolated from *fusarium tricinctum.* Soluble in methanol, ethanol.

effects

Caustic skin irritant and hemorrhagic, causing tissue necrosis on contact. Also causes blisters, nausea and dizziness, vomiting and diarrhea. Untreated, it may lead to death. Its systemic toxicity is proportional to dosage.

detection

(CHROMATOPOGRAPHY)

Primary extraction of T-2 toxin from organic solids

1. Extracted from organic matter with aqueous methanol.
2. Denature and precipitation of T-2 proteinaceous compounds with zinc acetate/aluminum chloride solution.

Refining

1. Toxin selectively partitioned into a benzene fraction and washed with a 1% potassium hydroxide solution to remove acidic compounds.
2. Extraneous materials removed by silica gel column chroma-topography using acetonitrile as an elutant. Acetonitrile removed by evaporation.
3. Hepafluorobutyryl imidazole (HFBI) added to form T-2 esters.
4. Esters seperated on 2% OV-1 6 foot glass column. Quantitated with nickel-63 electron capture detecter.

Analysis

Absolute T-2 recovery spiked at concentrations between 0.5 to 7.0 µg/gram was 100.62 + 10.24%. Sensitivity 0.1 µg/gram.

Refining from organic liquids

1. Blood plasma or urine selectively partitioned into benzene fraction.
2. Extraneous materials removed by silica gel column chroma-topography.
3. Hepafluorobutylryl imidazole added to form T-2 esters.
4. Esters seperated on 2% OV-1 gas chrom Q^R 6 foot glass column. Quantified with nickel-63 electron capture de-tecter.

Analysis

1. Recoveries of T-2 at concentrations between 0.1-3.0 µg/ml ranged from 89-98% and 91-99%. Sensitivity 0.01 µg/ml in blood plasma and urine.

Again, thanks to Dr Chalam for his help.

Military significance

Suspicians of chemical warfare in the phase of the war following the total U.S. withdrawal surfaced in the summer of 1975. Sufficient numbers of the Hmong minority in Laos had fled to Thailand suffering similar pathological effects to warrent suspicians (in many quarters) of chemical or biological agent use. Within a year, similar incidents were reported from areas in Cambodia (Kampuchea) as conflict insued between Khamer Rouge and Vietnamese elements.

In a number of seperate locations the same sort of report was made. First, light aircraft would circle an inhabited area, dumping a yellow-green powder. Within a minute or so, individuals inhaling the fine dust would stagger about, vomiting or defecicating. Then the aircraft would drop some sort of airbursting munition, leaving a dense red haze that drifted down into the yellowish green dust. Shortly thereafter oral hemorrhaging would be followed with asphyxiation. Mortality rates were usually described as high.

Initial theories included speculation of new types of nerve or blister agent, and toxins from cobra venom to bee venom.[1] Ideology and social views towards war and conflict entered into the debate from the first reports, many denying that such things even occur. A UN commission was formed on the matter by the early 1980s but UN investigatory personnel have repeatedly been denied access to the area by its Vietnamese military administration. The government of Thailand, which operates Lao and Khamer refugee camps, has no intention of being drawn into its neighbor's wars. Such autopsy data as it collects it does not release and the bodies of refugee dead are cremated according to public health laws.

1. Cartoonists had a field day, showing helicopters painted up like bees, with such captions as "We are approaching village, comrades. Everybody *BUZZ!*"

Reports of similar occurences beginning in the late 1960s in Yeman and continuing to include Ethopia and Afghanistan have only encouraged suspicians in the Western nations. Biological warfare is no more socially acceptable in polite circles than is chemical warfare.

General casualty-producing qualities

Tricothecene is less sensitive to the elements than is ricin without requiring special processing. Tricothecene can be bulk-produced with ease, and impurities in the origional fungal toxin mix do not diminish its lethality. Tricothecene could be deployed in much the manner as chemical nerve agents against the same sorts of targets.

Footnote: aflatoxins

A series of mycotoxins derived from *Aspergillus flavus*, a fungal parasite of the peanut plant. Although not considered as toxic as tricothecene, ricin, or botulinus it could be used as a serious incapacitating agent or even to "boost" concentrations or mixes of the former.

The aflatoxins are based around the following structure:

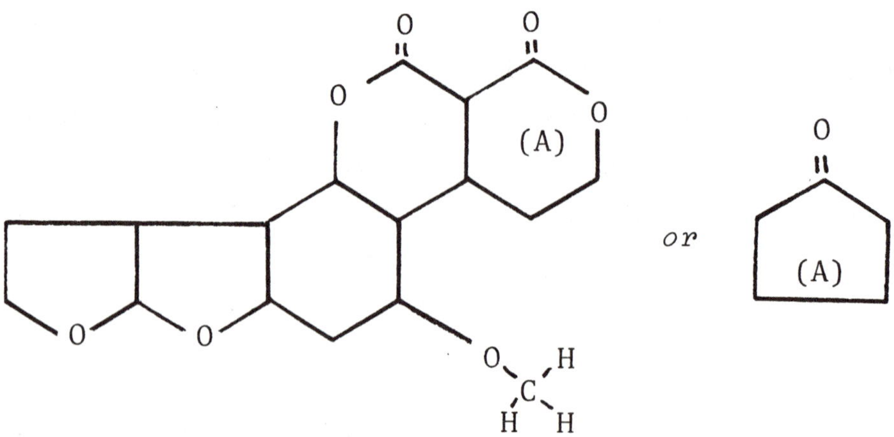

See Chapter Eight for combined references.

Chapter Eight

B I O L O G I C A L
P A T H O G E N S

some sample diseases

In December of 1969 the President of the United States, Richard Milhouse Nixon, renounced the principle of biological warfare. On his orders biological strategies were stricken from military doctorine and all stocks of biological agents were destroyed, save for those maintained for immunology development by the Public Health Service, a non military agency.

Definition

Biological pathogens are living organisms that attack the human body, disrupting its processes and endangering its health and well-being.

For purposes of discussion, these pathogens are divided into four categories:

- Bacterial
- Fungal
- Rickettsial
- Viral

Diseases and war have always been connected. In times of war normal patterns of life, especially food distribution and sanitation, are severely disrupted. Large bodies of people, both combatants and refugees, are thrown together in ways contrary to normal social patterns. Under these conditions diseases spread.

The notion of deliberately caused epidemics as a weapon of war is as old as organized conflict. Disease weakens an enemy's will to resist in ways which combat can not. The more open a society the less willing its leaders seem to use disease as a weapon.

New technologies: bioengineering

Since the early 1980s the United Nations has had an active program encouraging and assisting the spread of biotechnology and genetic engineering worldwide. The main UN motivation seems to be the development of new crop strains and more effective vaccines. Industry, government, and educational institutions are quite active in these new areas. The result has been a revolution in all the biosciences. Genetic engineering and gene-splicing kits for older children have been available since 1985, forming a sort of novel twist to the traditional chemistry set.

In February of 1983, the Washington DC columnist, Jack Anderson did a report on allegations of bioengineering in various places in the world being used to produce "superviruses more deadly than any known to man today.[1] In April of that year William Kucewicz began a five-week series in the *Wall Street Journal* entitled "Beyond Yellow Rain." In the series Kucewicz examined, in depth, the research institutes, the technologies, the personalities involved, and a general review of the scientific literature. Both the Anderson report and Kucewicz series were recieved with a thundering silence, interrupted by one or two muted protests that such things can not be, or if they could, modern cultured and scientific nations would never stoop to such acts.

Or would they?

1. quoted by Douglass & Livinstone, *America the vulnerable*, pp 57-58

New technologies: a final warning

Many, if not most, microorganisms have low survivability outside of a host organism and are susceptible to destruction by sunlight, hostile natural chemistry of the environment, or even to being eaten by other organisms. Only nature has ever succeeded in producing a first-rate epidemic and even those pass away.

The first biological warfare attempts began eons ago. Biblical injunctions against poisoning wells (at least those too close to home) are a commentary on the ancient practice of dumping human and animal bodies into water supplies in the hope that what killed them will go infect somebody else. A more scientific approach began in the 17th century when thoughtful people noticed that certain animals and their parasites were connected with contagion. More observant types also noticed that diseased tissue and other body by-products could be mixed with food and supplies (blankets were once a favorite method in the days before chlorine bleach) for the same desired effect. Twentieth century approaches until recently have ranged from the mundane (drop agar solutions of concentrated strains) to the ingenious (drop porcelain bombs filled with infected fleas).

Things began to change in world war two. The modern technique of freeze-drying things originated in about 1940 as a method of providing durable bacteria and other spores. This author has beat microencapsulation to death by now but nonetheless that technique which gives us safe powdered insecticides, and scratch-n'-sniff perfume (or dog food) samples in our magazines can be used for "bugs" as well.

And finally, there's the fact that any fool who doesn't mind dosing him or herself can culture this stuff at home.

Bacteria

Bacteria are the smallest living organisms having a complete cell structure and an independent metabolism. They are the most widespread of all organisms, although each of over 1500 seperate species thrives only in conditions related to its metabolism. Very few of them are able to capture and release energy from simple compounds. Most bacteria either feed off of living organisms (parasitic) or dead organic matter (saprophytic).

Bacteria come in three basic shapes:

1. BACILLI (rod-shaped)

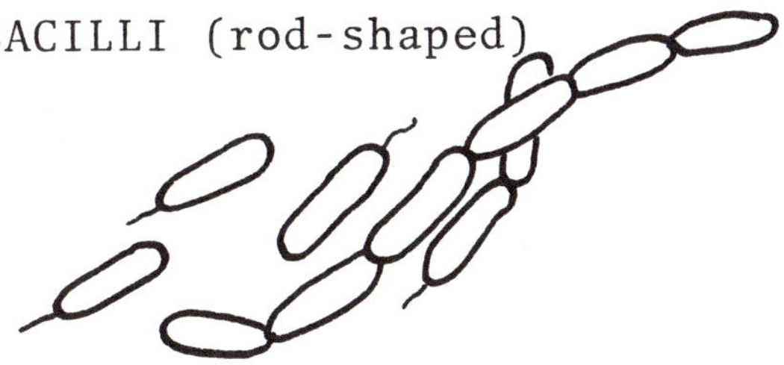

2. COCCI (spherical)

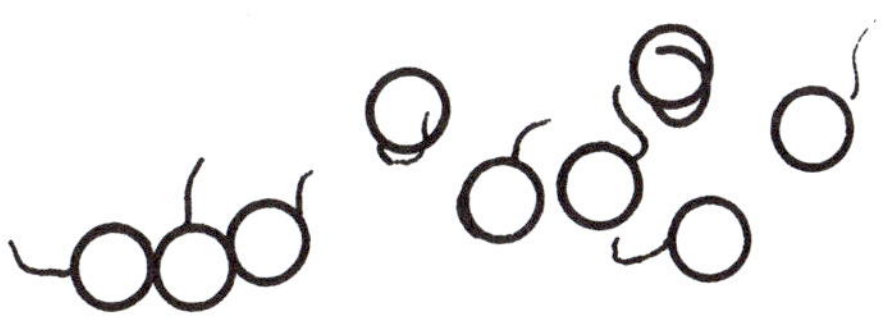

3. SPIRILLA (spiral)

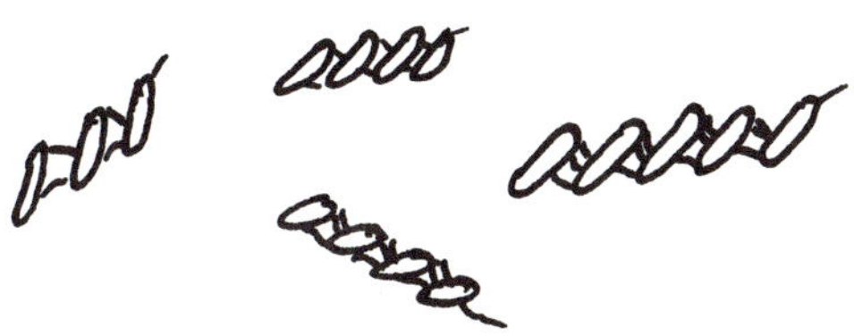

Most bacteria are benign. Their role in the great scheme of things is to decompose organic matter and to channel it back into the food chain. Bacteria have been incorporated into the higher life forms where they are used on a host-guest basis to metabolize foodstuffs. For example, the human intestines are filled with several distinct families of bacteria (bacterium, pl) which break down food to the point where the body's enzymes can absorb the by-products.

On the other hand, several classes of bacterium attack a human host, feeding off it at certain points when conditions favor its survival. In this manner such bacterium are diseases that damage human tissue, processes, and neuro-chemical processes.

Bacterium are more complex than viruses and hence present more of a challenge from the bioengineering aspect. It should be born in mind, however, that alterations to otherwise necessary bacteria strains (eg, those in the human intestines) would present a unique toxic hazard. Then, many of the more virulent diseases are bacteria caused. Examples include, anthrax, cholera, plague, and typhoid. In such cases these could be made more dangerous by developing strains just far enough from the origional to avoid control by existing vaccines. For this reason, immunologists must never rest on their laurels.

A SOMETIMES OVERLOOKED ASPECT

Certain bacteria have been developed capable of decomposing ~~waste~~ some waste plastics, and catalyzing the oxidation of some metals. It is not farfetched to imagine bacterial agents that would attack electronic devices.

Anthrax

once known as Agent N

class

Bacterial (bacillus).

areas of natural occurence

World-wide.

natural vectors

Common to sheep and cattle. The bacterium *bacillus anthracis* may be found in the meat, milk, hides, and hair of infected animals.

Quantities of the bacterium left exposed to light and air for over two hours at 20°C(68°F) will form into spore-like structures of great durability (see below).

artificial vectors

Anthrax bacteria can be cultivated in standard laboratory medium such as agar.

incubation period

1 to 2 hours, at most.

history

Anthrax is thought to have been the Fifth Plague of Egypt. The bacterium was isolated by Casimir Davaine in 1850. Louis Pastuer developed the first major Anthrax vaccine in 1877.

Anthrax was investigated by the Japanese in the mid 1930s for use in China against livestock, and then against large populations. On the Allied side, it was developed specifically for use against civilian populations (as a pre-atomic type of doomsday weapon) but never used. Enormous warstocks of the stuff were later destroyed following the war until by the 1950s it could be calculated in ounces.

Anthrax, especially in pseudospores, proved to be

too persistent. In the west, its principal test site was the island of Gruinard off the north coast of Scotland (in the Hebrides). A single mass exposure was made there in 1943, amounting to a pseudospore infestation that simulated a battlefield concentration. As of the late 1980s Gruinard Island (nicknamed Anthrax Island by the locals) is still too heavily infested with the pseudospores to allow humans on it. This is in spite of having been firebombed and burned over at least once. It would not be unfair to say that Gruinard has had something to do with the NATO disavowal of ever using such things as a weapon.

pathology

Anthrax is an acutely infectious disease of cattle and sheep which is readily spread among people, albeit on an individual basis. In its natural environment(s) those at risk are those persons who work with livestock. Under those conditions between 15 to 20% of persons seriously infected with the disease die. As a deliberately spread contagion those figures would be raised by a factor of at least two to three.

Contaminated meat causes coal-black watery malignant ulcers within two hours. Severe blood poisoning will follow. Pictures of persons whose arms were soaked in infected animal blood resemble partially blackened corpses with huge blisters. The disease is insidious. Inhaled, a similar sort of thing happens to the lungs. The mortality rate for pseudospore inhalation would probably exceed 90%.

Anthrax simply infests the human body and destroys its ability to function.

Brucellosis

once provisionally designated
agent US

other names

Undulant fever, Malta Fever, Mediterranean Fever; Bang's Disease.

class

Bacterial (bacillus).

areas of natural occurence

World-wide.

natural vectors

Caused by the several subtypes of *bacilli brucella: brucella abortus* (in cattle); *brucella suis* (in swine); *brucella melitensis* (sheep and goats); *brucella canis* (in dogs); *brucella ovis* (rams); *Brucella neotomae* (in desert wood rats). Brucella bacilli have also been isolated in deer, caribou, horses, cats, mice, chickens, and humans.

artificial vectors

Brucella bacteria can be cultured in most laboratory mediums, including agar.

incubation period

Within one to three weeks.

history

First isolated in the spleens of dying British soldiers on Malta in 1887. Before then this was thought to be several diseases until the particular brucella strains (see above) were isolated. As Mediterranean fever, it had built up a lethal reputation, especially given the lack of understanding of the disease and the often haphazard sanitary conditions which used to prevail in the area.

Studied as a war agent by the Japanese in the 1930s in China. Studied (under more benign conditions) by the Allies in the following decade. Prior to the end of the war it saw experimental production by the United States (hence its provisional code of "US") as a non-lethal or incapacitating agent. US stocks destroyed (processed into fertilizer) immediately following the war.

pathology

The unset of the disease comes slowly and the victim may not realize he or she is diseased. Gradually over a period of 2-4 days the victim will first feel chronic fatigue, a loss of appetite (leading to anorexia within a week), and a tendency to sweat when at rest. Aches and fevers intensify, then diminish ("undulate," hence the popular name for the disease), with a gradual rise in intensity.

The disease normally only presents 2% mortality, but damages to the liver, kidneys, spleen, lung, and heart may be permanent.

In its final stages the victim will suffer chronic muscle pains, constipation, nausea, eye pain, insomnia, and impotence in males. Less than 5% ever suffer relapse.

points of contagion

The disease occurs in man through contact with contaminated meat and unpastuerized milk. The majority of cases occur among slaughterhouse and packing plant workers.

The organism, which does not form spores, enters through broken skin, the membranes around the eyes, or via ingestion.

Cholera

class

Bacterial.

areas of natural occurence

South Asia and the Orient.

natural vectors

Cholera is almost exclusively an intestinal infection, caused by food and water contamination caused by *vibrio cholerae* and its El Tor biotype (with type O antigen) known as *vibrio cholerae 01* and similar organisms which have been designated *vibrio cholerae*. Contamination is almost always caused by comtamination connected with human wastes. Cholera is primarily a disease belonging to unsanitary conditions as it naturally occurs.

artificial vectors

Cholera bacteria can be laboratory cultivated in such standard mediums as agar with proper protein admixtures.

incubation period

Varies from between 24 hours and five days, depending on amount of initial dosage and the resistence of the victim.

pathology

Cholera is considered to be exclusively a disease of the intestines. Infection is always through the mouth and more immediate from contaminated water than from contaminated food mass, which remaining in the stomach is subject to attack from gastric acids.

The bacteria remain in the intestines and do not penetrate through to the blood or body fluids. In a sense cholera bacteria mimic the behavior of bacteria found naturally in the intestinal tract. However *vibrio cholerae* produces a toxin by-product. The toxin will enter the cells lining the intestine where it interferes with the digestive enzyme *adenylate cyclase* by preventing its complete metabolism. Normal absorption of sodium is blocked while full secretion of chloride ions is initiated (from salts metabolism). The result is that the intestines no longer absorb water, but actively excreet it. The result is diarrhea and general loss of water from the body.

The victim rapidly dehydrates and may go into vascular collapse and shock. Severe muscle cramps and neurovascular pain are the result of tissue dehydration. Treatment with proper antibiotics may rapidly destroy the bacterium, but its toxin must be flushed from the system at the body's own rate. Still, recovery may be well under way within two hours. And then, untreated cases involving massive ingestion have been known to kill victims within three to four hours after onset.

Glanders

other names

Equina

class

Bacterial (bacillus). ~~*Malleomyces*~~ PSEUDOMONAS *mallei*.

natural vectors

Primarily a disease of horses and mules. Infrequently communicable to dogs, goats, sheep, and man. Cattle are not affected.

artificial vecters

Occurence in humans would most likely be from cultured bacteria, as few persons live in unhygienic proximity to horses and mules. Glanders bacteria may be grown in standard laboratory medium containing the appropriate protein mix.

history

Accusations of deliberate spread of glanders among draft animals on the eastern front during world war one appear to have a basis in fact. Most supply transport and artillery was horse or mule drawn. Russian horses in great numbers suffered from the disease which may have been deliberately spread by agents of the Central Powers. Immunological efforts did bring the problem under control until the mid 1920s. This instance is a classical example of biological warfare directed not against personnel, but against animal populations.

Post world war two Allied investigation of Japanese biological warfare experimentation at the Pinfang (China) Instutute showed wartime use of Glanders against civil populations (animal and human) and against prisoners of war.

Allied studies of the war potentials of Glanders were briefly done at Camp Detrick, Maryland in 1943-1944.

pathology

Symptoms of the disease in humans are those of the disease in horses. At the onset, high fever and general malaise occur and the victim becomes prostrate.

The classical pathology involves inflammation of the mucus membranes of the nose and throat. Secondary lung infection is not unknown. Bacterial colonies in those areas precipitate the formation of pus which will drain through the nose and mouth.

In humans, skin eruptions supplement mucus inflammation. Pox-like nodules form on the skin which eventually break, leaving deep ulcers. Reinfection and coincidential infection(s) by other organisms may end in destruction to cartilage and bone.

Plague

other names

Bubonic plague (black death), septicemic plague, pneumonic plague, pharyngeal plague, cutaneous plague, endophthalmic plague. All of these are particular clinical forms of the same disease.

class

Bacterial (bacilli).

areas of natural occurence

World-wide.

natural vectors

Resulting from systemic infection by bacterium *yersinia pestis*. Generally blood-born from bite of infected animals or their fleas. Primarily engendered through *maintenance* hosts such as rats and mice, a portion of which have immunity to the disease but serve as continual carriers of the dormant bacteria. For as yet understood reasons, the bacteria become active after long periods of dormancy and are transferred to *amplification hosts*, which include non-immune rats and mice, squirrels, chipmonks, and prarie dogs. A third group, *incidental hosts*, (who may develop natural or clinical immunity through antibody production and do not harbor the bacterium as hosts) then acquire the disease. The latter group may include all mammals, including man, and may acquire the disease from any of the other catagories.

Clinical forms of plague arise from infections of various parts of the body where unique pathologies and means of transmission develop. For example, pneumonic plague involves plague infection of the lungs where blood mixes with lung mucous to form a unique series of protein bonds, which may cause infection by either airborn bacteria laden droplets or blood-to-blood contact (which may or may not revert to other pathologies).

Plague is classified as as *zoonosis*, a disease common to both man and animal. US Department of Health and Human Services data indicate that about 85% of US cases of plague are caused by flea-borne infection. The remaining 15% may be attributed to forms of direct contact.

artificial vectors

The disease is best cultivated through maintenance hosts, although the bacteria has been successfully cultivated in various laboratory media.

history

Plague, in particular bubonic plague is one of the most pandemic of diseases. Noted outbreaks in the West include the Athens epidemic of 430 BC, the Rome epidemic of 262 AD, and more recntly the world pandemic of 1334 to 1351 AD in which a sizable portion of the world's urban population died. Noted reoccurances include an on-again off-again epidemic in London between 1603 and 1665, the Hong Kong-to-India epidemics of 1894-1914, and sundry outbreaks in urban centers of South and North America dating to the 1890s.

Plague usually thrives in conjested urban areas. This is not due to septic factors often favoring disease pathogens but rather to the fact that rats multiply very well in cluttered, haphazard urban conditions.

incubation period

Within one to four days of infection.

pathology

Three major clinical forms of the disease are common among human populations:

Bubonic plague. So call because of of unique visible swelling of the lymph nodes, usually on one side of the body. Individual swellings are called *bubos* (late Latin word from which the English *bump* is derived), hence the term *bubo*nic. Containing a high percentage of oxidized blood with dead bacterium, these painful nodes in the lymph system are usually dark blue to black. Hence the popular name *black plague* and the more dramatic *black death*. This is the disease that wiped out a fourth of Europe by 1350. Its bacterium is often sub-catagorized as *Pastuerella pestis* after the man who devised an immune serium against it.

Bubonic plague develops its symptoms rapidly. Chills and fever are soon accompanied by the lymphatic swellings, noted above, which develop along the neck, armpit, and often the groin. The swelling often occurs along lymphatic ducts and is therefore near the skin surface. The swellings may burst open, becoming massive sores open to secondary infection. Complications may include plague meningitis or secondary pneumonia (not to be comfused with pneumonic plague). The victim typically goes into shock and respiratory arrest in the final stages of the disease. Plague infection responds slowly to most antibiotic therapy, so the patient will look and feel miserable for about two days subsequent. The bubos (being a by-product of a natural immunization process) may persist for about a week although lessening in size and pain. If the victim survives the disease complete recovery with no residual effects is almost universal.

Septicemic plague (primary). Plague infection without detectable bubos. May be confused with a number of other bacterial diseases characterized also by fever, malaise, overall weakness and secondary infection. Otherwise the progression of the disease is like bubonic plague. This underlines the need for trained medical personnel with proper diagnostic resources.

Pneumonic plague (primary). Spread from close contact

rather than from fleas. Airborne mucus will contain the bacterium and will keep them alive long enough to spread the disease to animals or persons in close proximity. Pneumonic plague engenders its own form of pathogenic lung congestion, or pneumonia, hence its name. Pneumonic plague develops rapidly, leaving its victims prostrate within hours of onset. Commonly confused with other forms or bacterial pneumonia and distinguished mainly by its virulent course.

Salomonella typhimurium

Salomonella typhimurium is one of a host of salomonella bacteria types, many of which cause diarrhea and other gasrointestinal disorders. It figures in food poisoning due to unsanitary conditions and is commonly mistaken for simple gastroenteritis. The bacteria is immune to cold but is destroyed by heat. The disease it engenders can be an extreme nuisance under normal conditions although, even with occasional vomiting and slight fever, it is not often debilitating. Most cases last no longer than 48 hours with treatment, although severe cases lasting over a week are not unknown.

Salomonella is included to illustrate the ease with which an unsuspecting community can be deliberately infected with a biopathogen.

On September 15th, 1984 an epidemic of salomonella began in the town of Antelope, Oregon. Within ten days about sixty clinically-treated cases had occured with no statistics available on minor or unreported cases. The outbreak was traced to four different restraunts, although Oregon public health officials could find no natural source for what they determined to be a common strain.

Near the town of Antelope there existed a religious community under the auspices of an Indian teacher, Bhagwan Shree Rajneesh. Tensions exusted between the town and the commune.

Following a series of events in 1985, Bhagwan Shree Rajneesh gave sworn testimony that his recently dismissed security aide, Ma Anana Sheela, had among other things "poisoned a nearby town." [1]

1. Douglass & Livingstone, *America the vulnerable.* p.32.

Tularemia

once provisionally designated
as agent UL

common name

Rabbit rever.

class

Bacterial (cocci).

areas of natural occurence

First isolated in Tulare County, California in 1911.

natural vectors

Caused by bacterium *francisella tularensis*, carried or active in infected rabbits, squirrels, or rats. May be transmitted by the fleas and ticks of same.

artificial vectors

May be laboratory cultured in mediums containing appropriate proteins.

incubation period

Depends on the extent of the origional infection and type of infection. Ulcerglandular and typhoidal: about one week. Pulmonary and oculoglandular: between 2 and 4 days.

history

First investigated as a biological incapacitating agent by the Allies during world war II and provisionally designated UL. Not deployed. War stocks destroyed following that war and last military stocks destroyed by Presidential order in the winter of 1970.

pathology

Tularemia is classified under four main pathologies, each reflecting a different path of infection for the same organism.

Ulcerglandular. Infection through animal (including fleas and ticks) bites or innoculation. Produces a reoccuring fever lasting several weeks. High concentrations of both live and dead bacteria are found in the lymphatic system, principally at or near the point of infection where the lymph nodes will be swollen. By the second week lesions and pus-filled abscesses will form at those points. Secondary influenza-like symptoms, chills, and headache are normal.

Ulcerglandular tularemia is the most common form the disease, although intentionally-spread tularemia would likely manifest as pulmonary or oculoglandular types. Ulcerglandular tularemia normally produces 3-7% mortality among untreated victims.

Pulmonary. Infection through inhalation of the organism. Typically creates an acute pathogenic pulmonary infection (ie, a pneumonia). Creates influenza-like symptoms like the ulcerglandular sort, only minus the external abscesses of the latter. Such ulceration as occurs is area, not point, within the lungs. Pulmonary tularemia is an intensely virulent form of the disease, characterized by bloody sputum (lung mucus), itself a highly infectious aerosol. The victim will be prostrate, with a reducued capacity of the lungs to oxygenate blood. As with all pneumonias, secondary infections may occur.

Pulmonary tularemia normally produces about 30% mortality among untreated vistims.

Thyphoidal (not to be confused with Typhoid fever) Inflection through direct ingestion of tularemia. Unlikely through eating infected animals, which would commonly be cooked. Water-borne infection has been repeatedly documented, and seems the most likely source.

Influenza-like symptoms occur, with the pronounced development of ulcerative lesions in the intestines. Misdiagnosed or untreated significant perforation and hemorrhage is expected.

Untreated victims should have about 30% mortalities.

Oculoglandular. Infection of the eyes and the mucous membranes surrounding the eyes. Causes severe pain, lacrimation, and light-sensitivity. Regional lymph nodes may be swollen. Although not particularly fatal, lack of immediate treatment may result in permanent damage to the cornea(s) through perforation and/or atrophy.

Typhoid fever

class

Bacterial.

areas of natural occurence

World-wide. Endemic in most third-world countries and periodic to all other areas. Current vaccines (paratyphoid A and B) give less than complete protection.

natural vectors

Origionally from cattle. Common in contaminated milk or milk products, and occasionally in infected meat and meat by-products. The bacterium readily contaminate water.

Some persons carry the disease bacterium but do not develop the active disease.

artificial vectors

Typhoid bacteria strains may be cultured in proper laboratory mediums, especially those containing appropriate protein bases.

incubation period

Generally one to two weeks. Known cases have incubated in less than 5 and as great as 21 days from known exposures. Children tend to develop the disease quicker than adults. Intensity of dosage and the general health of the victim directly influence the course and extent of the disease.

history

Typhoid fever has been known both to societies and to war for millenia, often causing more casualties than those associated with battle. For example, in the Anglo-Boer War (1899-1902) British forces incurred about 20,000 cases. In the mid-1930s the Japanese test facility at Pinfang, China developed typhoid as a weapon. In war-crimes trials it was alleged that typhoid was used against the Chinese civilian population and it was proven that it was tested on Allied prisoners of war. In the 1930s the Soviets devoted a new test facility on Vozrozhdeniya Island, in the Aral Sea, to examine typhoid fever, cholera, typhus, and other diseases under isolated laboratory conditions.

The specific class of bacteria causing this disease were isolated in 1880. The search for an effective vaccine continues.

pathology

Typhoid fever typically follows a four week course after incubation.

First week. A rapidly rising fever occurs, accompanied with a dull, aching headache. Pain occurs to the back and joints, not accompanied by swelling. Concurrent with the headache will be nausea with mild vomiting. A typical mental depression will be psychological and not physiological. Loss of appetite bordering on anorexia is common. Capillary nose-bleed has been reported in a great number of cases. The victim may be anemic and also suffer loss of feeling in the fingers and toes.

Signs on clinical admission commonly include: headache, joint and back pains, diarrhea without blood — or constipation, abdominal discomfort, vomiting, bronchial congestion, enlarged spleen, abdominal tenderness with puffiness of the skin , retention of urine, possible slight deafness, and a musty odor about the hips.

second week. Fever may have risen to as high as 105°F (possibly creating cerebrial neurodamage in some victims). Ulceration of the intestines may become pronounced, especially if untreated. Hemorrhage or puncturing of the intestines can be fatal of themselves. Rosy spots will have already developed on the chest. Abscesses may begin to develop in the inner regions of the buttocks. Severe bronchial congestion bordering on pneumonia may occur.

Third week. Weakness as the body's metabolism begins to decline. Muscle tone may have deteriorated and tremors occur with decline in motor response. Cardiovascular weakness (mycarditis) can occur. Severe fatigue accompanied with delirium can give way to coma in severe cases.

Fourth week. Recovery begins.

Screening of all patients and their contacts is essential. Some authorities recommend as many as six negative stool/urine and Vi blood antigen tests should be required before a patient be released back to the public. Some victims can remain carriers.

Fungii

These are single cell, colonial, or structural vegetable organisms having complete structure and organized activity. Unlike other plants they cannot (or at least cannot completely) metabolize certain proteins and enzymes essential to growth and reproduction in the manner of other plants. As a result, they obtain those substances from other living (or decaying) organisms, including man.

Coccidiodmycocis

other names

Desert rheumatism, the bumps.

class

Fungus. *Coccidioides immitis.*

areas of natural occurence

Endemic to the soil of the southwestern United States and the San Joaquin Valley of California.

natural vectors

Soil fungus common to the above areas.

artificial vectors

Easily cultured in appropriate laboratory medium.

pathology

Pulmonary (through inhalation). Naturally affects about 40% of infected persons (would be raised by artificieal spread of the contagion). Primary effect is a feverish illness resembling influenza with pronounced lung congestion lasting about 1 to 3 weeks. Accompanied with headache, muscle aches, and pains in the joints. About 95% of victims recover without bronchial damage. About 20% of active cases develop some form of skin rash, often accompanied with neural or arthritic pain.

Disseminated (whole body, through skin or ingestion). Characterized by persistent or recurrent fevers. Multiple skin lesions/rashes are normal, which in extreme infections often mimic the appearence of carcinomas. Swelling of the tissues around the brain (the meninges) may occur rapidly and is one of the most frequent manifestations of the disease. Bone tissue infection, with multiple lesions to long bones, the skull, and the spine occurs in 10 to 20% of acute cases.

Anti-plant fungii once classified as standard agents and used in world war two

- **Agent C.** *Sclerotium rolfsi.* Used against tobbacco plants, soya beans, sugar beets, sweet potatoes, and cotton.

- **Agent E.** *Helminthosporium oryzae van Brede de Haan.* Blights rice.

- **Agent IE.** *Piricularia oryzae.* Blights rice.

- **Agent LO.** *Phytophtera infestans (mort) de Bary.* Potato blight.

Rickettsia

Rickettsia are a group of microorganisms having limited metabolism but lack the complete structure of the bacteria. They live in the body tissues of land arthropods (insects and spiders) which in turn may infect animals and man. All the rickettsial diseases are spread to man by fleas and ticks, with the exception of Q fever which is normally contracted via aerosol inhalation from infected farm animals.

The class *rickettsia* was named in honor of Dr. Howard T. Ricketts who pioneered the study of this particular life form. He proved conclusively their being carried by arthropods, his initial work being with body lice transferrel of *tabardillo* strain typhus.

Q fever

other names

Query fever, la maladie de Derrick et Burnet

class

Rickettsial. *Coxiella burnetti.*

natural vectors

Occurs almost exclusively through the inhalation of aerosol sputum, commonly from domestic farm animals, cattle or sheep. In theory it can be passed between humans as a similar aerosol.

artificial vectors

Coxiella burnetti can be cultivated in laboratory medium containing appropriate proteins. It has also been cultivated in fertile chicken eggs.

incubation period

10 to 28 days.

history

Examined at Ft Detrick, Maryland during the 1950s and early 1960s along with other rickettsia for war potentials. Last military stocks were publicly destroyed by Presidential order in the winter of 1970.

pathology

Q fever is a non rash-forming, highly febrile disease of great virulence.

Following the onset of the disease the victim will experience severe fever (above 102°F), rapidly followed by intense headache and pains in the muscles and joints. Loss of appetite occurs accompanied by nausea. Either constipation or diarrhea accompanies gastrointestinal pains. There will be swelling of the tissues at the back of the mouth.

Q fever has serious systemic effects mostly absent in the other rickettsial maladies. It is not uncommon that the disease inflames the tissues of the heart, around the heart (with permanent heart valve damage common), of the brain, genitals, pancreas, liver, kidneys, and thyroid.

Prolonged convalescence lasting several months is normal among survivors.

Rocky Mountain Spotted Fever
Eastern hemisphere typhus (spotted)

common names

Spotted fever, tick typhus, fiebre manchada, fiebre petequial, fiebre maculosa, São Paulo typhus.

class

Rickettsial.

areas of natural occurance

Rickettsia was first isolated in Montana and Idaho, although most common to Atlantic seaboard, northeastern states and Canadian maritime provinces and Quebec. The total range is limited to North and South America. [For eastern hemisphere spotted fevers, see below.]

natural vectors

Caused by *rickettsia rickettsii* which is carried by several species of infected ticks (most notably wood ticks), which account for about 80% of clinically examined cases. Aerosol transmission is known to occur, especially to laboratory personnel who ignore basic safety precautions.

artificial vectors

Rickettsia rickettsii can be cultured in laboratory medium containing appropriate protein mixes.

incubation period

Depends on exposure and health of the victim. Commonly 7 days, but cases as early as 2 days and as late as 2 weeks have been recorded.

history

Examined at Fort Detrick, Maryland during the 1950s along with other rickettsia for war potentials. Last military stocks ordered destroyed by Presidential order in December of 1969.

pathology

Rocky mountain spotted fever has an abrupt onset following onset, although late incubation cases tend to be less intense than quick incubation cases. Severe headache followed quickly with muscle pains begin the pathology. The pains will be to the muscles of the neck, back, and legs. Loss of appetite will be immediate, accompanied by nausea and stupor. Related neurological abnormalities progressing from these symptoms include neck and shoulder rigidity, delirium, possible seizures (muscle) and, in extreme cases, coma. Sensitivity of the eyes to light is universal. As the disease progresses, liver and spleen enlargement will occur, although jaundice is almost unknown.

Infection through inhalation may result in a localized pneumonia, which may become a source of further contagion at the height of the febrile period. In the latter, body temperatures are normally at or above 102°F.

A rash due to blood congestion in the skin capillaries is the hallmark of this disease. In mild infections the rash may occur later in the disease, or in rare cases not at all.

Normally the rash begins to form on about the fourth day and its initial stages last between 2 and 6 days, beginning with numerous small dark spots along the palms, wrists, forearms, the soles of the feet and the ankles. In the next stage these slots progress up the legs and spread to the abdomen and face. These in turn may expand due to minor subcutaneous hemorrhage beginning as small reto to purplish blotches which turn blue or dark yellow.

Possible complications to the disease include hypotension and circulatory collapse through loss of circulating blood.

Recovery usually insures permanent immunity to the patient. Humans do not seem to become carriers.

other spotted fevers: Eastern hemisphere typhoid diseases

- **Fièvre boutonneuse** also known as African tick typhus, Kenya tick typhus, South African tick bite fever, Indian tick typhus. Caused by *rickettsia conorii*. Pathology similar to Rocky Mountain spotted fever.

- **Asian tickborne typhus** also known as North Asian tick-borne rickettsiosis. Caused by *rickettsia siberica*. Pathology similar to Rocky Mountain spotted fever.

- **Queensland tick typhus**. Caused by *rickettsia australis*. Pathology similar to Rocky Mountain spotted fever.

The above typhus diseases, having much the same appearence as Rocky Mountain spotted fever, have been discussed under that disease rather than under *murine* and *epidemic* typhus [below].

Reference to historical epidemics in Asia, Europe, and Africa will usually refer to the above three. All occur in crowded, unsanitary conditions and the first two are often known as *gaol (jail) fever*, *famine fever*, or *war fever*. Asian tickborne typhus was the epidemic that killed about 100,000 persons in Siberia in 1917-1918 and went on to kill over 3,000,000 more during the Russian Civil War (1918-1923), profoundly effecting the present course of history.

Typhus (non-spotted fevers)

• Epidemic typhus

common names

Louseborne typhus, European typhus, classic typhus, historic typhus, camp fever, war fever, ship fever, gaol (jail) fever, typhus exanthematique, tifus [sic] exantematico, tifus tabardillo, Fleckfieber, dermotypho. Note that several names are in common with Fievre boutonneuse and Asian tickborn typhus variants.

class

Rickettsial. *Rickettsia prowazekii.*

areas of common occurence

Endemic to third world areas in Africa, Asia and Latin America (see Brill-Zinsser disease variation).

natural vectors

Human lice, specifically louse feces or crushed infective lice entering the human body through cuts or incisions in the skin, or through the inhalation of infective louse feces. The rickettsia exist only in the digestive tract of carrier lice.

artificial vectors

Possibly cultured in laboratory mediums containing the proper protein mix.

incubation period

Between 5 and 23 days, averaging about 11 days.

pathology

A severe typhus disease manifesting with immediate high fever, chills, intense headache, back and muscle pains, and overall weakening. Constipation is usually present, although vomiting and nausea are rare. Flushed skin about the neck and face is common. There will be eye pain and photosensitivity.

A rash appears between the fourth and ninth day, erupting on the side of the chest in the form of small lesions which gradually spread to form larger, dark blotches by the tenth or twelfth day.

Epidemic typhus attacks the central nervous system with neurotoxic effects that may lead to coma. The liver and spleen will probably become enlarged and permanent damages to those organs are possible. Liver damage and subcutaneous hemorrhage may cause anemia with attendent hypotension and myocarditis. Diminished circulation has been known to contribute to gangrene of the appendages.

Infection can come through inhalation of infected lice feces or dust of crushed lice. The result will be a rickettsial pneumonia similar to that of Rocky Mountain spotted fever (qv). In addition, about 10% of clinical patients develop a secondary *bacterial* pneumonia.

Other complications may include purulent tonsolitis, throat infections, ear inflammation, and inflammation of the lymph glands of the head.

Sustained high fever may often result in personality alteration traits among survivors.

Typhus (non-spotted fevers)

• Murine typhus

common names

Endemic typhus, fleaborne typhus.

class

Rickettsial. *Rickettsia mooseri (rickettsia typhi).*

areas of common occurence

World-wide. Human infection highest in summer months, when flea and rat populations are at their peak. Rats tending to infest food storage areas, the disease tends to be more common to persons working or living in proximity to same.

natural vectors

Carried by fleas which typically infest rats. Fleas infect both rats and man. Not spread from human-to-human.

artificial vectors

Rickettsia mooseri can be cultured in laboratory medium containing the appropriate protein mix.

incubation period

Murine typhus has an incubation period between 6 and 14 days.

pathology

The onset of the disease is fairly rapid following incubation and it is often mistaken for mild Epidemic typhus. Fever, headache, muscle pains, pains in the joints. A rash usually appears on the sixth or seventh day after the onset of fever. The rash rarely forms the spotting pattern associated with the spotted fevers proper, spreading across the upper extremities and then fading to poorly delineated blotches. Systemic damage is infrequent. With proper treatment, recovery is rapid with no residual effects. Untreated, the disease may be severe and debilitating, requiring several months convalescence and producing about 2% mortality.

other typhus variants not involving whole-body spotting

• Brill-Zinsser disease

A milder-acting variation of Epidemic typhus (qv) and caused by the same organism, *rickettsia prowazekii*. Often refered to as *sporatic typhus, recrudescent typhus,* or *Brazillian typhus.*

Brill-Zinsser is a recurrent form of typhus, appearing anywhere from a few months to reported cases of 50 years following the initial infection. The factors that precipitate this are not known.

Brill-Zinsser presents an unusual contagion hazard, as the carrier is human rather than insect. In this case lice can pick up the disease from humans.

This disease produces a fever lower and/or shorter duration than Epidemic typhus. The rash is often absent. Complications may not occur. Mortalities are rare.

• Rickettsial pox

A form of typhus in which white blood cell matter, dead rickettsia and moribund tissue are expelled from the body through cutaneous eruption in the matter of the viral poxes (chicken pox, measles, etc). This phenomena may occur only at the point of infection or in a generalized eruption, depending on extent of infection and victim resistence. These vesticles form a crust which falls off, leaving a small pigmented patch without scars.

Rickettsial pox is caused by infection by *rickettsia akari* transmitted through the bite of the mouse mite. The incubation period lasts between 10 and 21 days. Sudden onset involves fever, loss of appetite, light sensitivity, headache, and the general malaise, or ill-feeling of the victim. The rash begins on about the third of fourth day (occasionally on the first) of the fever, beginning on the extremities and trunk, becoming vesicular rather than spotted.

The disease lasts about two weeks and does not have sequential effects.

• Scrub typhus

Scrub typhus is, strictly speaking, a spotted typhus but only between 40 and 60% of its victims ever develop whole-body spotting. Without the rash it is often mistaken for any number of typhoid-like illnesses, typhoid fever, infectuous mononucleosis, dengue, malaria, or many other infections.

Scrub typhus is a pronounced fever causing disease caused by chiggers (larval mites) infected with *rickettsia tsutsugamushi*. Its common extent is throughout eastern and southeastern Asia, and the islands of the western and couthern Pacific Ocean. Its synonyms include *tsutsugamushi disease, chiggerborn rickettsiosis, miteborne typhus, rural typhus, Japanese river fever, flood fever, Mossman fever.*

Scrub fever has an incubation period of between 6 to 19 days. Immediate onset is characterized by severe headache, commonly centered in both the frontal and rear of the head. A few hours later high fever (above 102°F) and shaking chills occur.In most cases swelling at the point of infection occurs often with formation of a lesion.

Pathology and symptoms are otherwise similar to those of Rocky Mountain spotted fever, save that spotting may or may not occur between the third and ninth day of fever.

Fever usually ceases after about two weeks of the illness. Convalescence is prolonged.

Viruses

The smallest and simplest forms of life, consisting principally of a protein jacket around a core of nucleic acid strands (DNA or RNA, but not both). They are charactorized by the lack of an independent metabolism and their being able to replicate only within the living cells of host cells. They are attracted and attach to specific areas within their host through chemical compatibility with specific enzymes of physiological processes. When a virus invades a host cell it redirects that cells activities towards its ends, to perform the metabolitic and reproductive functions which the virus is unable to perform of its own. The result is a disease pathology to the host organism.

A current controversy is whether or not a bio-engineered virus is capable of concentrating its activities in the nucleus of a host cell, to combine its DNA or RNA codings with that of the host cell. Such a virus/host relationship, although pathological to the host organism, would provide at least partial protection to the virus against the host's immune system. A bio-engineered virus could be protein-coded to attack a specific area or function of a host, and thus presents an extreme danger of pandemic proportions.

Viruses range in size from 15mμ[1] to 300mμ in length, and as such are not individually detectable

1. milimicron. A micron is 1/1,000,000th of a meter.

through optical microscopes. Their size and the nature of their protein coats enables them to penetrate most filters and cell membrances. Individual strains are heterogeneous in appearence. Various strains may occur as rods, spheres, polyhedrals, or elongated in shape. The spherical and polyhedral types may form into masses resembling crystals. Some of these latter forms may be extremely durable, capable of surviving in the environment outside a host body in a dormant stage, resistent to extremes of heat and cold and to many chemical combinations. Rod-shaped viruses may be difficult to cultivate and don't live long outside of their hosts.

Viruses are commonly divided into three catagories — bacterial, plant, and animal — according to the organisms they attack. They are further named according to their origion, mode of transmission, the disease they cause, or the geogrpahical locale they were first isolated in.

In recent decades viruses have come to represent a significant threat to the health of entire populations. Viruses, being mostly DNA or RNA, are the easiest of the living substances to manipulate in the laboratory. They are ideal subjects for gene-splicing and similar bioengineering techniques. Through painstaking efforts even otherwise viruses could be designed to attack certain areas in the human body, and even to graft onto human DNA or RNA belonging to their host cells, to the extent of eluding the body's natural defenses.

A majority of viruses are destroyed upon contact with chlorine compounds. Hexachlorophene in particular is a highly effective cleansing agent, especially where skin contamination has occured.

Dengue Fever

other names

Breakbone fever.

class

Viral (hemorrhagic).

areas of natural occurence

Indian subcontinent, Pakistan, Iran, Anatolian highlans, West Indies, Indochina, Indonesia, South Pacific. Will occasionally occur in Greece, and on the western peripheries of the Middle East.

natural vectors

Common mosquitos *aedes aegypti* and *aedes alpopietus.*

artificial vectors

May be artificially spread through pustulant materials containing viral colonies. Virus can be cultivated in fertile chicken eggs, then freeze dried.

incubation period

3 to six days.

pathology

Following incubation, fever, sore throat, running nose first occur although these will subside after the second day. On the fourth or fifth day skin errruptions (pustules) ~~will occur~~ and swelling will occur, accompanied ~~with~~ severe headache, pains in the joints and muscles, with inflammations of the nose and throat.

Seldom fatal, accept among infants, the elderly, and others with weakened immune systems. The disease may go into remission, although host antibodies will prevent a violent reoccurance.

Encephalitis

common names

By type. See pathology, below. Encephalitis is a *condition.*

class

Viral (hemorrhagic). Any of several.

areas of natural occurence

World-wide. Most pronounced in Asia. Occurances in the Pacific and East Africa.

natural vectors

Ticks are the most common. Various strains may be spread by fleas (Brazillian *Ilheus* strain), or mosquitos.

artificial vectors

May be extracted from blood from organs containing viral colonies. The virus can be cultivated in fertle chicken eggs. It may then be freeze dried.

pathology

General: most strains of encephalitis have a limited susceptibility among human populations, in their naturally occuring forms. Many other strains only seem to effect hooved animals. However, mortality rates in human populations may be as much as 50% of those stricken, especially if proper sanitation and medical facilities are not available. Major types likely to effect military populations are:

Japanese. Commonly occurs in the Far East and Pacific islands. First symptoms include a slight fever and stupor. Attacks the membranes surrounding the brain and spinal cord (*meningoencephalomyeltis*). Damages such tissues and spreads through the central nervous system. Spinal cord lesions like those caused by polio. All neurological damage permanent. Diminished mental capacity is to be expected, especially where the disease persists above a week.

Russian Spring-Summer. Commonly spread by ticks or from eating birds who have eaten infected carrion. Common to central and east Asia. First symptoms may include slight fever and stupor. Unlike the Japanese strain, in which the aches spread to the spinal cord and nerves, pains will center around the abdominal region. Russian encephalitis causes degenerative changes to body organs, often spreading along the line of the digestive tract. Permanent damage to the digestive, endocrine, circulatory, and reproductive systems may be expected among survivors, especially if the disease persisted over several days. Survivors will be susceptible to infection by other diseases in damaged organs.

Encephalitis lethargica. Referred to as a sleeping sickness, although not to be confused with African Sleeping Sickness, which is caused by a parasite. Encephalitis lethargica has initial symptoms which include the victim being irritable and sleepless, with accompaning fever and a slight paralysis of some part of the face. Sleeplessness will give way to langor, apathy, and drowsiness. The victim will not sleep so much as be in a deep stupor, with extreme confusion and delusion bordering on hallucination. Mental changes merging into insanity are common among survivors of severe bouts, as is a certain susceptibility to Parkinson's Disease.

Influenza

other names

The flu. The grippe (archaic). Various strains are named after areas of origion or specific attributes, symptoms.

class

Viral. New strains and sub-types develop frequently as older strains seem to fall by the wayside.

natural vectors

Person to person contact. Virus is present in secretions and discharges from the nose and mouth of a victim, often airborne from coughing or sneezing. Often present in body wastes.

artificial vectors

May be spread from virus cultivated in fertile chicken eggs. Then it may be freeze dried.

incubation period

Usually a week to ten days.

pathology

Strains of influenza commonly occur as epidemics or pandemics, although some strains are suspected of being able to go into remission within their host victims.

The disease(s) last from between two days and two weeks. Victims are left weak for periods often exceeding the actual length of infection, and may be subject to other diseases , most notably pneumonia and various ear, eye, nose, throat, respiratory, and intestinal infections both during and following influenza.

Influenza begins with fever and shortly involves acute inflammation of the nose, larynx, and bronchial tubes. Present are racking neuralgic and muscular pains, gastrointestinal disorder, severe headache, insomnia, and possible convulsions and delirium. The principle danger is through the above mentioned complications, although victims may die of fever itself.

The most militarily significant occurrence of influenza occured in the pandemic of 1918-1919. Sweeping up from North Africa, the "Spanish Flu" passed through the dying engagements of world war one and then swept around the world several times. It left in excess of twenty million[1] dead out of a human population then of a little over a billion.

1. Some sources place the figure as high as 50 million.

Meningitis (viral and aseptic)

other names

Acute lymphocytic meningitis; benign lymphocytic choriomeningitis; nonbacterial meningitis; serious meningitis; viral meningoencephalitis.

definition and causes

Meningitis is not a specific disease onto itself, but is rather a condition which may be brought on by any of several organisms, most notably viruses. In this catagory would be included:

Paramyxoviruses:
- mumps
- measles (may cause encephalic symptoms first)

Picornaviruses:
- echoviruses
- coxsackieviruses
- enterviruses

Adenovirus (types 3 and 5)
Herpes simplex(1 and 2)
Arboviruses (attack the CNS more than the brain)

pathology

Meningitis is an acute inflammation of the meninges, the three membranes that surround the brain and spinal cord (known as the dura matter, pia matter, and the arachnoid). This pathology causes the body to produce excess quantities of cerebrospinal fluid, which is rich in white blood cells. The result is a swelling of those tissues around the brain and spinal cord, causing extreme discomfort to the victim and impairing some neurological functions. Headache and stiffness of the neck and back occurs, usually accompanied by vomiting and fever. Fever and pressure on the brain may often cause personality changes.

As this condition is caused and abetted by any number or viruses the meningital symptoms may be submerged in any number of others.

Psittacosis

once provisionally designated
agent SI

other names

Parrot fever, ornithosis

class

Viral (coccoid). In appearence like a miniature rickettsia, although lacking complete metabolism.

areas of natural occurence

Originates in tropical forested areas; most notably in Central or South America, as pertains to most studies.

natural vectors

Caused by coccoid virus *chlamydia psittaci* found active or dormant in tropical parents. Infectuous to pigeons and poultry. Caught by humans handling infected birds, poultry products, or sputum, blood, or lung tissue from infected birds.

artificial vectors

May be cultivated in laboratory mediums with compatable protein bases and in some instances in fertile eggs of susceptible species.

incubation period

About 1 to 4 days.

history

Examined by the Allies during world war two for possible use as a biological incapacitating agent, although further studies of the disease in Central and South America suggested that a 20% mortality rate was probable. The program was cancelled at the end of the war and further work was limited to immunological studies. The war stocks were processed into (inert) fertilizer.

pathology

Normally causes nausea and diarrhea concurrent with

chills and fever. Severe infection causes a pneumonia (pathologic lung congestion) indistinguishable from most common viral pneumonias. This latter effect poses the greatest hazard.

Rift Valley Fever

class

Viral (hemorrhagic).

areas of natural occurence

Common to east Africa and the Nile River valley, with occasional outbreaks in bordering areas.

natural vectors

Common mosquitos *aedes aegypti* and *aedes alpopietus.* As the virus is found in the lungs it can be transmitted as an aerosol (coughing or sneezing). Cases of other personal contact transmission are not uncommon.

other vectors

May be artificially spread through pustulant materials containing viral colonies. The virus can be cultivated in fertile chicken eggs, then freeze dried.

incubation period

Possibly in as little as 24-36 hours.

pathology

The disease runs its most virulent course in about 2 to 4 days. Severe fever is common, to about 104°F. This fever may cause significant mental and motor/muscle-nerve aftereffects. Bloody diarrhea should be expected. Liver damage followed with jaundice may occur during the latter febrile period.

After the fever subsides, two complications may or may not occur. First is an acute inflammation of the retina (retinitis). One or both eyes may be effected. Vision loss may be temporary, or permanent where retinal scarring has occured. The second takes the form of an acutely altered state of consciousness (perhaps personality change) due to the course of neuronal inflammation and destruction. This is an effect similar to that of viral encephalitis (qv).

Smallpox

class

Viral.

areas of natural occurance

World-wide. Acutely infectious. Widely vaccinated for.

natural vectors

Person to person contact. Virus is present in secretions and discharges from the nose and mouth of a victim. Skin eruptions and resulting scabs contain viral colonies.

artificial vectors

Dried scab material can be spread through clothing, bedding and onto tools and utensils. Smallpox was one of the first diseases used as a weapon of war in the modern era. The virus can be cultivated in fertilized chicken eggs. Then it may be freeze dried.

incubation period

One to three weeks.

pathology

First to occur is a three to four day period of severe chills, headache, nausea, and pains in the back, arms, and legs. On the fourth of fifth day the first skin er-ruptions occur, along with a high fever which slowly goes into remission. The erruptions first take the form of small red spots on the forehead, face, and wrists. Within a day these change into papules, which feel like lead shot under the surface of the skin. These spread all over the body, as they soften into vestules with depressions on the top.

The virus is most active in the layer of fat under the skin (subglutinus cells). As the virus migrates up through the skin, it liquifies fat and skin cells into

? SUBCUTANEOUS

pus, which wells up into the vestules, making them pustules. At this time the high fever returns. The pustules increase in size and gradually dry to form soft, yellow smelly scabs containing concentrations of the virus. After about seven days these scabs fall away, leaving pitted scars.

Fever and secondary infections may cause death.

Yellow fever

class

Viral.(hemorrhagic).

areas of natural occurence

World wide.

natural vectors

Common mosquitos *aedes aegypti* and *aedes alpopietus.*

artificial vectors

The virus can be cultivated in mice or fertle chicken eggs. The virus may then be freeze dried.

incubation period

One to six days.

pathology

Yellow fever is an infectious viral disease which attacks the liver and digestive tract. The disease runs through three stages. The first symptoms include severe headache, high fever, and pains in the back, arms, and legs. Rapid pulse rate is common during the initial stage although it subsides into the second day. Nausea occurs, causing vomiting. A white residual protein mass (albumin) appears in the urine. The second stage is a false remission. During this period the virus is multiplying in the fatty tissue under the skin (subglutinous). As the virus rises up through the skin, the third stage occurs, accompanied by fever and muscle spasms. The skin of lighter skinned persons will appear to have turned yellow at this point. Massive sweating occurs. Oxidized blood will occur in vomit.

Fever and secondary infections may cause death.

RECOMMENDED READING

Agnew, L.R.C., ed. *Dorland's illustrated medical dictionary, 24th edition*. Philadelphia. W.B. Saunders. 1965.

Clarke, E,G,C,, ed. *Isolation and identification of drugs*. London. The Pharmaceutical Press. 1974.

Conn, Rex B., ed. *Current diagnosis*. Philadelphia. W.B. Saunders. 1985.

Douglass, Joseph D. and Livingstone, Neil C. *America the vulnerable, the threat of chemical/biological warfare*. Lexington, MA. Lexington Press. 1987.

Griffith, H. Winter. *Complete guide to symptoms, illness, and surgery*. Tucson, AZ. The Body Press. 1985.

Harris, Robert and Paxman, Jeremy. *A higher form of killing, the secret story of chemical and biological warfare*. New York. Wang and Hill. 1982.

Thomas, Clayton L, ed. *Tabor's cyclopedic medical dictionary*. Philadelphia. F.A. Davis Co. 1973.

Urdang, Laurence, ed. *Mosby's medical and nursing dictionary*. St. Louis, MO. C.V. Mosby Co. 1983.

Urdang, Laurence, ed. *Urdang dictionary of current medical terms*. New York. John Wiley & Sons. 1981.

Windholz, Martha, et al, eds. *The Merck index, an encyclopedia of chemicals, drugs, and biologicals, 10th edition*. Rahway, NJ. Merck & Co. 1983.

CONFLICTING VIEWS ON THE "YELLOW RAIN" CONTROVERSY: scholarly dissertations

American Medical Association. *Chemical-biological warfare in Asia*. JAMA (Journal of the American Medical Association). July 22/29, 1983, vol 250, no. 4. editorial

British Medical Association. *Chemical and bacteriological weapons in the 1980s*. The Lancet. July 21, 1984.

Chapter Nine

THE HERBICIDES

Official definition

Herbicides are chemicals that possess a high potential for destroying or limiting the production of food and defoliating vegatation. These chemical compounds kill or limit the growth of plants. They may be subdivided into the following catagories:

(1) Plant growth regulators that promote, inhibit, or otherwise modify physiological processes in plants — sometimes causing plant death.

(2) Defoliants that prematurely remove leaves from plants.

(3) Desiccants that dry up plant foliage.

(4) Soil sterilants that prevent the growth of green plants when present in that soil.

(5) Surface-active agents that enhance the wetting, sticking, or spreading of antiplant compounds on plants and facilitate their dispersion.

FM 3-9

The agents discussed in this chapter have all at one time been standard military compounds.

- Agent Blue (cacodylic ~~oxide~~ ACID)
- Bromacil
- 2,4-D : 2,4-dichloroxypehnoxy acetic acid
- 2,4,5-T: 2,4,5-trichloroxyphenoxy acetic acid
- Agent Orange

hydroxymethylarsine oxide

active component

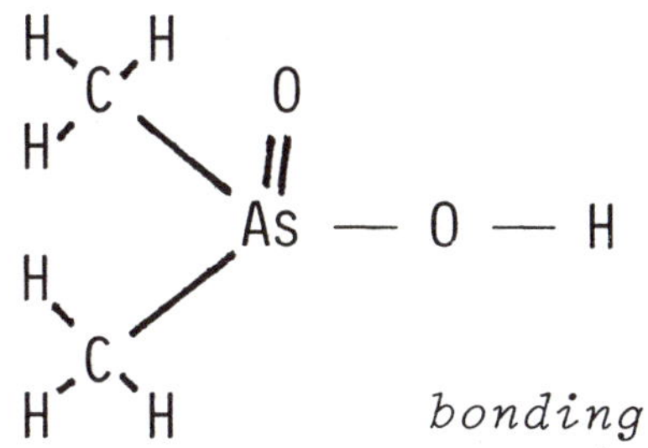

bonding around pentavalent arsenic ion

AGENT BLUE

Common names: cacodylic acid; dimethylarsenic acid

Family: herbicide (dessicant)

In pure form a colorless, odorless crystalline solid. In solution with water, ethanol, or acetic acid it forms a dark brown liquid.

Military applications

Agent Blue was so called because of a US Army color coding system used on the 55-gallon drums in which pre-mixed chemical herbicides were purchased.

Cacodylic , or dimethylarsenic, acid was first developed in the early 1920s for use against certain skin diseases. Its property of water molecule absorption led to its use as a plant desiccant and insecticide by the early 1960s.

The military solution consisted of 3 pounds of cacodylic acid salts per gallon in an aqueous solution, with a neutralizer to prevent the corrosion of brass of steel hose nozzles.

Blue was used where herbicides less virolent than Bromacil or the 2,4-D/2,4,5-T based types were required. In particular, Blue was used against rice crops in southeast Asia. At concentrations below $\frac{1}{2}$ gallon per acre Blue will prevent the growth of fruiting bodies (grain) in rice crops without destroying the plants themselves.

Otherwise, Blue is a specialized herbicide which is more effective against grasses than broadleaf plants. It kills the plant body through absorption of water through the leaves. Low-growing foliage may die within 2 to 4 days although regrowth can occur within 30 days.

The Blue formulation of cacodylic acid is more stable than the parent compound. Whereas pure cacodylic acid may be attacked by oxidizers, the Blue formulation seems immune to both strong alkalies and acids and decomposes primarily through hydrolysis.

Toxicity

Cacodylic acid contains about 54% arsenic by weight. Arsenic is a systemic poison. It displaces calcium in bone matter. It will have detrimental effects on the production of new blood cells. It destroys the action of the blood enzyme cytochrome oxidase, degrading blood hemoglobin. As arsenic is removed from the system through the liver and kidneys, those organs may in turn be damaged. Only the fact that cacodylic acid already contains two very strong arsenic-oxygen bonds prevents it from being a more toxic substance in the above regards. Blue does not appear to remain in the environment for any extended length, as might be the case of other herbicides in this chapter.

Persons in the area where Blue is stored, transported or used should avoid eating, drinking, or smoking. Persons with Blue on their skin should flush it off at the first opportunity.

NIOSH studies (# CH 7525000) report that skin and eye irritation are common and that prolonged dosages may lead to pre-carcinogenic conditions. Pure cacodylic acid, when heated, omits arsenic gas and unstabilized solutions may react violently with iron, aluminum, and zinc alloys.

Blue, being a stabilized solution, probably presents less of a physiological and environmental hazard than its parent compound.

Molecular weight of Blue is 137.99, based on hydro-methylarsine oxide. Solubility of the field solution is about 80 grams per 100 grams of water. Other specific data of this superceeded herbicide mixture lie outside the general public domain.

5-bromo-6-methyl-3-(1-methylpropyl)-2,4 (1H,3H)-pyridinedione

(Bromacil)

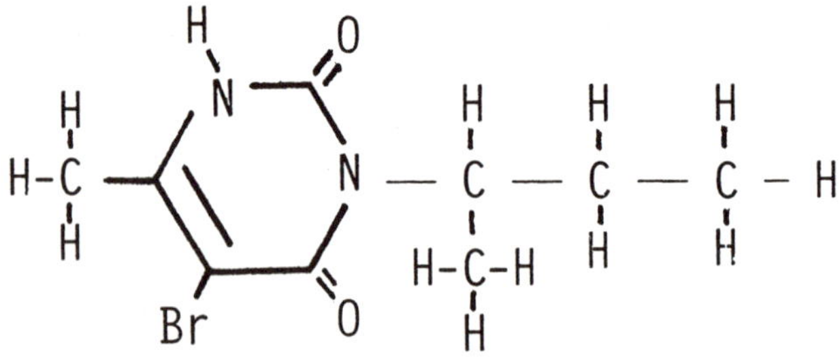

Other chemical names: 5-bromo-3-sec-butyl-6-methyluracil
Trade names: Bromacil, Hyvar, Uragon, Urox B

Type: herbicide (soil sterilant)

In pure form a white, odorless crystalline solid. Usually found in solution with water, acetonitrile, acetone, ethanol, or diesel oil. Formula copyrighted by Du Pont.

Military applications

Bromacil is a commercial herbicide used in its origional (commercial) formulation for tactical military purposes. It is effective in retarding the growth of annual and perennial grasses and broadleaf weeds. Recommended commercial usages range from citrus orchards to pineapple fields. Bromacil has also been used to retard the growth of broadleaf brush growing in heavily wooded areas.

Bromacil would be used in areas where removal of undergrowth is desired without causing any significant damage to forest or crop lands. Such purposes could range from denying an enemy concealment to the selective reduction of brush fire hazards.

Toxicity

Bromacil has shown itself to have little, if any, toxic effect on mammals when used according to manufacturer's guidelines. The pure chemical has shown itself not to be carcinogenic, nor causing birth defects in laboratory animals. Bromacil in and of itself has extremely low vapor pressure. Its probable hazards would probably be due more to its solvent base than to the chemical itself. Solutions based on acetone or diesel oil would offer the greatest toxic hazards while a water base solution would offer the least toxic. The former type would be used where persistency and immediate penetrability are required, the latter for more general applications.

Specific data

permissible exposure limit

10 mg/m^3.

protection required

For personnel applying Bromacil, civillian filters or respirators sould be used. They would conform to the following OSHA standards: CCROVFDPest/ DMOVDMPest/ SAF/ SA:PD, PP, CF/ SCBAF for maximum protection.

decontaminants

Personnel: use water and soap/ mild detergent. Alcohol solutions are also effective.
Terrain: water and detergeant solution. Any strong acid.

vapor pressure

.0008 mm Hg at 100°C(212°F).

liquid density

water: 815 ppm. Will decompose slowly in wet soil.
xylene: 3.2 g/100 ml
acetone: 16.7 g/100 ml
strong base: 8.8 g/100 ml
ethanol: 13.4 g/100 ml

melting point

157-160°C(314.6-320°F)

fire and explosion hazard

Pure Bromacil is nonfalmmable. Its solvents may be.

decomposition point

Above melting point

stability in storage

Stable in metals, plastic, or glasss.

action on metals and other materials

None of significance.

molecular weight

161.1

action on metals or other materials

No effect on metals. Softens paint and most natural and man-made rubber on contact.

DO NOT apply using rubber hoses or allow splashed liquid on equipment with exterior rubber gaskets or on tires.

molecular weight

221

2,4-(dichlorophenoxy) acetic acid

(2,4-D)

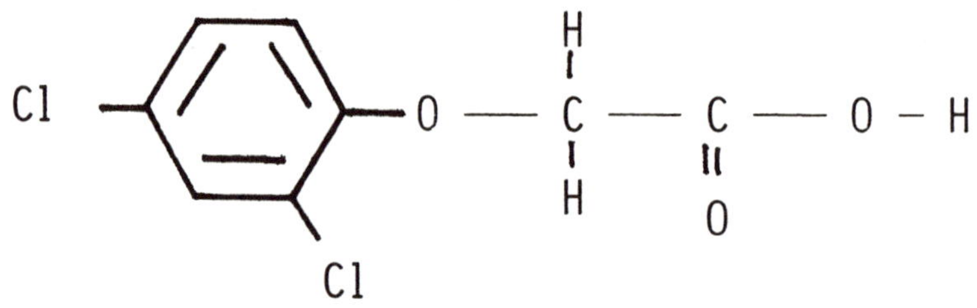

Trade names: active ingredient in: Agrotect; Amidox; Amoxone; Aqua-clean;Chipco Turf Herbicide D; Crop Rider; Chloroxone Crotylin; Decamine; Ded-weed; Desormone; Dicopur; Dicotox; Dinoxol; DMA-14; Emulsamine; Envert 171 & DT; Esteron 99,76BE,44; Estone; Fernesa; Fernimine; Fernoxone; Foredex 75; Formula 40; Hedonal; Herbidol; Ipaner; Krotline; Lawn-Keep; Macrondray; Miracle; Monosan; Moxone; Netagone, 600; NSC 423; Pennamine, D; Phenox; Pielik; Planotox; Plantgard; Rhodia; Salvo; Spritz-Hormin; 2,4 D; Super D Weedgone; Superormone; Transamine; Tributon; U46 DP; RHAP; Visco-RHAP Low, Drift & Low Volatile 4L; Weed Ag-Bar; Weedar, 64; Weed-B-Gone; Weedeze Wonder Bar; Weedone, LV4; Weed Tox; Weed Trol.

Type: herbicide (growth regulator)

In pure form a colorless, odorless crystalline solid. Most commonly found in solution with alcohols, or in various petrochemical solutions where it forms dimethylamine salts or various alkyl esters. May form up to 50% of the active ingredients in the above commercial solutions. Often found together with minute quantities of a related compound 2,4,5-T. Its ester is used in the formulation of Agent Organge, an altogether different substance.

Military applications

2,4-D was introduced in 1942 as a herbicide for the control of broadleaf plants and as a general plnat growth regulator. It first saw large-scale tactical use in the British Malay campaign of 1955-1957 where it was used as a general defoliant. Later applications included use by both United States and Australian forces in Vietnam.

In all of its military usages, 2,4,-D was purchased as an off-the-shelf item from commercial sources. It was used in jungle warfare to deny an enemy the use of terrain by limiting plant growth which would otherwise provide concealment. In its use in the 1950s through the early 1970s, other applications such as its use against crops were developed.

Plant effects

2,4-D produces results against smaller, more sensitive plants within one hour. Serious systemic damage against larger plants and small trees will be evident within 24 hours.

2,4-D is most effective against broadleaf plants. These include plam, nut, and fruit trees. The broadleaf plants also include cotton, sugar beets, potatoes, sweet potatoes and yams, flax and soy beans. Not as effective against larger trees as 2,4,5-T.

The first effects of 2,4-D are the drying or shrinking of leaves. In the more woody plants the stalks or stems may remain green while developing cracks and callous tissue. The latter may be compared to blistering in humans. It becomes obvious at joints and at the crown portions of plants where height growth would have been. On larger shrubs, and notably on trees, the protective bark over the roots may crack away leaving swollen or stringy tissues which will either rot or dry up.

Toxicity

Detailed studies of the toxic hazards of 2,4-D did not come to fruitation until the late 1960s. First indications of toxicity came from the agricultural sector. U.S. agencies such as OSHA (Occupational Safety and Health Administration) and professional bodies as NIOSH (National Institute for Occupational Safety and Health) have published much updated material on 2,4-D since the early 1980s.

2,4-D will penetrate the human body through the skin and eyes. It may be ingested through the lungs or gastrointestinal tract.

Full effects on human long-term exposures are not yet fully known.

Short-term exposure effects are documented. Exposures of 10 mg/m^3 over an eight-hour period, or of 0.09 mg/liter liquid solution may cause weakness, stupor, muscle twitching, and convulsions. Developments of chloracne rashes are common. Liver and kidney damage is documented; 2,4-D is removed from the body via the liver and kidneys and residuals there should be a prime medical concern. Eating, drinking, and smoking should never be permitted where 2,4-D solutions are stored, processed or used.

Damage to the eyes beyond initial irritation does not appear to be the case. Pure 2,4-D forms no vapors. Any vapor hazard is a product of the solution base. Although 2,4-D usually forms about 50% of solution active ingredients, active ingredients only form between 0.5% and 15% of the total mass.

Specific data

median lethal dosage (LCt_{50})

28 grams (pure); 500 mg-min/m^3 (solution)

median incapacitating dosage (ICt_{50})

20 mg-min/m^3 (solution)

permissible exposure limit

10 mg-min/m^3 (inhalation); 0.03 mg/liter (ingestion)

rate of detoxification

Major symptoms of mass dosage, such as stupor, hyproflexia, fibrillary twitching of some muscles and urinary incontinence subside after about 24 hours; profound muscle weakness and exhaustion may subside after another 24 hours (based on US Public Health Service report or patient recieving 3.6 grams of 2,4-D)

protection required

Protective mask/respirat in open areas. In close concentrations protective overclothing would be advised. Civilian filters or respirators must meet following standards: CCROVFDPest/ DMOVDMPest/SAF/SA:PD,PP,CF/ SCBAF.

decontaminants

(Personnel) water and soap or mild detergent. (Equipment) water and soap or mild detergent, alcohol, alcohol keytone solution. (Terrain) water and detergent solution or fire. Pure 2,4-D destroyed by heat over 160°C (320°F). NEVER USE OXIDIZERS!

vapor pressure

Insignificant when pure.

liquid density

1.1 weight of water.

melting point

160°C (320°F) with decomposition

explosion hazard

Fire and explosion with strong oxidizers.

decomposition point

160°C (320°F).

stability in storage

Stable in metal or plastic canisters.

Go To Page 417

(2,4,5-trichlorophenoxy) acetic acid

(2,4,5-T)

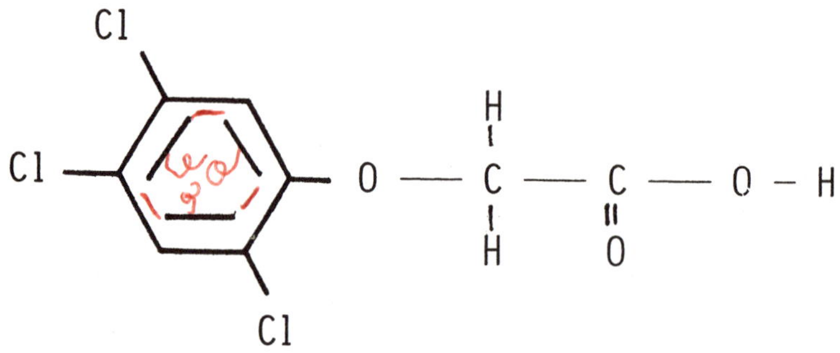

Trade names: Esterone 245; Trioxone; Weedone
Type: herbicide (growth regulator)

In pure form a colorless, odorless crystalline solid. 2,4,5-T solutions are commonly based on water or ethanol, or in oil-based solutions where it forms methylamine or alkyl esters. Chemically related to 2,4,-D , which may be found in 2,4,5-T solutions.

Background

2,4,5-T predates 2,4-D by a year, being reported in the Journal of the American Society (vol 63, p. 1768) in 1941. In the strict sense, 2,4-D is only a refined version of 2,4,5-T. This explains in part why concentrations of either one are found in solutions of the other. Having a single chlorine atom more than 2,4-D, 2,4,5-T has a more stable phenyl group than the former. It comes as no surprise that most sources consider 2,4,5-T less reactive (and less toxic) than 2,4-D.

Military applications

2,4,5-T is a general plant-growth regulating herbicide which, like 2,4-D, has seen military usage from the second world war to the present. It was first used in large quantities in the British Malaysian campaign of 1955-1957. In the Vietnam War, it was used by United States and Australian forces as a general defoliant, to deny covering terrain and foliage to Viet Cong and North Vietnamese troops.

Other than being more effective against woody plants and trees than 2,4-D, the two solutions were often used interchangably.

Plant effects

2,4,5-T produces rapid destruction of small, sensitive plants within an hour. Systemic damage against bamboo, large shrubs, and trees will be apparent within 24 hours. It dries or shrivels the leaves of all plants. Woody plants and trees will develop cracked stems or stalks and calloused, canker-looking, pockets in joints and around the crowns, (tops) where new growth would normally occur.

2,4,5-T is effective against broadleaf shrubs and trees, including palm, nut, and date trees. It will kill cotton, sugar beets, potatoes, sweet potatoes and yams, flax and soy beans. More effective against Irish potatoes and trees than 2,4-D, although generally not as quickly or as thoroughly toxic as the latter.

Toxicity

Toxic studies of the long-term effects of 2,4,5-T were limited until the late 1960s, following complaints from the agricultural sector, where 2,4,5-T has seen continuous use since the early 1940s. US.S agencies such as OSHA and professional groups such as NIOSH have published much updated material on 2,4,5-T since the early 1980s.

2,4,5-T will penetrate the human body through the skin and eyes. It may be ingested through the lungs or the gastrointestinal tract. Damage to the eyes does not appear to pose any significant threat. Effects on the skin may include rashes and chloracne outbreaks.

Short-term exposure effects are documented. 2,4,5-T is removed from the body primarily through excretion through the kidneys. Like 2,4-D, no metabolites are known.

Acute overdosages are not unknown in the agricultural industry. Effects include muscular weakness and stiffness, nausea, vomiting, and diarrhea. Liver and kidney damages may result from chronic exposures.

Like 2,4-D, 2,4,5-T does not appear to directly cause the development of tumorous or cancerous tissue in humans, although some sources claim it as a contributing factor to certain precarcenoma conditions.[1]

1. Journal of the American Medical Association, vol 256 no.9 (September 5, 1986. Hoar, et al. *Agricultural herbicide use and risk of lymphoma and soft-tissue sarcoma.*

Specific data

lethal dosage

5000 mg-min/m^3.

incapacitating dosage

20 mg-min/m^3 (inhalation).

permissible dosage

10 mg-min/m^3 (inhalation); 0.7 mg/liter (ingestion).

rate of detoxification

Average of 89% of total dose excreted within 4 days; Blood plasma bonding broken down in liver and excreted through kidneys (OSHA).

protection required

Protective mask/respirator in open areas. In close concentrations, protective clothing would be advised but is not OSHA mandated. Civilian filters or respirators to meet the following OSHA standards: CCROVPest/ DMOV-Pest/SAF/SA:PD,PP,CF/ SCBAF.

decontaminants

Personnel: water and soap, mild detergents. Equipment: water and soap, mild detergents, alcohol, alcohol-keytone solution. Terrain: water and detergent solution or fire. Pure 2,4,5-T destroyed by heat over 158°C(316°F).

vapor pressure

Insignificant when pure.

liquid density

1.1 weight of water.

melting point

158°C(316°F) with decomposition.

fire or explosion hazard

None

decomposition point

158°C(316°F).

stability in storage

Stable in steel, plastic, or glass.

molecular weight

255.5

Agent ORANGE

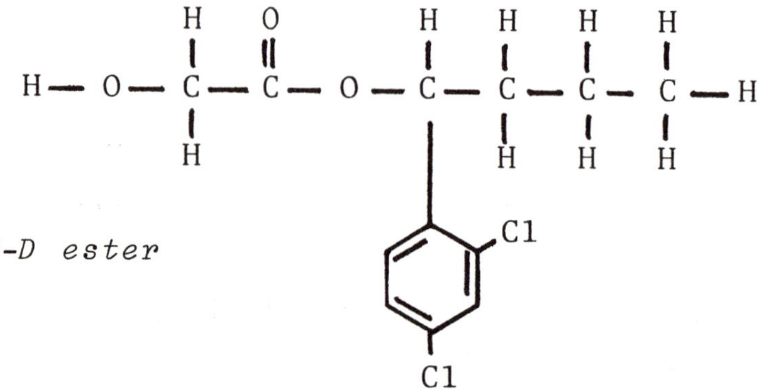

2,4-D ester

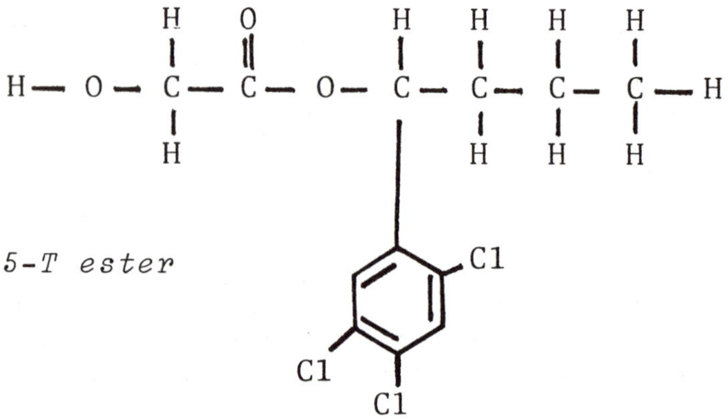

2,4,5-T ester

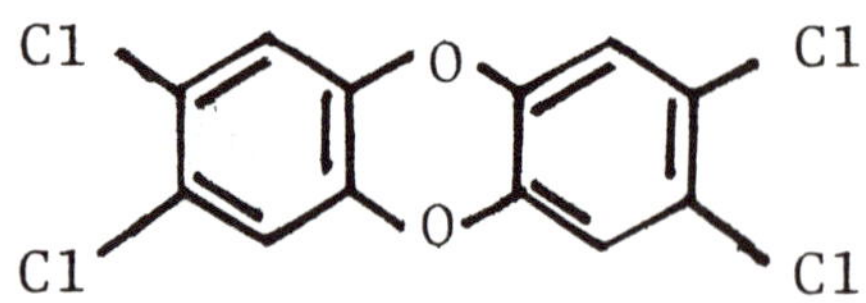

Dioxin
(contaminant?)

AGENT ORANGE

Standard NATO agreement (STANAG) code: (none common)

Common name: Agent orange

Formula: mix of 2,4-D ester & 2,4,5-T ester & dioxin (proportions varied)

Family: herbicide

Military applications

Agent orange was a specific formulation designed for military use. It is no longer in United States military use.

Orange was designed to defoliate entire forests, thus denying their use, concealment, and cover to enemy forces. It was effective in its application, but appears to have been a highly persistent, and somewhat indiscriminate biocide as well.

Controversies

Agent Orange was designed to be a mixture of the esters of 2,4-D, and 2,4,5-T, two general use herbicides which were developed in the early 1940s. The combined esters of those two compounds, it was felt, would make an effective substance for use against grasses, broadleafed plants, and trees.

Either the manufacture of the esters, or their chemical reactions in the drum[1], gave rise to a contaminant, dioxin, which was not supposed to be in the formulation. Dioxin is extremely toxic and, even in the infinitestimal quantities later discovered in Orange, is a known carcinogen and mutagen.

Orange was applied to the southeast Asian landscape with all the due precautions (at least in official orders) as applied to 2,4-D and 2,4,5-T. There appears to have been much unofficial casualness in the way some ground troops sprayed this herbicide onto foliage, resulting in personnel often soaking themselves with the stuff. Likewise, troop movements through Orange contaminated areas were common.

Within a few years after American involvement in the war ceased, the federal courts were involved in litigation from former servicement who had been exposed to Orange.

1. Color-coded orange, hence the name of this agent.

Plant effects

Orange acts differently than its components, and here the dioxin admixture cannot be ignored, in that instead of diminishing plant growth it encourages it. Absorbed through the leaves, Orange causes a growth frenzy throughout the entire organism. Such food reserves the plant has come out of root and stem storage and go into the accelerated growth of leaf and stem strcutures. As these reserves are used up, so are the plant fluids which are not replaced. Hence, the plant is forced to dry up as it gets bigger. At this point the plant dries out from top to bottom as it rots from the roots upwards.

Effects on equipment

Orange is highlyreactive with many woods, natural fibers, and petrochemical derivatives. It will slowly dissolve the hoses it is sprayed through, the uniforms and boot soles of those who use those hoses, and the interior diaphrams and seals of the pumps that move it. It will remove paint from vehicles and aircraft within days of contact. It will damage vehicle tires, seals, hoses, and upholstery. It will deteriorate the fabric aileron surfaces on aircraft.

Toxicity

In manuals published in the mid 1970s, the toxicity of Agent Orange is listed as *unknown*. The advent of dioxin and the tort claims aspects are likely to cloud this issue for many decades before thorough-going studies can establish an an impartial and detailed analysis of this agent.

For that reason, there are no Specific Data.

RECOMMENDED READING

American Conference of Governmental Industrial Hygienists, Inc. *Documentation of the threshold limit values, fourth edition.* Cincinnati. American Conference of Governmental Industrial Hygienists, Inc. 1980.

Christensen, H.E. and Luginbyhl, T.L., eds. *NIOSH toxic substances list, 1974 list.* HEW Publication Nr. 74-134, 1974.

Clayton, George D. and Clayton, Florence E., eds. *Patty's industrial hygiene and toxicology, third revised edition.* New York, John Wiley & Sons. 1978

Crone, Hugh D. *Chemicals and society, a guide to the new chemical age.* London. Cambridge University Press. 1986.

Daintith, John, ed. *Dictionary of chemistry, derived from the Oxford University Press concise science dictionary.* New York. Warner Books. 1986.

Deichmann, M.N, et al. *Clinical toxicology of commercial products.* Baltimore. Williams and Wilkins . 1969

Harris, Robert and Paxman, Jeremy. *A higher form of killing, the secret story of chemical and biological warfare.* New York. Wang and Hill. 1982.

Hoar, Shelia K., et al. *Agricultural herbicide use and risk of lymphoma and soft-tissue sarcoma.* In the Journal of the American Medical Association (vol 256, no.9, p.1141). Sept 5, 1986.

Lewis, Richard and Sweet, Doris, eds. *Registry of toxic effects of chemical substances.* US Department of Health and Social Services, Centers for Disease Control. National Institute for Occupational Safety and Health. 1985.

Mackison, Frank W., et al, eds. *Occupational guidelines for chemical hazards.* US Department of Health and Human Services. Public Health Services. Centers for Disease Control, National Institute for Occupational Safety and Health. US Department of Labor, Occupational Safety and Health Administration. 1981.

Meyer, Eugene. *Chemistry of hazardous materials.* Englewood Cliffs, NJ. Prentice-Hall. 1977.

Sax, N. Irving, ed. *Dangerous properties of industrial materials.* New York. Van Nostrand Rheinhold. 1984.

Sax, N. Irving and Lewis, Richard J. *Rapid guide to hazardous chemicals in the workplace.* New York. Van Nostrand Rheinhold. 1986.

Windholz, Martha, et al, eds. *The Merck index, an encyclopedia of chemicals and drugs, 10th edition.* Rahway, NJ. Merck & Co. 1983.

Winter, Ruth. *Cancer-causing agents, a preventive guide.* New York. Crown Publishers.

Chapter Ten

STANDARD DECONTAMINANTS

- sodium hypochlorite (STB, etc)
- sodium hydroxide (caustic soda)
- sodium hydroxide-alcohol solution (caustic alcohol and DS2)

sodium hypochlorite

Na - O - Cl

Formula: NaOCl (ClNaO)

Common names: chlorine bleach, eau de Labarraque (in aqueous solution) (main component of standard military decontaminant Supertropical Bleach, or STB)

Molecular weight: 74.44

Pure sodium hypochlorite is a pentahydride prepared from sodium hydroxide (NaOH) and chlorine gas in the presence of water. Liquid NaOCl bleaching solutions are made by NaOCL stabilization in water at 0°C(32°F) with 29.3 grams NaOCl to 100 ml H_2O. Solid mixes such as STB are made by treating NaOCl with a 5% aqueous solution of sodium bicarbonate ($NaCHO_3$) and mixed (diluted with chloronated lime (calcium oxide; CaO/Cl^-) and sodium bicarbonate ($NaCO_3$).

Sodium hypochlorite is commonly used in the form of a pre-mix for slurry, dumped into a heating/mixing/spray apparatus. Proportions vary with each brand of mix. As a liquid decontaminant, this compound should be used in a mix no more dilute than 2 parts liquid bleach to one part water.

Sodium hypochlorite is mildly corrosive to animal and vegetable tissues (the latter including cloth, rope, etc). Although not caustic like sodium hydroxide, this compound will cause skin irritation with exposure.

DO NOT MIX OR USE WITH SODIUM HYDROXIDE (CAUSTIC SODA) OR CAUSTIC ALCOHOL (DS2). EXPLOSION OR FIRE WILL RESULT.

use: against the following agents, by code: CG, DP, GA, GB, GD, GF, VX, VE, VR, MD, LD, ED, PD, HN1, HN2, HN3, CX, HL, T, Q, all biologicals.

sodium hydroxide

Na – O – H

Formula: NaOH (HNaO)
Common names: caustic soda; soda lye; sodium hydrate
Molecular weight: 40.01

Produced by combination of calcium hydroxide with sodium carbonate; from sodium chloride by electrolysis; sodium metal and water vapor at low temperatures.

Rapidly absorbs CO_2 and water vapor from the air. One gram dissolves in 0.9 ml cold water or 0.3 ml warm water. Caustic alcohol (the main proponent of standard decontamination solution DS2) is produced at the ratio of 1 gram NaOH into 7.2 ml methyl or ethyl alcohol.

Sodium hydroxide generates considerable heat while dissolving into water or when reacting with acids.

Mixture with sodium hypochlorite (NaOCl-STB, bleach) causes immediate anhydration of the latter. FIRE OR EXPLOSION IS POSSIBLE. DO NOT MIX THE TWO COMPOUNDS.

use: against the following agents, by code: L, MD, ED, PD, HD, HN-1, HN-2, HN-3, CX, T, Q, HL, HT, GA, GB, GD, GF, VX, VE, CG, DP, DA, DC, DM, CA, CN, CNB, CNC, CNS, CS (All), all biologicals

Sodium hydroxide is a highly caustic compiund in pure form. In aqueous solution it remains so.

pH scale

% in aqueous solution	*pH of that solution*
0.05	12
0.50	13
5.00	14

characteristics

% in aqueous solution	*density (g/cc)*	*precipitation (freeze) temp*	*boiling temperature*
5	1.056	-4°C(24.8°F)	102°C(215.6°F)
10	1.111	-10°C(14°F)	105°C(221°F)
20	1.222	-26°C(-14.8°F)	110°C(230°F)
30	1.333	1°C(33.8°F)	115°C(239°F)
40	1.434	15°C(59°F)	125°C(257°F)
50	1.530	12°C(53.6°F)	140°C(284°F)

preparation: use pre-mixed solutions from stock whenever possible. Solutions above 0.05% should not be used where human contact will occur. Use where gross area contamination has occured and future environmental safety would be at risk.

Be cautioned that NaOH is highly caustic to all animal and vegetable tissue (the latter including cloth, rope, etc). NaOH strips paint from surfaces and aqueous solutions corrode aluminum and its alloys. Do not use on or near electronic equipment. DO NOT USE WITH OR NEAR SODIUM HYPOCHLORITE (STB, bleach). EXPLOSION OR FIRE MAY OCCUR.

sodium hydroxide-alcohol mix

$$\left[\; Na - O - H \; \right] \begin{matrix} C_2H_5OH \\ \text{or} \\ CH_3OH \end{matrix}$$

Formula: NaOH in alcohol solution.

Common names: caustic alcohol (main component of standard military decontaminating solution DS2)

Produced by dissolving up to one gram of sodium hydroxide (NaOH) in 7.2 ml of alcohol, usually either methanol or ethanol. Other alcohols may be used.

General characteristics are those of sodium hydroxide, with the noted exception of caustic alcohol being a more efficient organic solvent. Dilute solutions may be used for cleaning of equipment and similar tasks where sodium hydroxide is simply too caustic.

Caustic alcohol generates little heat when combining with water or acids, and is to be preferred over the parent compound (NaOH) in delicute decontamination tasks.

Mixture with sodium hypochlorite (STB, bleach) causes immediate anhydration of the latter. FIRE OR EXPLOSION IS POSSIBLE. DO NOT MIX THE TWO COMPOUNDS.

use: against the following agents, by code: HD, L, HN1, HN2, HN3, MD, ED, PD, CX, HL, HT, T, Q, GA, GB, GD, GF, VX, VE, BZ and most pharmaceutical types; all biologicals.

RECOMMENDED READING

Clayton, George D. and Clayton, Florence E. *Patty's industrial hygiene and toxicology*. New York. John Wiley & Sons. 1978.

Dainith, John. *Dictionary of chemistry, derived from the Oxford University Press concise science dictionary*. New York. Warner Books. 1986.

Godman, Arthur and Denny, Ronald. *Barnes & Noble thesaurus of chemistry*. New York. Barnes & Noble. 1985.

Parker, Sybil P. *McGraw-Hill dictionary of chemical terms, third edition*. New York. McGraw-Hill. 1984.

West, Robert C. *CRC handbook of chemistry and physics, 67th edition*. Boca Raton, FL. CRC Press. 1987.

Windholz, Martha, ed. *The Merck index, an encyclopedia of chemicals, drugs and biologicals, 10th edition*. Rahway, NJ. Merck & Co. 1983

INDEX OF AUTHORS

GENERAL SUBJECT

INDEX